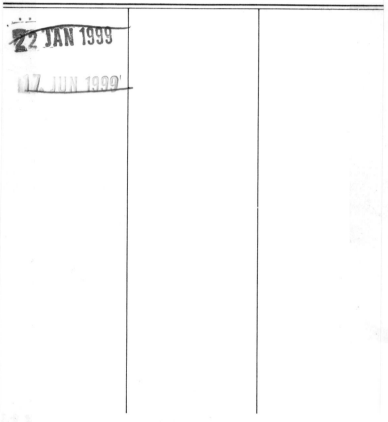

Color Atlas of Pediatric Surgery

Second Edition

Color Atlas of Pediatric Surgery

Second Edition

Peter S. Liebert, M.D.
Associate Clinical Professor of Surgery
Columbia University College of
   Physicians & Surgeons
Associate Attending Surgeon
Babies and Children's Hospital of New York

With a contribution by
Thom E Lobe, M.D.
Professor of Surgery and Pediatrics
Chairman, Section of Pediatric Surgery
The University of Tennessee
Memphis, Tennessee

W.B. SAUNDERS COMPANY
A Division of Harcourt Brace & Company
Philadelphia   London   Toronto   Montreal   Sydney   Tokyo

W.B. SAUNDERS COMPANY
A Division of Harcourt Brace & Company

The Curtis Center
Independence Square West
Philadelphia, Pennsylvania 19106

Library of Congress Cataloging-in-Publication Data

Liebert, Peter S.
Color atlas of pediatric surgery / Peter S. Liebert. — 2nd ed.

    p. cm.

Includes index.

ISBN 0-7216-5885-7

1. Children—Surgery—Atlases. I. Title.
    [DNLM: 1. Surgery, Operative—in infancy & childhood
    —atlases. WO 517 L716c 1996]
RD137.3.L54 1996
617.9′8′00222—dc20

DNLM/DLC   95-33478

Color Atlas of Pediatric Surgery, 2nd edition   ISBN 0-7216-5885-7

Printed in the United States of America

Last digit is the print number: 9   8   7   6   5   4   3   2   1

To my wife, Mary Ann Liebert
For her love and support, during the writing of this book—
and always.

Foreword

The development of pediatric surgery has been a microcosom of the experience in the broader disciplines of surgery and pediatrics, and, in a sense, of medicine itself. Pediatric surgery came late in the succession of specialties that split off from the parent disciplines, and for that reason, perhaps, established itself—with journals, societies, textbooks, and an accreditation board—faster than might have been possible half a century earlier.

Initially, the specialty of pediatric surgery was a response to the need for better outcomes in the management of surgical problems in children. The real need was for a better understanding of physiology, pharmacology, anesthesiology, and pathology as it pertained to children, but especially to infants, including neonates.

It was inevitable that as the pediatric surgical specialist mastered the challenges of the field's requisite supportive skills, there was improvement in morbidity and mortality. It was soon perceived that the general pediatric surgeon was developing more familiarity and better results with some of the pediatric lesions traditionally treated in long-established anatomical surgical specialties. The reception of the pediatric surgeon was cordial by pediatricians but with surgeons varied from skepticism to hostility.

I have always felt extraordinarily fortunate to have been on the scene at the visible beginnings of this saga and to have participated in its evolution for 35 years in the active academic practice of the surgery of children. All these historical musings are to introduce the thought that this *Color Atlas of Pediatric Surgery* by Dr. Liebert (whom I was privileged to train) has something for all the aforementioned categories of those interested in the diagnosis and treatment of surgical problems in children.

For the pediatrician, photographs of both common and unusual lesions can only help in instant recognition and diagnosis when the time comes. For surgeons not familiar with the various procedures, one good proven method of surgical technique can be visualized that can only improve the comfort of dealing with the unfamiliar as well as contribute to a good result. For the practicing pediatric surgeon, the techniques displayed in clear photographs will confirm or deny the numerous intricacies of technical procedure that make surgery such a personal endeavor. For the surgeon in training, here is a treasure trove of diagnostic and surgical technical photographs between two covers of a book.

Thirty or 40 years ago, no such atlas would have been possible, but had one been undertaken, the contents would have been much more inclusive—lips and palates, meningomyelocele, a variety of urologic procedures and pediatric cardiac surgery—for the early pediatric surgeon was a surgeon of the skin and all of its contents.

Today, as many as a dozen pediatric surgical subspecialties have developed, and that is as it should be, because children now get fair surgical treatment as they compete for attention in an adult world. This atlas should contribute to that effort in many ways. I know that is why Dr. Liebert compiled it. I compliment him on his scholarship and for this outstanding contribution to the further unfolding of the field of pediatric surgery.

C. Everett Koop, M.D., Sc.D.
(Reprinted from the first edition)

Preface

This atlas has been designed as a concise clinical reference for the significant anatomic and functional problems in pediatric surgery and for the surgical techniques used in correcting those problems. It is organized in a logical progression from patient presentation to diagnostic confirmation to therapeutic intervention. The text and illustrations should be of interest and practical value to those at all levels of experience, from novice student to specialist practitioner.

For all but the pediatric surgeon or trainee in pediatric surgery, it is difficult to have extensive direct experience with the variety of clinical material seen in a major children's hospital center. Yet, in many institutions, general surgeons and surgical subspecialists are called upon to recognize and to treat both simple and complex problems in the pediatric patient. The surgical resident is expected to learn about many pediatric surgical conditions, and today most certification examinations in surgery include questions about pediatric surgery. Although there is no substitute for individual experience, a reference for the clinical diagnosis and treatment of congenital and acquired conditions requiring surgery in children can be most valuable.

The best reference is one that demonstrates actual clinical situations as they appear to the operating surgeon. Medical illustrations can enhance and clarify the progress of an embryologic process or a surgical technique, but there is no substitute for clear, color photographs to demonstrate a surgical lesion or an operative procedure.

During a career of 30 years devoted exclusively to pediatric surgery, I have used my camera in the office, clinic, hospital, and operating room to record the details of pediatric surgical diagnosis and therapy. Most often I was both surgeon and photographer; occasionally I was able to record the procedures of my talented colleagues or to duplicate some of their photographs. The object was always to have teaching material that would interest and educate medical students, physicians and surgeons in training, and my fellow practitioners. The best of that clinical material has been incorporated in this book.

The second edition of the *Color Atlas of Pediatric Surgery* contains much updated and new material. There is a completely new chapter on laparoscopic and thoracoscopic surgery in children. A considerable number of new color photographs and imaging studies have been added, introducing new techniques and replacing older illustrations. To clarify the steps of a greater number of surgical techniques, additional original drawings were commissioned; they are especially useful to illustrate procedures and techniques that do not lend themselves to photography. They also improve understanding of the anatomy and surgical repair of other problems, for which the drawings are alternated with operative photographs.

This text continues to provide valuable diagnostic and therapeutic information for pediatric and general surgeons in their practices, for fellows in pediatric surgical training programs, for medical students, and for parents who are being educated concerning procedures recommended for their children.

Peter S. Liebert, M.D.

Acknowledgments

The author wishes to acknowledge the contributions of many colleagues in the preparation of this atlas. Photographs, radiographs, illustrations, and permission to use personal clinical material were provided by Drs. Sarah Abramson, R. Peter Altman, Walter Berdon, Robert H. Connors, Carol Hilfer, Leif Holgersen, William McCann, Joseph Murphy, Ira Novich, Alberto Pena, and Judson Randolph. Dr. Barry Sachs—pediatric surgical colleague, good friend, and sailing companion—reviewed the entire original manuscript; many of his excellent suggestions and additions have been incorporated in the text.

Dr. Thom Lobe has contributed the new chapter on laparoscopic and thoracoscopic surgery in children. No one has better clinical experience or is a better teacher in this area of pediatric surgery. Additional operative photographs for that chapter were contributed by Dr. Steven Stylianos.

A great debt is owed to Dr. C. Everett Koop. His encouragement of his chief surgical residents at the Children's Hospital of Philadelphia to photograph their clinical experiences has provided the basis for this book. When I told him of my plans for this atlas, Dr. Koop sent me all of the printed notes compiled from his clinical lectures at the Children's Hospital, with permission to draw on them for the text. Lastly, he wrote the Foreword to the first edition of this book, a significant honor from a distinguished teacher, surgeon, friend, and former Surgeon General of the United States.

The editorial and production staff at W.B. Saunders have been a pleasure to work with—cooperative, understanding, and efficient. Medical Editor Lawrence McGrew has kept me on schedule and has supervised all the important stages in the publication of the *Atlas*. Arlene Chappelle has been a thorough and careful copy editor. Linda R. Garber, in charge of production for the book, has done an exceptional job in keeping proofs flowing into my office. Steven Stave is responsible for arranging the text and illustrations for easy reading and smooth transitions.

I want to extend a special thanks to Joel Herring, the talented medical artist who produced the excellent line drawings for both editions of this book. He worked with me through carefully crafted step-by-step illustrations for both common and complex procedures. His collaboration is much appreciated.

My secretary, Donna Kischowski, handled the correspondence to colleagues and editors, and supervised the return of galleys and page proofs. Most important, she kept my surgical office running smoothly during the hectic phases of production of this volume.

In the care of patients and in the preparation for this edition of the *Color Atlas of Pediatric Surgery,* I wish to acknowledge the contribution of surgical residents and fellows in pediatric surgery, with whom I am privileged to work and who continue to open my eyes to new ways of doing and seeing things. It is their hands that appear in many of the operative photographs.

My family, as always, has been supportive during the time and effort required in the production of this second edition. I also thank my wife, Mary Ann, an experienced editor and publisher, for her own suggestions to improve the *Atlas.* And I hope that sons Peter, Jr. and Lewis continue to take pride in this book, which they have watched come to fruition.

Pediatric surgery is constantly fascinating and tremendously rewarding. It is broad enough to interest the worker, difficult enough to satisfy the ambitious, and new enough to stimulate the imagination. The infant "with no language but a cry" and the child with no words to express the desire to be well and normal ask that we make available to them the benefits of increased knowledge of their surgical diseases.

Willis J. Potts, M.D., *The Surgeon and the Child,*
W.B. Saunders Co., 1959

Contents

Chapter 8

Chapter 9

Chapter 10

Chapter 11

Chapter 12

Chapter 13

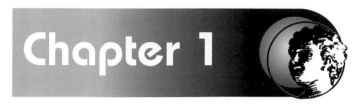

Chapter 1

General Considerations in Pediatric Surgery

Examination

The surgeon's powers of observation are challenged by the patient who cannot describe his or her symptoms or provide an accurate history of his or her illness. The patient's posture at rest or when moved, willingness to walk or hop, alertness, and responsiveness to stimuli are subtle observations that may help to tell a story.

Except in extreme emergency situations, the physician's approach to children must be gentle, starting with those portions of the physical examination that produce least discomfort or fear. Most children feel more secure with a parent standing by. Some cannot be comforted or consoled, and the examination must proceed despite squirming, resistance, and crying. A sympathetic, yet firm, approach works best.

The examination should progress from areas of least to those of greatest discomfort. The child in pain has voluntary muscular resistance to abdominal palpation, which may be overcome by the surgeon's moving the examining hand imperceptibly deeper with each respiration. Slow rectal insertion of a well-lubricated finger is tolerated by most children. When the patient's inability to cooperate prevents evaluation of an urgent problem, sedation is indicated. The author prefers barbiturates, which do not interfere with response to pain or depress respirations when given in appropriate doses (pentobarbital 3.0–4.0 mg/kg).

Laboratory Studies

Laboratory studies should be limited to those necessary for the safe conduct of anesthesia and surgery and to those indicated by the patient's diagnosis and clinical condition. In recent years, pediatric surgeons and anesthesiologists have completely eliminated the requirement for "routine" laboratory tests prior to uncomplicated surgical procedures, such as inguinal herniorrhaphy, in which little or no blood is lost. A complete blood count (CBC) is indicated when there is a reason to suspect that the patient is anemic or thrombocytopenic; in addition, the white blood count and differential may help if there is a question of active infection. If a single screening urinalysis has been normal in the past, it should be repeated only for specific clinical indications. Urine specific gravity is a simple measure that may be obtained to assess the adequacy of hydration. Serum electrolyte determination is indicated for the child with severe or prolonged vomiting, diarrhea, enteric fistulas, urinary diversions, renal abnormalities, or large fluid losses; these losses may include third-space fluid shifts associated with burns, peritonitis, and ascites formation. It is mandatory for patients with certain endocrinopathies, such as the adrenogenital syndrome. In cases of nonspecific acute severe abdominal pain, and following blunt abdominal trauma, serum amylase levels are measured. Teenage girls being evaluated for abdominal pain should have a pregnancy test (serum hCG level).

Blood urea and creatinine levels are important when evaluating a child with known renal disease or large fluid losses. They are also indicated in children receiving total parenteral nutrition or medications with potential renal toxicity. In children, determinations of liver chemistries and serum clotting factors, electrocardiograms, and radiographic and other imaging studies all are dictated by known or suspected abnormalities in specific organs or body systems; they should *not* be ordered as a "routine."

A specimen for blood typing and crossmatch is drawn in all cases of major trauma and in those with the potential for significant blood loss. The well-publicized potential for transmission of the human immunodeficiency virus (HIV) and hepatitis virus in transfused blood has frightened parents, many of whom would like to be the donors for children who need surgery. All accredited blood banks now use only blood that has been screened for HIV and hepatitis. Parents need to know that if they wish to donate blood for a child, it must be done long enough before the date of elective surgery to allow thorough screening of their blood.

Preoperative Preparation

Physiologic Preparation

The achievement of normal homeostasis and anticipation of perioperative needs are the aims of preoperative preparation. Restoration of fluid and blood volume and correction of abnormalities in electrolyte balance, clotting factors, hormone levels, and nutrition are carried out as clinical circumstances permit. Anti-infective measures include cleansing of the skin, mechanical and antibiotic bowel preparation, and preoperative parenteral antibiotics when indicated. High fever is brought down with salicylates and cool compresses or baths. The stomach should be empty before administration of general anesthesia. Fluids may be given by mouth up to 4 hours prior to elective surgery in infants, with 8 hours of restriction in older children. In acute emergencies, when there may be a full stomach, and in all cases of intestinal obstruction, there must be decompression with an adequate-sized nasogastric tube. In newborns, especially premature infants, great care must be taken to avoid hypothermia and hypoglycemia—before, during, and after surgery.

Psychological Preparation

Psychological preparation of the child (and parents) alleviates some of the trauma of hospitalization, manipulation, and surgery. For younger children (younger than 8 years of age), the rules of preparation are (1) tell the truth, (2) keep the explanations simple, and (3) describe innocuous experiences that the child can confirm. ''You will blow into a mask, like astronauts wear, and will see a rubber balloon get bigger and smaller when you blow'' describes induction of anesthesia for a child. Older children need to know about pain relief and to be assured that they will not ''wake up'' in the middle of the procedure. A preoperative hospital orientation is helpful. A number of fine illustrated children's booklets are available to assist in preoperative preparation.

Anesthesia

General Anesthesia

General anesthesia is indicated for all but the most minor procedures in infants and toddlers, and for all intraabdominal, intrathoracic, and intracranial operations, as well as deep dissections of the head and neck and the extremities. In the past, some procedures were carried out under local anesthesia or regional block because of an individual child's unusual cardiac or respiratory problems. Current anesthetic management of infants and children—with modern anesthetics, well-trained anesthesiologists, precise control of oxygenation, and sophisticated monitoring—makes general anesthesia the preferred choice for those children.

General anesthesia is best conducted in a child who is calm and cooperative or moderately sedated, has a normal body temperature, is adequately hydrated, and is free of respiratory and metabolic impairment and systemic infection. Preparation and patience are the best ways to allay fears. In elective situations, the toddler or young child may be assured by the supportive presence of a parent in the operating room during induction of anesthesia. Preoperative sedation is appropriate for those children who cannot be calmed. Many anesthesiologists choose to administer atropine, preoperatively or at the onset of anesthesia, for its drying of secretions and vagolytic effect.

The choice of anesthetic agent is determined by the age and condition of the child and the nature of the surgery. One may induce inhalation anesthesia by wafting it from an open tube under the child's nose, rather than by clamping a mask on the face of a struggling patient. Other children feel more comfortable sitting up, on the operating table or on a parent's lap (Fig 1.1). In children younger than 10 years who require an intravenous line, it is placed with less emotional trauma once the child is asleep. Major procedures require the placement of one or more intravenous needles or catheters of adequate diameter for blood and fluid administration.

During induction of anesthesia, as well as throughout the procedure, the child's temperature must be kept within normal range. The smaller the child, the more rapid the heat loss. Placement of a heating blanket under the child and a radiant heater overhead helps significantly. Wrapping the extremities in cotton batting or Webril and covering the head with a stocking cap are useful additions, especially in cool operating rooms. The ideal operating room temperature for neonates and infants is 76–80° F; heat loss can be minimized further by covering

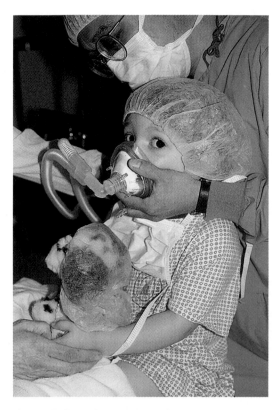

Figure 1.1 A 4-year-old girl undergoes anesthesia induction while sitting up on the operating table. This is a less threatening position for many children and allows a smoother induction.

the baby with an adhesive plastic drape directly on the skin. In special situations, the child's temperature may be maintained with the use of commercially available hollow plastic blankets or wraps into which warm air is constantly circulated. Antiseptics used to cleanse and prep the skin and solutions for irrigating body cavities should be warmed. Core temperature is monitored with a rectal or esophageal thermistor probe. For prolonged procedures, humidification of the anesthetic gases minimizes heat loss and insensible water loss.

The conduct of pediatric anesthesia utilizes monitoring devices for heart rate and electrocardiogram (ECG), blood pressure, pulse oximetry, expired CO_2, and—in critical situations—arterial blood gases, central venous and pulmonary artery pressures, and urinary output. The anesthesiologist notes changes in skin color, nail-bed perfusion, the quality of breath sounds, and the strength of heart tones. Accurate estimates of blood loss are made by measuring blood suctioned from the operative field and by weighing sterile gauze sponges before and after use. Refrigerated blood is warmed prior to administration. It is important to correct any acidosis, hyperkalemia, and dilution of clotting factors that may result from the rapid infusion of a large volume of bank blood.

During prolonged procedures, it is important to pad bony prominences, such as the heel and the elbow, to prevent pressure injury to the skin. In addition, the position of the patient's trunk and extremities must be adjusted to avoid tension on nerves and nerve roots and to avoid compression of blood vessels.

Local Anesthesia

Local anesthesia may be used for repair of skin lacerations and for many minor superficial elective procedures in cooperative children. The surgeon's impression of the child's maturity and ability to cooperate, bolstered by parental confirmation, determines suitability. For lacerations, a local anesthetic may first be dripped into the wound, numbing it sufficiently to allow painless injection of additional anesthetic. A combination of lidocaine, epinephrine, and tetracaine (LET) has been popularized for such topical use. For injections into the intact skin, only the first needle stick will be felt if, with subsequent infiltration of anesthetic solution, the needle is advanced slowly into an area already anesthetized by the previous injection. EMLA (2.5% lidocaine in 2.5% prilocaine) is a topical anesthetic that may be applied to normal intact skin to block pain at the site of even the first injection or intravenous needle insertion; however, to be effective, it must be applied at least 45 minutes prior to the injection.

Fluids and Electrolytes

Maintenance of adequate circulating blood volume, good organ perfusion, proper urine output, and normal acid-base and electrolyte balance is part of the surgeon's responsibility to the patient. Even the child taking full feedings must be monitored for volume and content of those feedings. When oral feedings are withheld for any appreciable time (more than 6 hours in an infant younger than 18 months, or more than 12 hours in a toddler of 2–4 years), maintenance levels of water and salts must be given parenterally, preferably in an isotonic (5%) glucose solution. The premature newborn, with a tendency toward hypoglycemia, may require a 10% glucose infusion. Replacement of fluid and electrolyte losses depends on an accurate assessment of prior losses, measurement of continuing loss, and serial electrolyte determinations. In infants, significant enteric losses are replaced every 8 hours.

Basic fluid requirements, to replace urine and insensible losses, are determined by the child's normal weight or calculated body surface area according to the following table:

Body Weight (kg)	24-h Volume: D_5 in ¼ or ⅓ Normal Saline	
First 10 kg	100 mL/kg	
10–20 kg	add 75 mL/kg	OR 1500 mL/m² surface area
20–40 kg	add 50 mL/kg	

The nature of certain losses allows good estimates concerning their correction. The following are common examples:

1. Prolonged vomiting, such as that of infants with pyloric stenosis, leads to dehydration and alkalosis, with losses of sodium, potassium, chloride, and hydrogen ion (acid). Low body stores of extracellular potassium are rapidly exhausted. Prior to surgery, a solution of at least 75 mEq/L of sodium and chloride (D_5 in ½ normal saline) and 30–40 mEq/L of potassium—even in the presence of a serum potassium in the low-normal range—must be given until the imbalances are corrected.

2. The postoperative replacement of fluid losses from gastric drainage from a nasogastric tube or gastrostomy should utilize a similar intravenous solution, but with less potassium (15–20 mEq/L), unless previous hypokalemia must be corrected.

3. Enteric fistulas, such as ileostomies, may lead to excessive sodium, potassium, and bicarbonate loss. Biliary drainage contains considerable bicarbonate. These losses must be replaced, with correction of the associated acidosis, using a solution in which the primary anion is bicarbonate, not chloride.

Postoperative Care

Respiratory Care

Following prolonged inhalation anesthesia, all patients have areas of microatelectasis of the lungs that they must clear. The infant does so by vigorous crying. Older children must be encouraged to cough and breathe deeply. The internal diameter of the child's airway is already narrow (3.0 to 3.5 mm in the newborn's trachea); any aspirated material or tenacious secretions may dangerously impede respirations. Humidification of inspired air or oxygen loosens secretions for easier clearing. Chest physiotherapy, with postural drainage and percussion, is helpful in treating postoperative pulmonary problems in infants and children. Thick secretions and mucus plugs call for nasotracheal suctioning, suctioning through an endotracheal tube, or even bronchoscopy.

Infants who were premature at birth—especially those less than 48 weeks' gestational age at the time of surgery—or those who have had neonatal cardiorespiratory problems are more likely to develop apneic episodes immediately following surgery under general anesthesia. Therefore, they are hospitalized overnight for observation, even after routine surgery, and are kept on an apnea monitor and pulse oximeter.

Putting a child on a respirator poses other potential problems. The endotracheal tube inserted must be of proper size, and uncuffed, to avoid tracheal mucosal damage. The tube should be securely taped in place and its position checked periodically with chest radiographs. One regulates the respirator settings according to clinical indices and arterial blood gases. Continuous monitoring of oxygen saturation by pulse oximetry has proved helpful. Complications of long-term ventilation include oxygen toxicity and barotrauma to the lungs, and granulomas or stenosis of the trachea from intubation.

Tracheostomy is reserved for situations requiring tracheal intubation for more than 4–6 weeks, and for congenital and acquired upper airway obstruction (see pages 11 and 12 for technique).

Pain Relief

The adequate relief of pain, especially in those children who cannot communicate their pain, is an important aspect of postoperative care. Simple peri-incisional block with a long-acting local anesthetic such as bupivacaine (Marcaine) can offer considerable comfort for many operations. The pain of limited deeper procedures, such as herniorrhaphy, is adequately diminished by acetaminophen or aspirin in appropriate doses (6–8 mg/kg every 4 hours). Major thoracic, abdominal, spinal, or orthopedic surgery requires parenteral narcotic analgesia. Children fear intramuscular injections; regular intravenous (IV) administration of morphine or meperidine will alleviate anxiety, as well as pain, in the immediate postoperative period. Younger children must have the analgesic administered by a physician or nurse. For children of adequate age and competence (8–10 years and older), patient-controlled analgesia (PCA) may be used after major surgery. By pressing a button that activates a pump delivering narcotic solution, the patient may self-administer small doses of intravenous narcotic up to a set limit.

Antibiotics

Antibiotics are advised in infants and children to treat known or suspected infection or to prevent a likely infection, either as a consequence of the clinical situation or in a susceptible patient. The *routine* use of antibiotics in pediatric surgery should be condemned.

Parenteral antibiotic therapy is clearly indicated in treating known serious infections; examples are systemic sepsis, meningitis, peritonitis from a perforated viscus, an undrained abscess or empyema, and spreading cellulitis—especially cellulitis of the head or face, which may seed infection to the cavernous sinus of the brain.

Susceptible patients include newborn infants, especially premature infants, who are known to be deficient in some immunoglobulins and to have low resistance to certain infections. Perioperative antibiotic prophylaxis is used frequently in these infants. Most oncologists ''cover'' with antibiotic therapy their immunosuppressed patients who are undergoing surgery. Children with congenital and acquired immunodeficiencies (see page 7, HIV-Infected Children) are particularly susceptible to infection with common and uncommon organisms. Patients with cardiac malformations or implanted foreign material receive antibiotic prophylaxis, particularly before surgical or dental manipulation; and children after splenectomy all are given a prolonged course of oral prophylactic antibiotic because of the known risk of overwhelming sepsis in the asplenic child.

Human or animal bites that puncture the skin must be assumed to be contaminated with a variety of aerobic and anaerobic pathogens; broad-spectrum treatment is indicated. Similar therapy must be considered for ''dirty'' puncture wounds. Any injury that produces a large area of devitalized tissue is a potential site for infection. Gas gangrene, resulting from *Clostridium perfringens* infection, produces a rapidly spreading myonecrosis that requires wide debridement of the wound, high-dose systemic antibiotics, and even hyperbaric oxygen therapy to prevent a fatal outcome (Fig 1.2).

Similar tissue-destructive infections, some fatal, have been reported recently, caused by a microaerophilic group A streptococcus. Most patients with this infection have been adults with a preexisting condition that compromised their resistance to infection, either locally or systemically. Early recognition of the infection, debridement, and prompt treatment with massive doses of intravenous antibiotic are necessary.

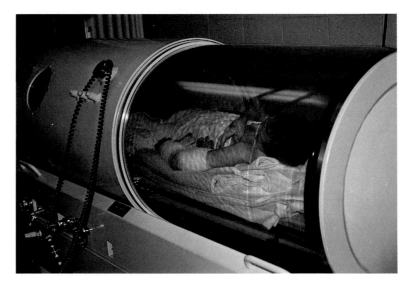

Figure 1.2 A 13-year-old boy with an anaerobic, tissue-necrosing infection is seen receiving oxygen therapy in a hyperbaric capsule. With this therapy, the infection resolves rapidly.

Antibiotics are used, singly or in combination, to treat specifically identified or suspected organisms. The following common examples are illustrative.

A penicillin is generally used to treat streptococcal infection (50,000–100,000 U/kg/d) and for prophylaxis (250 mg/d) against encapsulated organisms in cardiac or asplenic patients.

Oxacillin or nafcillin (50–100 mg/kg/d; neonates, 60–80 mg/kg/d) is effective for staphylococcal infections; mature abscesses respond best to surgical drainage.

The peritonitis of perforated appendicitis may be treated with a combination of an aminoglycoside (gentamicin 7.5 mg/kg/d) for coliform organisms and clindamycin (40 mg/kg/d) or metronidazole (30 mg/kg/d) for anaerobes; a single cephalosporin, cefoxitin (150 mg/kg/d), is used by some to achieve the same therapeutic range. The addition of a penicillin (ampicillin 100–150 mg/kg/d) to treat associated enterococcus infection is a matter of individual choice.

Deep or extensive animal bites should be treated with intravenous ampicillin/sulbactam (Unasyn 160 mg/kg/d) after open cleansing and debridement. This combination is effective against streptococcus, staphylococcus, and *Pasteurella multocida,* common canine oral flora.

Complications of antibiotic administration include allergic reactions, toxicity, development of resistant organisms, and colitis resulting from suppression of normal enteric flora. *Clostridium difficile* is the organism responsible for the pseudomembranous colitis that may follow prolonged antibiotic administration. Vancomycin is the currently recommended therapy for this condition. Intestinal candidal infection may also follow prolonged antibiotic therapy. Aminoglycosides do not tend to produce renal toxicity in children as compared with adults, and higher relative doses (5–7.5 mg/kg/d) are used; however, periodic peak and trough serum aminoglycoside levels are obtained to ensure that they are in a safe therapeutic range.

Catheters and Tubes

It is important in treating the small patient to know what size and type of catheter or tube to use for a particular purpose.

A #24 gauge needle-catheter is appropriate for IV fluids in the smallest premature infant. For rapid blood administration, however, a peripheral cutdown using a #22 gauge polyvinyl or Silastic catheter—or a percutaneous #19 or #20 gauge internal jugular line—is preferred. Older children need larger-gauge IV lines, or more than one line, for massive volume restoration.

For gastric decompression, a #8–#10 Fr nasogastric tube will pass readily in most newborns; premature infants may require oral placement. A double-lumen #10 Fr sump catheter is used in the upper pouch of a newborn with esophageal atresia (see Chapter 4). The following nasogastric tube sizes are appropriate: #12 for ages 1–3, #14 for ages 4–8, and #16 for ages 8–14.

Urinary catheterization in the newborn is best accomplished with a sterile #6 or #8 Fr straight tube, which can be taped to the lower abdomen. The smallest available Foley catheter is #8 Fr. Long-term indwelling balloon catheters are generally avoided in boys younger than 6 years of age because of possible urethral injury and subsequent scarring.

A #12 Fr chest catheter is appropriate to decompress a pneumothorax in a newborn; a #16 Fr tube may be used to drain fluid and blood following thoracotomy. Too large a chest tube through the intercostal space in any child may erode the ribs and neurovascular bundle. When a thoracostomy tube is placed, to avoid puncturing the lung or mediastinal structures, it is recommended that a small skin incision be made, that the ribs be spread with a small mosquito hemostat, and that the catheter be passed directly into the chest between the blades of the hemostat. The author never inserts chest catheters by introducing them through the skin using the sharp-pointed stylet that accompanies some.

Monitoring

Postoperative monitoring of a child's cardiorespiratory status and temperature is always indicated in the premature infant and for the critically ill child. The electrocardiogram, respiratory excursions, oxygen saturation by pulse oximetry, and central venous and arterial pressures all may be seen on a monitor screen as well as read—and recorded—in digital form. Audible and visible alarms are set for acceptable upper and lower limits. Monitoring is an adjunct to the evaluation of a child after surgery; it is no substitute for experienced nursing observation and care.

Special Considerations

Children with Sickle Cell Disease

For surgery in sickle-cell patients, there may be a need for preoperative transfusions and special operative management. The deoxygenation of abnormal hemoglobin S (HbS) in patients with sickle cell disease causes red blood cells to distort and become rigid. These cells then clog the microcirculation, causing thrombosis, infarcts, and hemolysis. For elective surgery under general anesthesia, children with sickle cell disease are transfused preoperatively with normal blood to achieve a HbS level of less than 30%. This level can be achieved by rapid exchange transfusion for major emergency surgery. During anesthesia, specific precautions are taken to maintain oxygenation (40%–50% FIO_2) and hydration (125–150 mL/hr/m^2) and to avoid acidosis.

HIV-Infected Children

Children with HIV infection may need the help of a surgeon to make or confirm the diagnosis of a specific opportunistic infection. Because a large number of children with acquired immunodeficiency syndrome (AIDS) have pulmonary infection with *Pneumocystis carinii,* bronchoscopy with lavage or lung biopsy may be necessary before initiation of treatment. Lung biopsies may be performed through a limited thoractomy or by thoracoscopy (see Chapter 8). These patients also frequently require central venous access for parenteral nutrition and for administration of medications. In all procedures on HIV-positive patients, the surgeon should be protected from the patient's secretions, needle punctures, and cuts with sharp instruments; eye protectors, double gloves, and waterproof gowns are mandatory.

Special Procedures

Peripheral and Central Venous and Arterial Access

Peripheral and central venous access is essential for the administration of fluids, blood and blood products, medications, chemotherapeutic agents, and nutritional support. Additional help in managing the seriously ill patient has been afforded by the monitoring of central systemic and pulmonary venous pressures. The techniques for venous access in children are important ones to master.

When central lines are placed for short-term use, they may be inserted percutaneously directly into a large vein (subclavian, internal jugular, or femoral) and threaded into a central location. There is available for neonates and tiny infants a fine (#24 gauge), flexible, central venous Silastic catheter (PIC) that is placed peripherally through a needle, usually into the antecubital basilic vein (Figs 1.3–1.8).

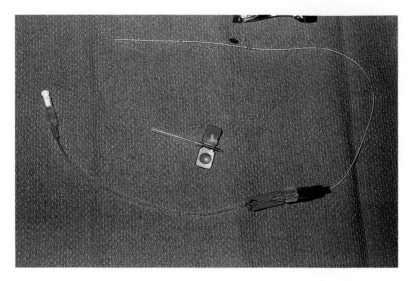

Figure 1.3 The sterile butterfly needle and fine, flexible Silastic catheter are prepared for use. The catheter is filled with heparinized saline solution and is plugged prior to insertion.

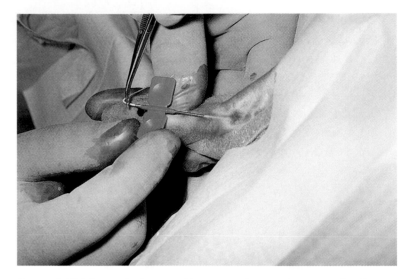

Figure 1.5 Through the needle inserted into the vein, the fine Silastic catheter is threaded to place the tip in the superior vena cava or right atrium.

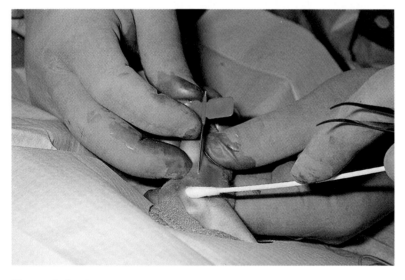

Figure 1.4 The infant's arm is prepped and draped, as for any sterile procedure. Proximal pressure with a sterile cotton-tipped applicator distends the basilic vein.

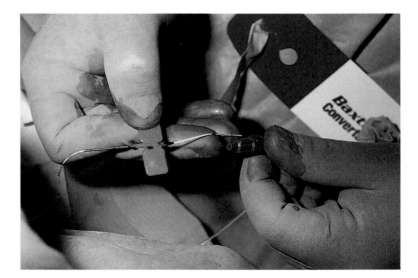

Figure 1.6 The Silastic catheter is disconnected from its hub to allow the needle to be withdrawn. It is then reconnected and flushed gently with heparinized saline.

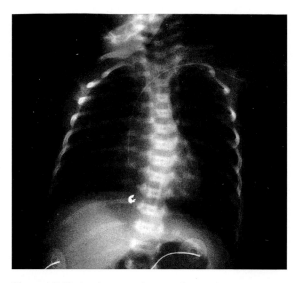

Figure 1.7 A chest radiograph, with 0.5 mL of intravenous contrast material injected into the catheter to enhance visualization, shows the catheter tip in the right atrium.

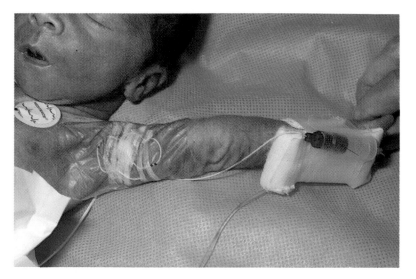

Figure 1.8 The catheter is then carefully secured in place. This infant's catheter is placed into the axillary vein.

For total parenteral nutrition and chemotherapy, long-term indwelling central venous catheters are needed; they are generally of a larger size (#3.5–#9 Fr), have a porous cuff incorporated into the wall to prevent inadvertent removal, and are tunneled subcutaneously before entrance into the vein. They may be inserted percutaneously or via cutdown (Figs 1.9–1.13). Strict antiseptic care is necessary to prevent infection of the catheter and entry site.

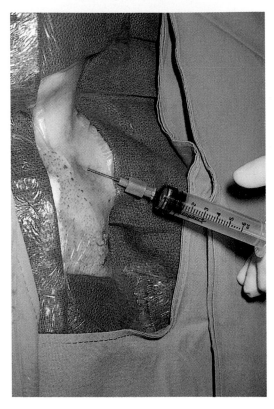 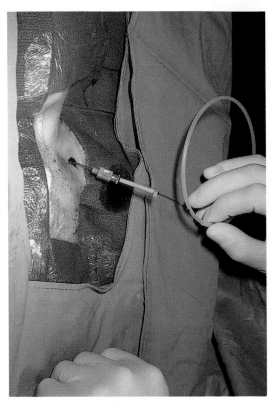 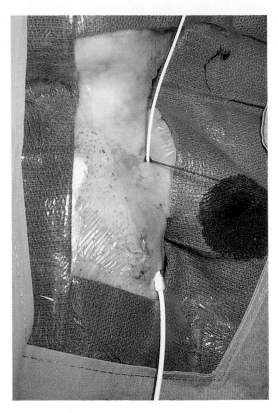

Figure 1.9 Subclavian Vein Catheterization The patient is placed supine, in Trendelenburg position, with a small support behind the shoulders. The chest and neck are prepped and draped with sterile towels. The needle is directed deep to the clavicle and is aimed medially, parallel to the clavicle and slightly superiorly. Return of venous blood into the syringe confirms entry into the subclavian vein.   **Figure 1.10** A flexible guide wire is passed through the needle into the vein. Proper passage into the right atrium may stimulate premature contractions, seen on the cardiac monitor. It is advisable to check the wire position with portable fluoroscopy (C-arm).   **Figure 1.11** When the guide wire is seen to be properly placed, the needle is withdrawn over the wire, and a small skin incision is made at the wire entry site. The catheter is brought through a tunnel created under the skin from an incision on the chest wall to the subclavian incision. The porous cuff, seen here outside the entry site, is then positioned in the subcutaneous tissue 1.5 to 2.0 cm superior to the entry site. The catheter is then trimmed to a length that will place the tip in the right atrium or superior vena cava.

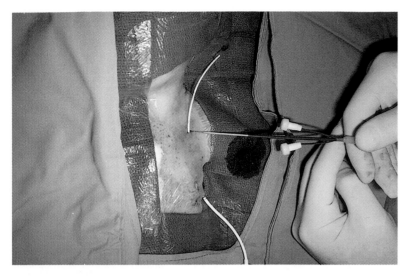

Figure 1.12 The split sheath and dilator are placed over the guide wire into the subclavian vein, as seen here, and the wire is removed. The head-down Trendelenburg position increases venous pressure in the upper body and prevents venous air embolism through the open sheath.

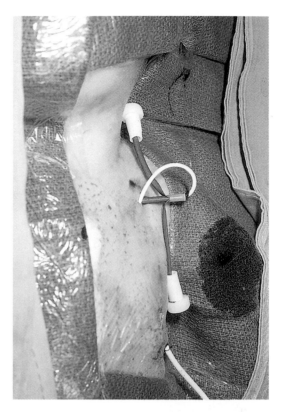

Figure 1.13 The catheter is shown being passed into the split sheath. Its final position is confirmed by fluoroscopy. The sheath is peeled away by traction on the two white knobs. The entry site is closed with interrupted sutures, which are tied to help secure the catheter. The subclavian stab wound is closed with subcuticular sutures. A sterile, occlusive dressing with antibacterial ointment is placed at the catheter entry site.

Arterial lines facilitate the monitoring of blood pressure and blood gases. Percutaneous placement is possible in experienced hands; however, a superficial artery—radial or temporal—is always accessible by cutdown when monitoring is essential (Figs 1.14–1.16).

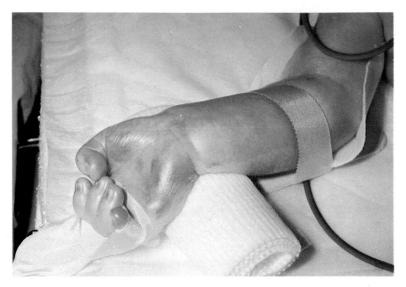

Figure 1.14 Arterial Cutdown The infant's arm is restrained on a board with the wrist extended over a soft pad.

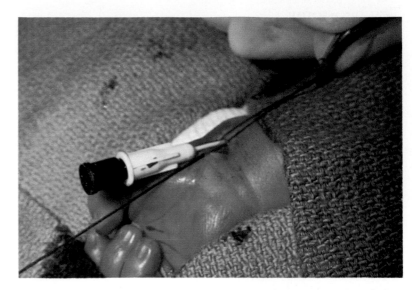

Figure 1.16 The catheter needle is passed into the arterial lumen under direct vision. The artery is not ligated. A small dressing is applied, and the catheter is secured well with tape.

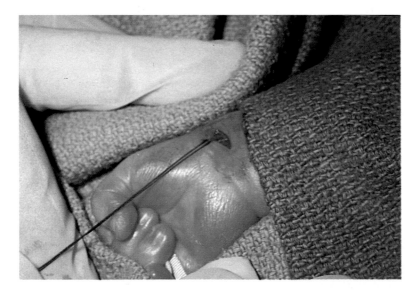

Figure 1.15 A small incision over the palpable artery allows exposure. Ligatures of silk are passed around the artery after it is isolated.

Tracheostomy

Tracheostomy is indicated when intubation is needed for more than 4–6 weeks and for congenital and acquired upper airway obstruction. Whenever possible, the child is intubated first. The technique in children is illustrated in Figures 1.17–1.20.

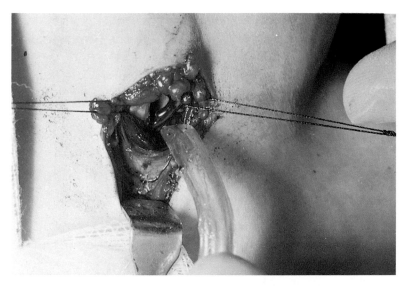

Figure 1.19 The uncuffed tracheostomy tube is being placed under direct vision and will be tied in place around the neck.

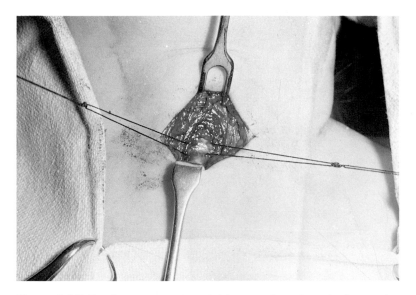

Figure 1.17 Tracheostomy The child is intubated, with the neck extended. A transverse incision over the trachea is made 2 cm above the sternal notch and is carried to the trachea. A 3-0 silk suture is placed through the anterior wall around a tracheal ring on each side of the midline.

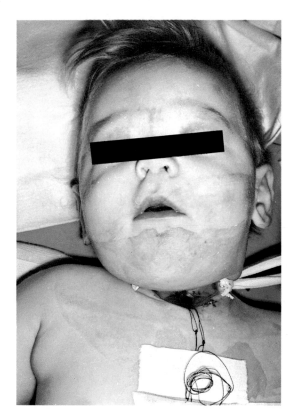

Figure 1.20 The child's tracheostomy tube is secured. Should it dislodge, gentle traction on the silk sutures will expose the tracheal opening for ease in replacement.

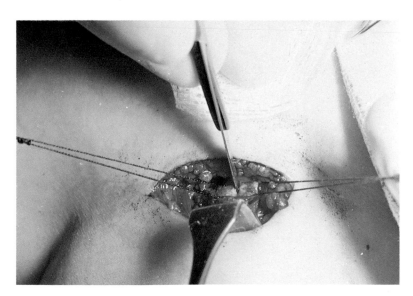

Figure 1.18 With traction placed on the silk sutures, a vertical incision is made through two tracheal rings in the midline. Cartilage is not excised.

Extracorporeal Membrane Oxygenation (ECMO)

In the patient with potentially reversible pulmonary or cardiac insufficiency, temporary circulatory bypass through an extracorporeal artificial "lung" may be lifesaving. ECMO is now used to treat newborns with persistent fetal circulation (pulmonary artery hypertension), congenital diaphragmatic hernia, respiratory distress syndrome, and meconium aspiration. It is also used for children in cardiac failure, especially after corrective cardiac surgery.

The patient's internal jugular vein is cannulated to drain venous blood into the primed ECMO circuit. In the venoarterial bypass, a cannula is placed into the internal carotid artery for blood return. For venovenous bypass, a double-lumen venous catheter is used for drainage and blood return. Systemic anticoagulant is administered. A continuous roller pump draws the venous blood through an artificial lung consisting of a silicone rubber membrane around which 100% oxygen is circulated (Fig 1.21). As the blood is oxygenated, CO_2 removal occurs; a small amount of carbon dioxide (2%–5%) is actually added to the oxygen mixture to prevent hypocapnia.

The usual time on ECMO is 2–5 days, although patients have been maintained for twice that time. As the patient's pulmonary and/or cardiac function improves, the flow rate may be decreased and the patient eventually weaned from the circuit, with removal of the cannulae.

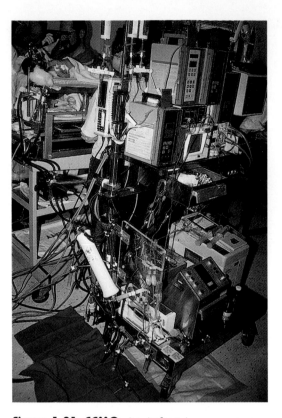

Figure 1.21 ECMO An infant is seen on extracorporeal oxygenation. The white cylinder in the lower left contains the gas exchange membrane. The stainless steel roller pump and controls are seen on the bottom of the cribside cart. Monitors and intravenous pumps for fluids and medication are mounted above.

Nutrition

The need for adequate nutrition in pediatric surgical patients has been well established. Children must satisfy the metabolic demands not only of tissue repair and healing but also of rapid and continuing growth and development. Preparation for major elective surgery should include assessment of nutritional status and correction of nutritional deficiencies. Postoperative patients need continuing nutritional support, even in the face of prolonged inability to use the gastrointestinal tract or to absorb nutrients from a short or malfunctioning gut.

In the assessment of nutritional status of a child, clinical history, height and weight for age, triceps skin fold thickness, and serum albumin and transferrin levels all are helpful. The state of hydration is important, because children have a higher percentage of body water and more rapid water turnover than adults. Calorie and protein requirements are especially high in the "growing years." Infants to the age of 1 year need 90–120 kcal and 2–3.5 g protein daily per kilogram of body weight. From 1–7 years, 75–90 kcal/kg and 2–2.5 g/kg protein are considered normal requirements. These needs increase with fever, sepsis, major surgery, major trauma, and extensive burns.

Two significant advances in the past 25 years include the formulation of elemental enteral diets and the development of central and peripheral venous hyperalimentation, also known as total parenteral nutrition (TPN). Elemental diets consist of protein hydrolysate or amino acids, glucose as the carbohydrate, and fat in an easily absorbable form such as medium-chain triglycerides (MCT). They are especially useful in patients with gastrointestinal tract disease and are given directly into the stomach or intestine by tube. Bolus feedings are generally used, but the child without gastroesophageal reflux may safely be fed by mechanically regulated continuous drip feeding. Because of the high osmolality of most enteral feedings, they must be diluted when first given to the infant or child; the concentration is subsequently increased progressively to full strength, as tolerated.

TPN is used when the gastrointestinal tract cannot be used because of intestinal obstruction, prolonged ileus, severe inflammatory disease, enteric fistulas, necrotizing enterocolitis, or severe prematurity. Current solutions consist of a balanced mixture of purified amino acids and hypertonic glucose to which appropriate electrolytes, vitamins, and trace elements are added. Intravenous fat emulsion provides additional calories and essential fatty acids. Commercially prepared solutions of 25% glucose and 3.5%–5% purified amino acids can be used in the child older than 10 years old. Younger children need to be started on lower concentrations of solute. Neonates and infants must have specifically formulated TPN solutions; they start with 10% glucose and 1.5%–2.0% amino acids, and concentrations are increased to 15% glucose and 2.5%–3.0% amino acids. Even low amino acid concentrations may produce cholestatic jaundice in some neonates, especially after the repeated administration of diuretics. In these infants, TPN must be discontinued until the jaundice clears.

In tiny premature infants and in some older children in whom central lines cannot be placed, peripheral parenteral nutrition (PPN) may be given through peripheral intravenous lines. Because high concentrations of solute would rapidly cause venous thrombosis, glucose concentrations are limited to 10%–12%. Nevertheless, premature infants have been shown to gain weight on PPN and to develop until they are physiologically able to tolerate enteral feedings.

Chapter 2

Skin and Subcutaneous Tissue

Warts

A viral infection in the skin, the verruca vulgaris (wart) frequently disappears spontaneously. When it does not, removal by freezing, electrocauterization, or careful acid application is indicated. The base must be treated as well, to destroy the virus and prevent recurrence. The author prefers curettage of the wart and electrocauterization of the base. This procedure can be carried out under local anesthesia in most children older than 8 years.

Pigmented Nevi

Pigmented nevi, especially those in areas of frequent skin irritation, are of greatest concern when there are changes in color, size, or configuration—especially at puberty (Fig 2.1). Malignant changes are rare in children; what is called a "juvenile melanoma" is not a dangerous tumor. However, nevi on the soles, palms, fingers, genitalia, and belt or bra line are frequently excised for diagnosis and to relieve future concern. Wide local excision is indicated for proven malignant melanoma (Fig 2.2).

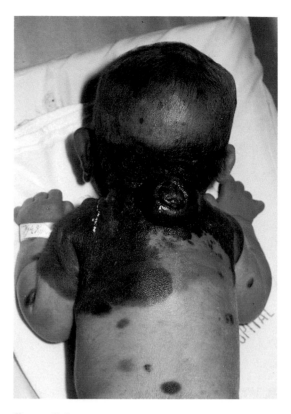

Figure 2.2 The extensive nevus of the head, neck, shoulders, and back in this newborn girl contains a firm, raised, central mass, which is a congenital malignant melanoma.

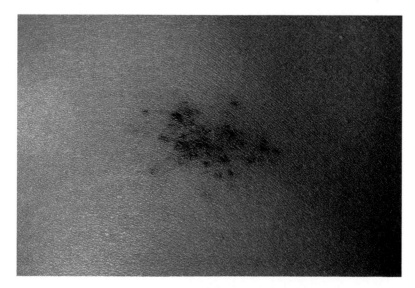

Figure 2.1 Nevus Despite its multiple, small, dark foci of pigmentation, this is a benign juvenile nevus.

Giant Nevi

Giant nevi, frequently covered with hair (Fig 2.3), are of cosmetic importance (Fig 2.4) and are potentially pre-malignant. Current surgical approaches to the giant nevus include (1) excision with skin grafting, (2) serial excision, and (3) the use of subcutaneous tissue expanders and subsequent primary excision.

Keloids

The formation of massive overgrown scars (keloids) in areas of skin trauma or previous surgery is an individual characteristic, more common in black people. Keloid formers should avoid unnecessary skin trauma, such as ear piercing (Fig 2.5). The author has found the most effective treatment of mature keloids to be (1) careful excision of the keloid, (2) meticulous subcuticular closure using fine (5-0) absorbable polyglycolic acid sutures or a ''pull-out'' monofilament of nylon or Prolene, and (3) intradermal injection of the excision site with corticosteroid (dexamethasone) at surgery and every 4 weeks thereafter for 6–12 months (Figs 2.6, 2.7). Steroid infiltration alone may be attempted early in the development of a keloid. Good results can never be ensured with any treatment.

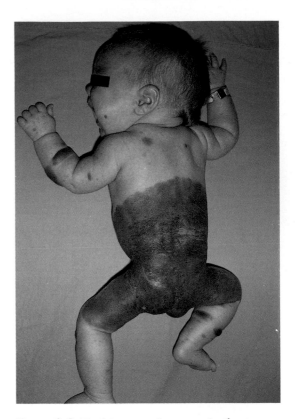

Figure 2.4 *Bathing-trunk nevus* is the term for this circumferential, benign giant nevus, which extends from midtrunk to knees.

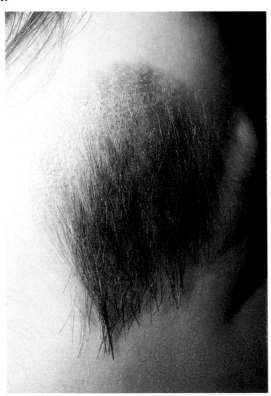

Figure 2.3 The large, hairy nevus of the frontal scalp is cosmetically unacceptable and will be excised.

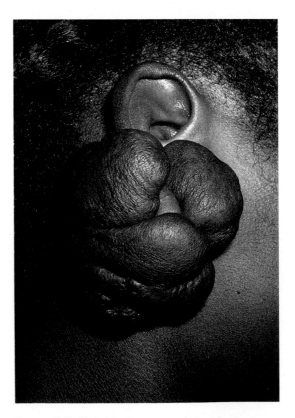

Figure 2.5 Keloid The site of simple ear piercing in this susceptible girl developed into a cauliflowerlike keloid.

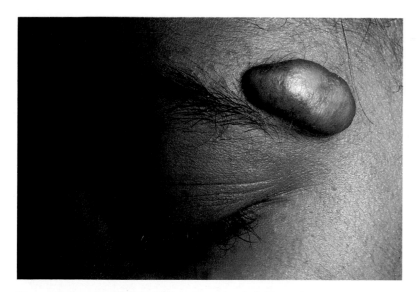

Figure 2.6 A small laceration over the left brow led to this keloid.

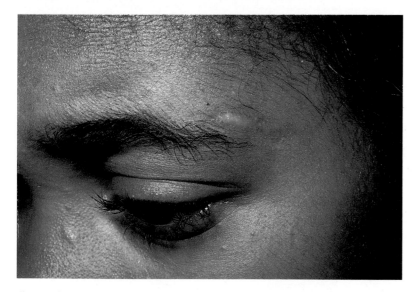

Figure 2.7 The result of excision and monthly infiltration of the scar with dexamethasone is seen after 7 months.

Ehlers-Danlos Syndrome

Ehlers-Danlos syndrome, or ectodermal dysplasia, is characterized by lax skin (Fig 2.8), gaping of even minor lacerations, and poor healing. Elective surgery in these patients requires careful hemostasis and delayed suture removal. Inguinal hernias are more common in children with Ehlers-Danlos syndrome.

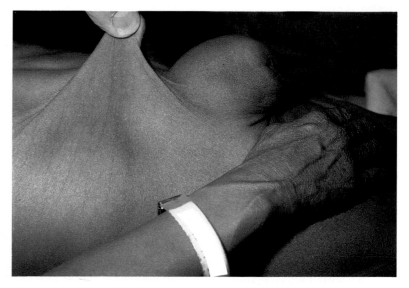

Figure 2.8 Ehlers-Danlos Syndrome The skin of a child with Ehlers-Danlos syndrome is elevated from the abdomen. Her umbilical hernia is repaired, and the skin incision is approximated with great care.

Hemangiomas

Hemangiomas are benign vascular lesions that appear as tumors, birthmarks, and malformations. The classification of hemangiomas has undergone recent revision, based on the time of appearance and biologic behavior of the lesion. Those that are considered to be purely vascular malformations, such as cutaneous port-wine stains, are always present at birth, grow with the child, have an equal male:female distribution, and do not disappear or fade spontaneously. All other true hemangiomas have the following characteristics: they have a period of rapid proliferation, whether or not they appear at, or after, birth; they are more common in girls by a ratio of 3:1; involvement is most often of the skin and subcutaneous tissues, but they may infiltrate into muscle and fascia and are sometimes found in other internal organs, such as the intestine and liver; there may be associated other vascular anomalies, such as a lymphangioma or arteriovenous malformation; and they generally involute slowly after the period of proliferation.

Capillary hemangiomas ("strawberry marks") are limited to the skin surface. They blanch with pressure and can be observed to involute as the pink color changes to skin color, starting in the center and spreading to the periphery of the hemangioma (Fig 2.9). A rare type of capillary hemangioma, termed a "fire-field" hemangioma, grows very rapidly, leading to local tissue necrosis (Fig 2.10); it requires prompt treatment to control the lesion.

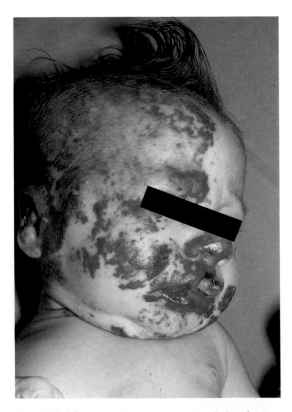

Figure 2.10 Small hemangiomas of the face coalesce and spread, with subsequent necrosis and tissue destruction of the upper lip. This "fire-field" hemangioma requires immediate treatment to induce regression.

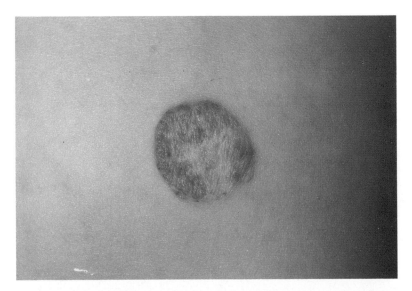

Figure 2.9 Hemangioma This "strawberry mark" in a 2-year-old was once pink. The central portion is fading to normal skin color; the rest of the hemangioma will regress, as most do, by the age of 5 years.

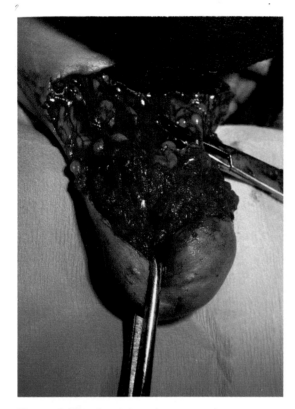

Figure 2.11 The large cavernous hemangioma is being excised from the neck of an 18-month-old girl; note a sizable draining vein identified by the hemostat.

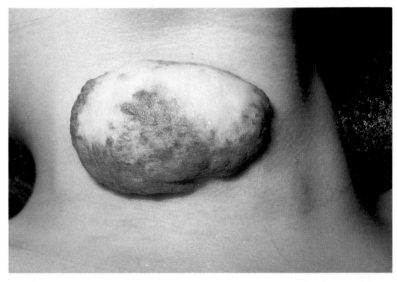

Figure 2.12 The capillary portion of this hemangioma is fading. There is a firm, underlying mass.

Cavernous (venous) hemangiomas are subcutaneous, with a bluish tinge and ''bag-of-worms'' consistency. Some involute, but prominent ones that do not do so must be excised (Fig 2.11).

Composed of compact masses of endothelial cells, the hemangioendothelioma is a solid lesion that may involve the skin, subcutaneous tissue, or deeper layers (Figs 2.12, 2.13). Although spontaneous regression is the rule, the residual loose skin is often excised for cosmetic reasons.

Mixed lesions may contain any of the other types of hemangioma (Figs 2.14–2.17).

Complications of hemangiomas include (1) rapid increase in size with tissue necrosis; (2) platelet trapping and thrombocytopenia—the Kasabach-Merritt syndrome; (3) recurrent or severe bleeding; (4) infection, with and without erosion; and (5) residual cosmetic defect. Systemic steroid therapy is the first choice of treatment when there are the complications of persistent bleeding, necrosis, or platelet trapping. Interferon administration has been used with some success when steroid therapy has

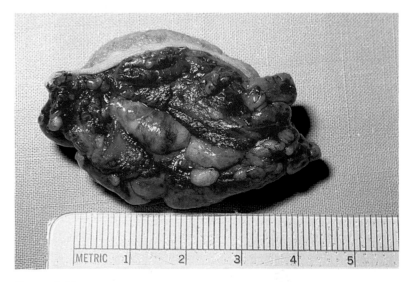

Figure 2.13 The excised mass is a hemangioendothelioma.

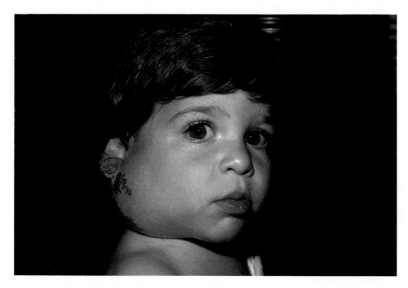

Figure 2.14 Present at birth, this lesion rapidly grew to occupy the posterior half of the right face of this boy, seen here at age 2.

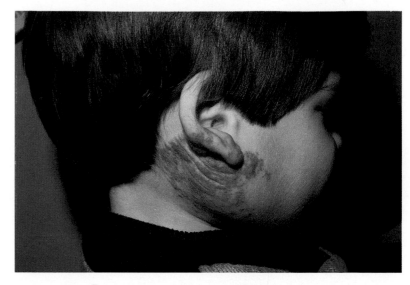

Figure 2.16 The capillary portion is beginning to fade, and the cavernous hemangioma is stable in size 18 months later.

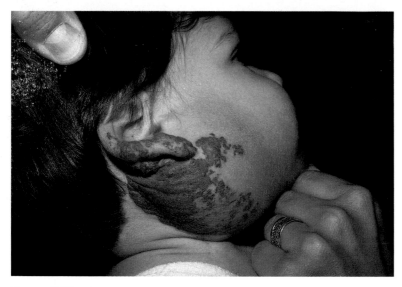

Figure 2.15 The protruding mass is a mixed capillary and cavernous hemangioma involving the face, neck, and ear.

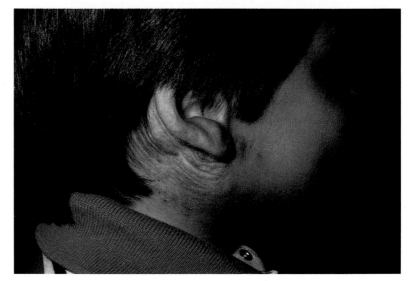

Figure 2.17 After 20 months of additional observation, the capillary part of the hemangioma is almost completely faded, and the cavernous part is no longer visible and is barely palpable—an unexpectedly favorable result.

failed to shrink the lesion. Surgical excision, where possible, is indicated in emergency situations or for cosmetic considerations. Intracutaneous malformations, such as port-wine stains, are now being treated successfully by laser therapy. Treatment of hemangiomas with dry ice and electrocautery is to be condemned, because these methods produce unnecessary scarring; and superficial ionizing radiation should be used in children only for tissue-destructive proliferation that cannot be controlled by other means.

Localized hemangiomas associated with arteriovenous malformations should be excised (Figs 2.18, 2.19). Large hemangiomas and multiple arteriovenous fistulas of the extremities (Klippel-Trenaunay syndrome) may lead to hemihypertrophy (see Fig 2.67); a number have been reported to respond well to intermittent pneumatic compression.

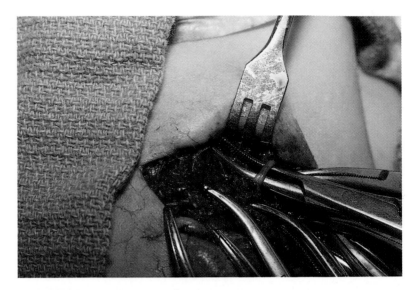

Figure 2.19 At surgery, a sizable arterial vessel is seen feeding the malformation. The draining veins are also large, as would be expected in an arteriovenous malformation.

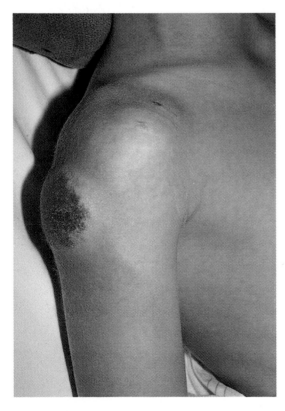

Figure 2.18 The hemangioma of this 7-year-old boy's upper arm is noted to be growing in size, with increasing prominence of the adjacent veins. An arterial pulsation is felt in the hemangioma.

Pyogenic Granuloma

Pyogenic granuloma is an acquired, proliferative, cutaneous vascular lesion that resembles a capillary hemangioma. It is not, as the name implies, an infectious process; it is thought by some to be the result of minor trauma. Children have a greater tendency to develop these lesions, most often on the face, neck, and scalp (Fig 2.20). The granuloma begins as a small erythematous papule, which grows rapidly, may form a crust (Fig 2.21), and bleeds easily. Initial treatment is by cauterization or electrocoagulation. Persistence or recurrence of this benign lesion requires surgical excision.

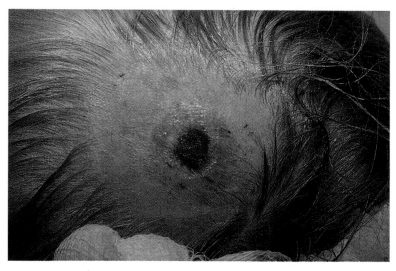

Figure 2.20 Pyogenic Granuloma A tiny red papule on the scalp of this 3-year-old has grown rapidly to the lesion seen here.

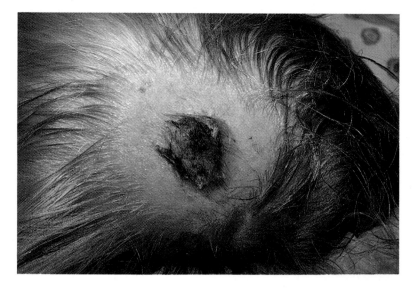

Figure 2.21 The granuloma develops a crust and then bleeds profusely when the crust sloughs or is avulsed. It does not respond to cauterization and requires surgical excision.

Lymphangiomas

Lymphangioma is a hamartomatous malformation with cystic dilatation of the lymphatic vessels. It may present as a single cyst (Fig 2.22), a locally infiltrating lesion (Figs 2.23–2.25), or a process involving an entire extremity (Fig 2.26). Occasionally it is associated with a hemangioma in a ''hemolymphangioma.'' A lymphangioma of the neck is called cystic hygroma (see Chapter 3).

Unless they produce functional or cosmetic impairment, lymphangiomas of the trunk and extremities are best left alone and frequently involute spontaneously. The two complications are infection and sudden bleeding into the cysts. Intraabdominal lymphangioma may be seen in association with large mesenteric cysts (see Chapter 9).

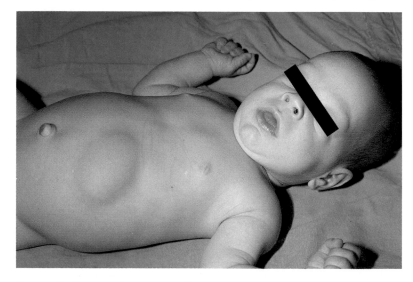

Figure 2.22 Lymphangioma There is a single lymphangiomatous cyst on the abdomen of this 2-month-old boy.

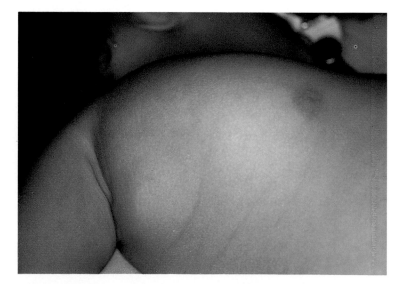

Figure 2.23 The cystic mass of the right shoulder and chest is demonstrated.

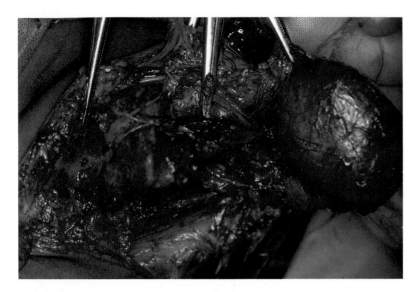

Figure 2.24 Dissection of the mass shows it to invade the pectoral muscle and chest wall.

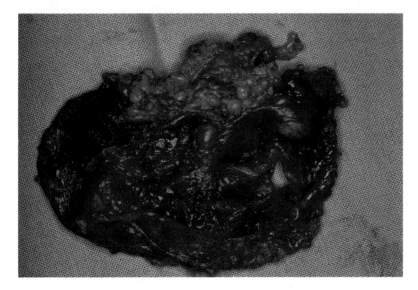

Figure 2.25 The specimen of the extensive lymphangioma is excised, after many of the cysts have been emptied of fluid.

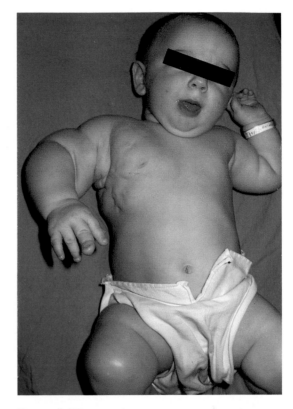

Figure 2.26 Lymphangioma involves the entire right arm in this 9-month-old boy. There is an associated macrodactyly of the middle finger.

Lipomas

Lipomas are well-demarcated, subcutaneous fatty masses. Mature lipomas are benign and generally have only cosmetic significance (Figs 2.27, 2.28). If not completely excised, they can recur locally. Lipoblastomas are well-circumscribed lesions, usually found in infants; despite the histologic appearance of malignancy, they do not metastasize and tend to mature with the child. Other tissue elements may be found in mixed lesions, such as fibrolipoma and angiolipoma (Figs 2.29–2.31).

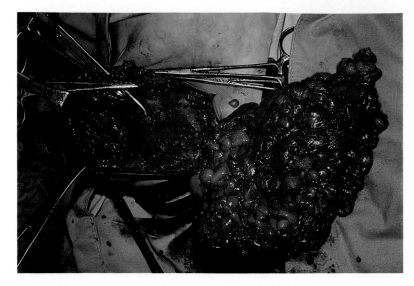

Figure 2.28 The huge mass of subcutaneous fat is excised to the fascia.

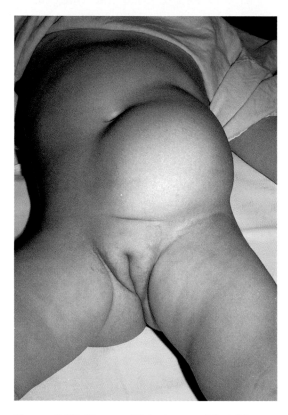

Figure 2.27 Lipoma This 2-year-old girl has a fatty mass that occupies the entire left mid and lower abdominal wall.

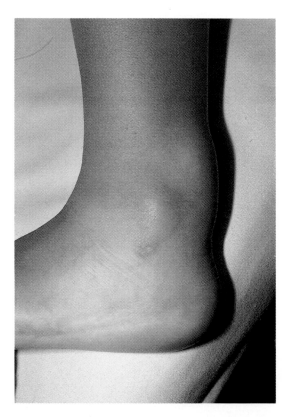

Figure 2.29 Angiolipoma A firm mass overlying the Achilles tendon of this 3-year-old girl has been growing slowly.

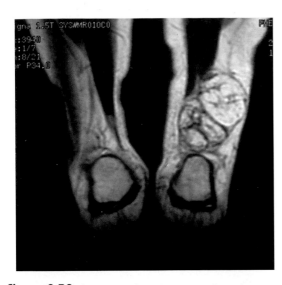

Figure 2.30 A magnetic resonance imaging scan shows the extent of the well-encapsulated tumor mass, displacing but not invading local structures.

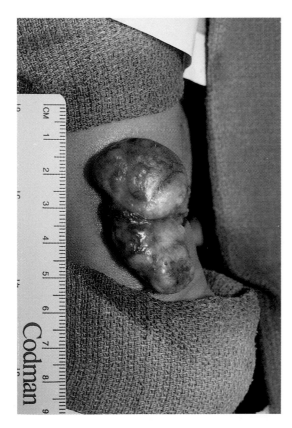

Figure 2.31 The tumor mass is seen at surgical excision. The histologic diagnosis is angiolipoma.

Neurofibromas

Neurofibromas are hamartomatous growths that may occur in the skin and subcutaneous tissue (Figs 2.32–2.34), along nerve trunks, in the viscera, in the orbitofacial area (Fig 2.35), and in the central nervous system. Neurofibromatosis—von Recklinghausen's disease—is transmitted as an autosomal dominant trait. It is characterized by café-au-lait spots on the skin, which increase in size and number at puberty. Tumors should be excised if they become large, painful, or deforming. The rapid growth of a tumor mass may signal malignant degeneration to neurofibrosarcoma; immediate excision is advised.

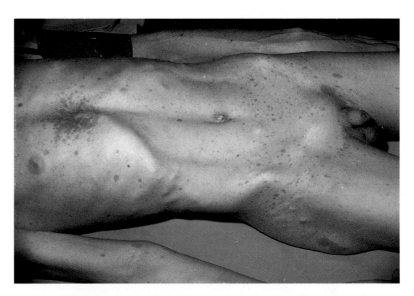

Figure 2.32 Neurofibromatosis Multiple subcutaneous neurofibromatous nodules are seen in this thin 15-year-old. He has café-au-lait spots on the chest and left thigh.

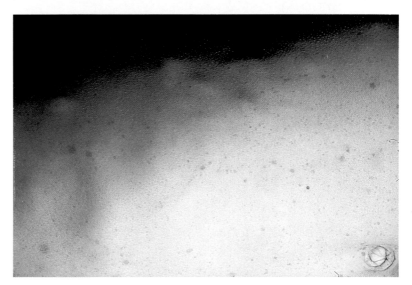

Figure 2.33 The neurofibromas are seen clearly in this close-up photograph.

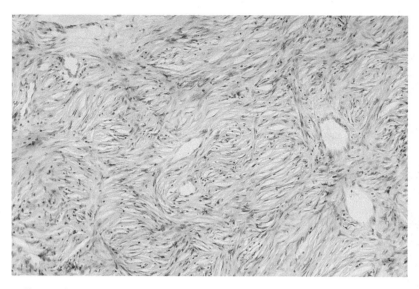

Figure 2.34 This photomicrograph is of an enlarging mass in the popliteal space of the same patient. Neural elements are seen in the fibrous tissue matrix.

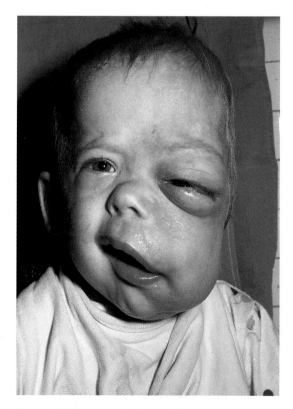

Figure 2.35 A single neurofibroma distorts the left side of the face of this 14-month-old boy.

Epidermoid Cysts

Cysts in children are frequently of congenital origin. Epidermoid inclusion cysts (dermoids) containing typical waxy sebum are most common at the corner of the brow (Fig 2.36) and in the midline of the head and neck (Figs 2.37–2.39); midline scalp lesions may extend through the bone, and their extent should be delineated by preoperative imaging studies. Other cyst locations include the posterior neck, scalp, external ear (Figs 2.40, 2.41), and dorsum of the nose. Cosmetic appearance is the usual indication for excision, although some cysts become abscessed, requiring drainage and subsequent excision.

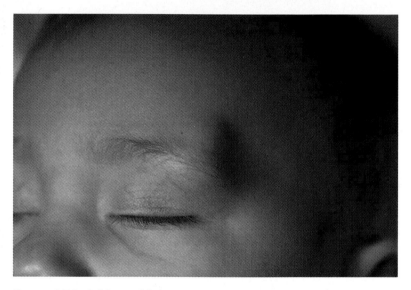

Figure 2.36 Epidermoid Cyst The lateral corner of the brow is a common site for epidermoid cysts. The incision for removal is placed at the edge of the brow and is closed with subcuticular sutures for the best cosmetic result.

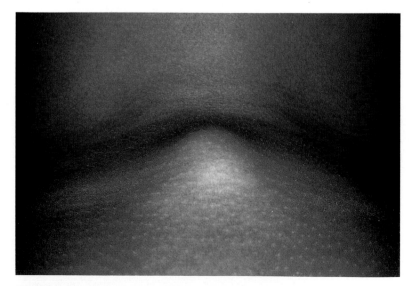

Figure 2.37 This 2-year-old has a round cystic midline neck mass.

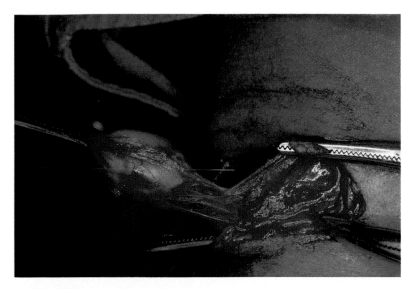

Figure 2.38 A transverse incision exposes the mass for dissection. There are no deep sinus tracts from the cyst and no attachment to the hyoid bone.

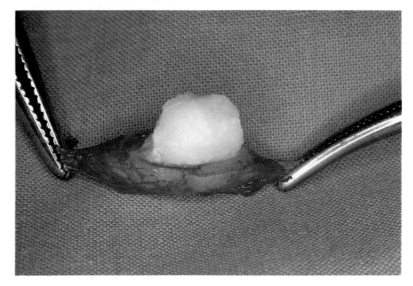

Figure 2.39 The excised cyst contains the waxy sebaceous material characteristic of epidermoid cysts.

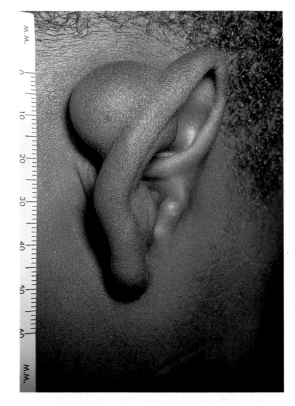

Figure 2.40 This cyst of the posterior ear was present for many years. It grew in size and is seen just prior to excision.

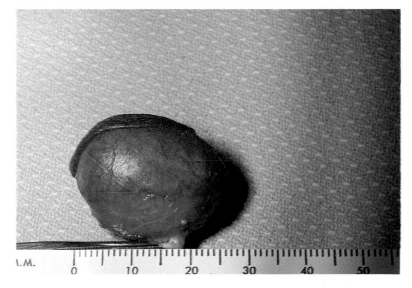

Figure 2.41 The specimen measures 2.5 cm and is filled with waxy material.

Neck Abnormalities

Midline Cervical Cleft

This unusual fault of embryologic development leaves a midline skin defect in the neck, covered with shiny membranous tissue (Fig 2.42). Repair includes excision of the skin defect and associated subcutaneous scar and Z-plasty to break the vertical incision (Figs 2.43, 2.44).

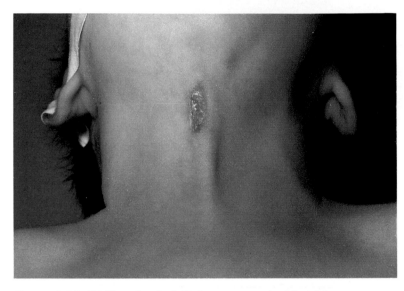

Figure 2.42 Midline Cervical Cleft A 2½-week-old girl has a congenital midline skin defect and a tight subcutaneous fibrous tissue band.

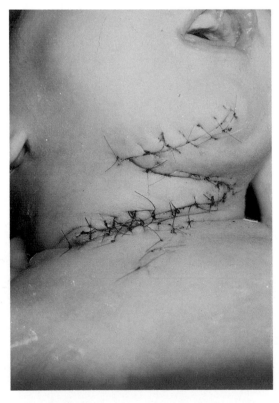

Figure 2.43 The shiny skin lesion is excised, and a double Z-plasty is performed.

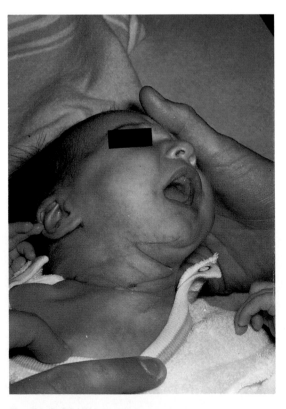

Figure 2.44 Following suture removal, the operative site is healing well and a satisfactory cosmetic result is anticipated.

Branchial Remnants

Remnants of the early embryologic branchial (gill) arches and clefts include branchial cleft cysts and sinuses (see Chapter 3) and protruding skin tags; some skin tags contain cartilage, a "leftover" of the branchial arch (Fig 2.45, 2.46). When these facial remnants are found bilaterally, there is an increased likelihood of associated renal anomalies. Occasionally, one or more small, firm subcutaneous masses without an associated skin tag are felt in the mid or low neck; these also represent residual cartilaginous rests. These branchial remnants are excised, with care taken to remove all of the contained cartilage, part of which extends into the subcutaneous tissue (Figs 2.47, 2.48).

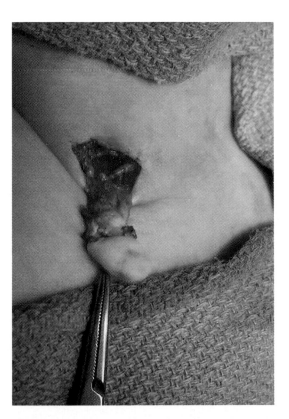

Figure 2.47 The contained cartilaginous remnant extends into the subcutaneous tissues. It is completely excised.

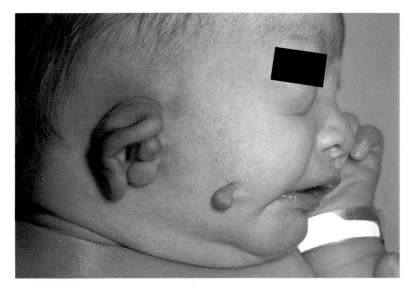

Figure 2.45 Branchial Remnant The skin tag containing a spicule of cartilage is a remnant of the embryologic branchial arch. There is an ipsilateral ear deformity.

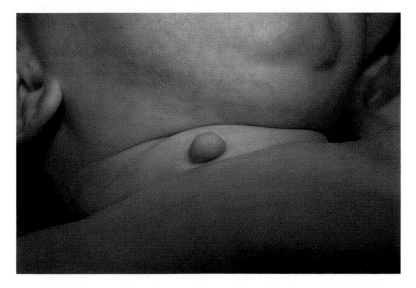

Figure 2.46 The protruding skin lesion of the neck, at the anterior border of this infant's sternocleidomastoid muscle, is a branchial remnant containing cartilage.

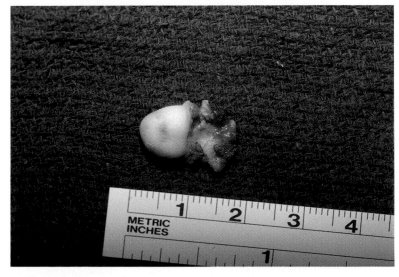

Figure 2.48 The excised specimen and excised cartilage are demonstrated. A plastic repair with subcuticular sutures is performed.

Lymph Nodes

Enlarged lymph nodes in children almost always result from local or systemic infection, and most deserve simple observation and treatment of the infection. Some may become acutely abscessed, requiring drainage (Fig 2.49).

An indolent cervical abscess in a child may result from atypical mycobacterial infection or cat-scratch disease; in both infections, incision may lead to a chronically draining sinus. In many cases of atypical mycobacterial infection, the diagnosis can be confirmed by acid-fast stain of the needle-aspirated contents. In both diseases, the involved node should be completely excised (Fig 2.50). Microscopic examination of the node proves the diagnosis in cat-scratch disease. The finding of firm, fixed nodes in the cervical and supraclavicular areas raises the suspicion of lymphoma. They should undergo excisional biopsy (Figs 2.51–2.53).

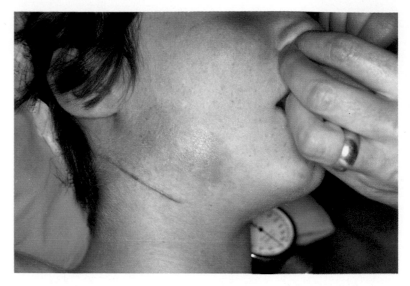

Figure 2.50 A chronic infection of the submandibular nodes with an indolent abscess is seen in this 13-year-old girl; she has a positive skin test for Battey's atypical mycobacterium. Excision of an involved node on the same side had been performed a year previously.

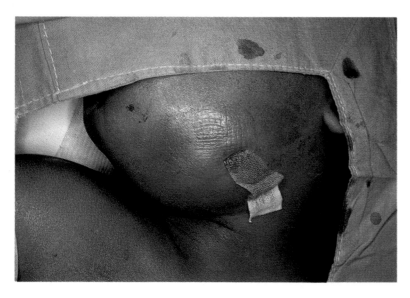

Figure 2.49 Lymph Node Abscess The abscessed submandibular lymph node is seen at the time of incision, drainage, and packing with iodoform gauze.

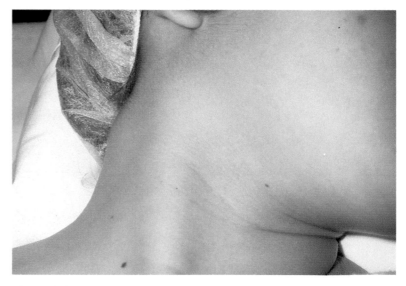

Figure 2.51 Hodgkin's Disease An enlarged lymph node protrudes in the posterior triangle of the neck of this 14-year-old girl.

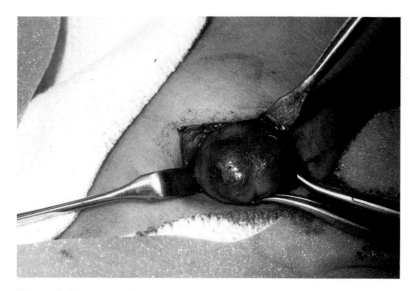

Figure 2.52 The entire node is dissected and excised.

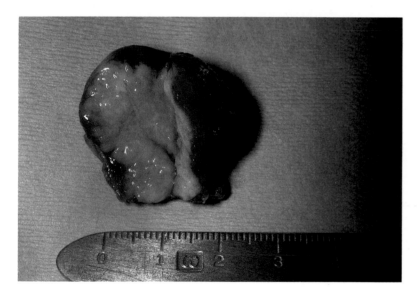

Figure 2.53 A fleshy uniform consistency of the node on cut section is consistent with the subsequent diagnosis of Hodgkin's lymphoma.

Extremities

Ganglion

A ganglion is a subcutaneous cyst that arises from a tendon sheath or joint capsule and contains a clear, viscid fluid. In the popliteal space it is called a *Baker's cyst*. Interference with function and cosmetic appearance are the reasons for excision (Figs 2.54, 2.55). Direct trauma to the cyst may cause it to rupture, but many subsequently recur.

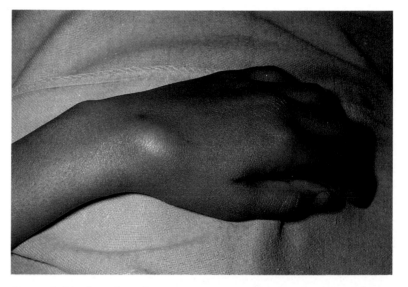

Figure 2.54 Ganglion Cyst The cystic, well-defined mass of the left wrist of this 9-year-old is a typical ganglion.

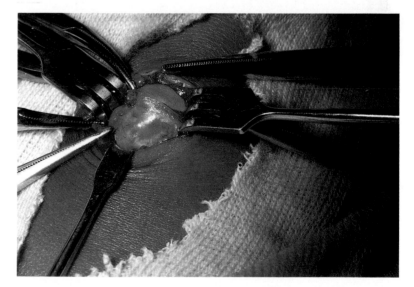

Figure 2.55 At the operative dissection, the shiny cyst is found to communicate with the joint capsule of the wrist. The cyst is excised and the communication with the joint is sutured closed.

Polydactyly

Frequently familial, extra digits on the hands and feet are removed for the sake of appearance (Figs 2.56, 2.57). Only those rudimentary digits with a very thin skin attachment (2 mm in width or less) should be ligated. All others should be excised surgically, with careful plastic repair at the base. Interference with function is associated with more complex hand abnormalities, which require careful evaluation of bony and soft tissue anatomy, as well as function, prior to any surgery (Figs 2.58, 2.59).

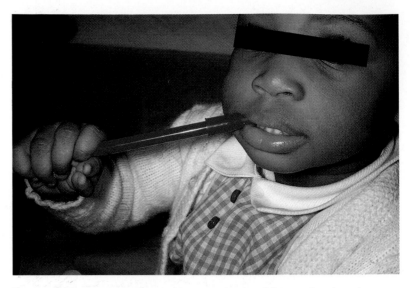

Figure 2.58 This 15-month-old uses both of her right thumbs to grasp. Future repair must consider appearance and function.

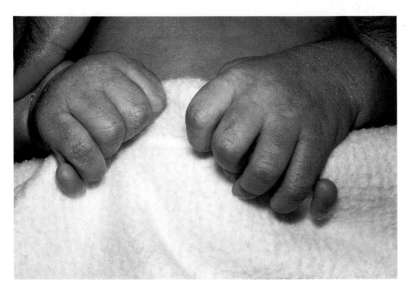

Figure 2.56 Polydactyly The most common form of polydactyly is shown, with rudimentary extra digits attached by a small skin bridge. Those pictured here have too wide an attachment for ligation and are excised.

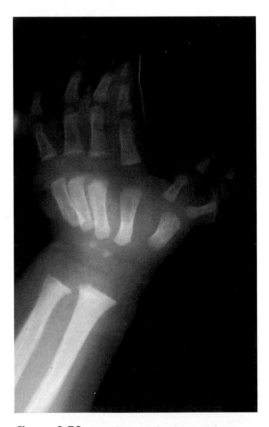

Figure 2.59 A radiograph shows the phalanges of both thumbs articulating with the first metacarpal.

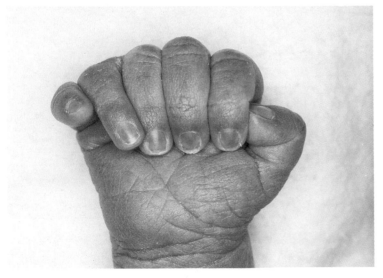

Figure 2.57 The sixth finger of this infant's hand has full sensation and motion and a normal appearance. It is not removed.

Syndactyly

Syndactyly may occur as an isolated deformity or in association with a particular syndrome, such as Apert's syndrome. Fused digits, especially fingers, must be separated for adequate function (Figs 2.60, 2.61). Skin webbing is repaired with plastic technique, which avoids longitudinal scars across joints. Most repairs require skin grafts. Bony syndactyly (Fig 2.62) requires more careful planning for functional repair.

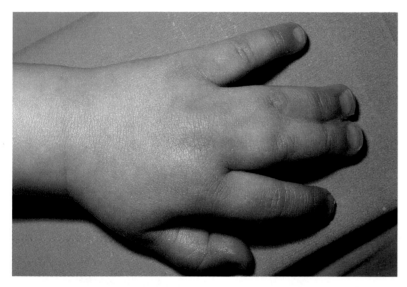

Figure 2.60 Syndactyly Skin and subcutaneous tissue bridge the proximal part of this 1-year-old's third and fourth fingers.

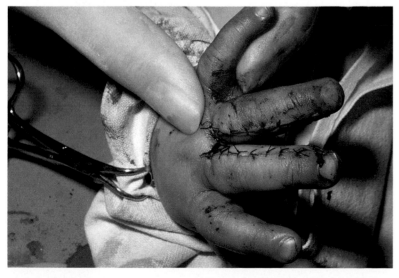

Figure 2.61 The syndactyly is divided, with creation of a web space and skin grafts to the bare finger surfaces.

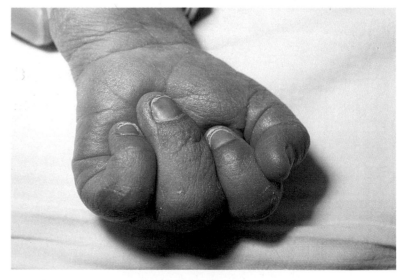

Figure 2.62 Bony syndactyly of the third and fourth fingers forms a single middle digit in this newborn infant.

Annular Bands

Congenital annular bands (constriction of the skin and subcutaneous tissue) of the extremities are attributed by some to constricting amniotic bands in utero. In the most extreme form, they are associated with distal limb deformity—Streeter's dysplasia (Fig 2.63). Z-plasty of the constricting band (Figs 2.64, 2.65) is performed in infancy to allow growth of the extremity; distal deformities are repaired later.

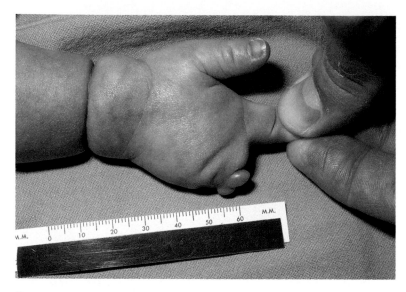

Figure 2.63 Streeter's Dysplasia A congenital annular band of the wrist is associated with agenesis of the fingers; this combination of anomalies is called *Streeter's dysplasia*.

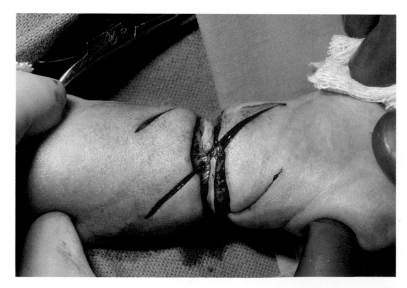

Figure 2.64 The band of tight skin and subcutaneous tissue is excised, and multiple Z-plasties are created to break the scar and prevent future constriction.

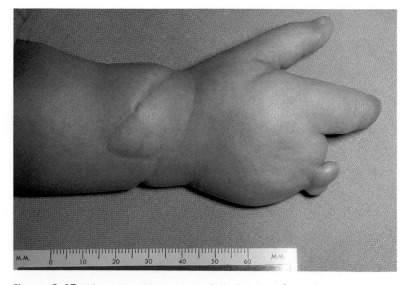

Figure 2.65 The operative site is fully healed 6 weeks later.

Tourniquet Syndrome

In infants, it is not unusual to find a strand of maternal hair wrapped around a finger or toe. The distal redness and swelling has the appearance of a paronychia (Fig 2.66). Removal of all the constricting hair is sufficient treatment, unless there has been severe vascular impairment.

Vascular Anomalies

Vascular hamartomas of the extremities may include hemangiomatous and lymphangiomatous elements. Arteriovenous fistulas often lead to hypertrophy of the extremity (Fig 2.67); most are not amenable to surgery, and intermittent pneumatic compression currently offers the best result. Congenital lymphedema (Fig 2.68) may resolve spontaneously or may require a compressive elastic garment; complete subcutaneous excision and grafting is a last resort procedure. Congenital varicosities (Figs 2.69, 2.70) are best palliated by elastic support.

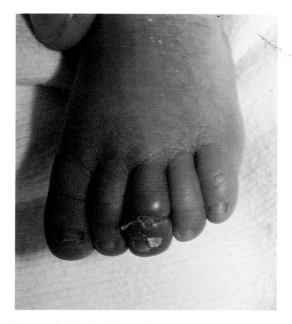

Figure 2.66 Hair Tourniquet The deep impression in the skin made by a constricting strand of maternal hair around the middle toe and the resulting inflammation are seen following removal of the hair itself.

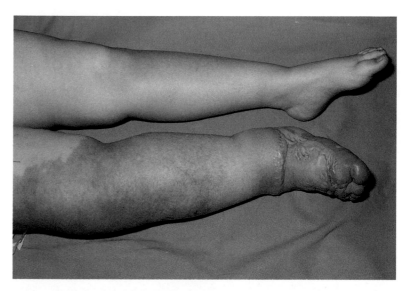

Figure 2.67 Vascular Anomaly Hemihypertrophy and macrodactyly are seen in the right leg of this girl with a hemangioma and small arteriovenous fistulas.

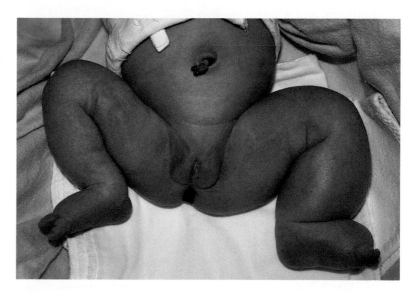

Figure 2.68 This 2-day-old has congenital lymphedema of the left leg.

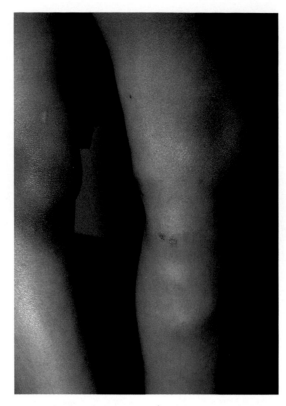

Figure 2.69 An unusual congenital venous
anomaly with varicosities of both legs is
seen in this 7-year-old boy.

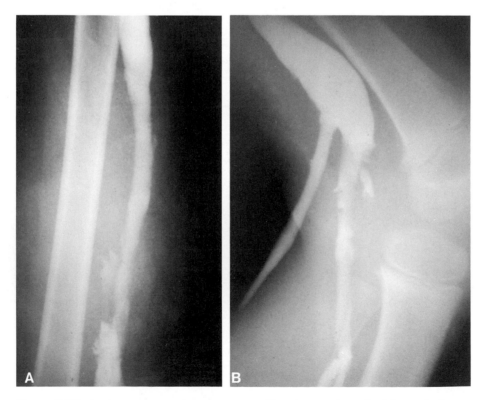

Figure 2.70 A. A venogram demonstrates dilatation and marked irregularity
of the saphenous vein. **B.** The deep femoral vein has an area of dilatation
just above the knee on this lateral view.

Sacroperineal Area

Pilonidal Cysts and Sinuses

Thought to originate as either a congenital cyst or the ingrowth and infection of a hair follicle, the pilonidal cyst is common in adolescence. It presents as a painful, inflamed midline sacral cyst with one or more visible skin sinuses (Fig 2.71). The infection may regress under local heat application and antibiotic therapy or may form an abscess that drains spontaneously or requires surgical drainage. Within 6–8 weeks after complete resolution of the inflammation, the entire cyst should be excised to the presacral fascia, along with all sinus tracts (Figs 2.72, 2.73).

Although the common treatment is excision and open packing to allow slow filling in of the defect, the author has performed a modified primary closure in nondiabetic patients when there is no evidence of residual inflammation at the time of surgery.

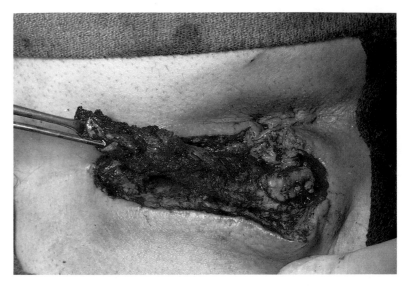

Figure 2.72 The inflamed cyst and sinus tracts are dissected in their entirety to the depth of the sacral fascia.

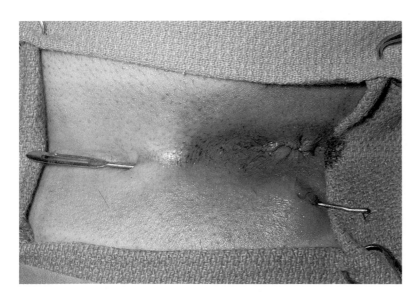

Figure 2.71 Pilonidal Cyst and Sinus A probe enters the skin sinus over a pilonidal cyst and exits through another sinus next to the anus, where this 17-year-old had chronic purulent drainage.

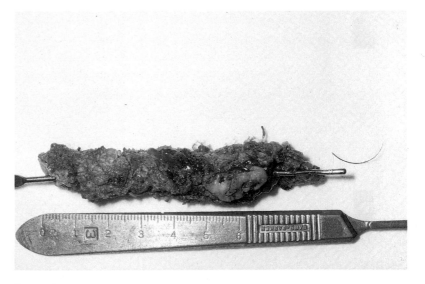

Figure 2.73 The excised specimen is more than 8 cm long.

Chapter 3

Face, Head, and Neck

Tumors

Nasal Glioma and Encephalocele

When the embryologic space (glabella) between the nasal and frontal bones fails to close during early intrauterine development, dura may protrude into the space, forming a meningocele; if brain protrudes with the dura, it is an encephalocele (Fig 3.1). Neurosurgical repair is indicated. If neural tissue alone is trapped anteriorly during embryologic bony closure of the glabella, a nasal glioma results (Fig 3.2). It is excised for diagnosis and for reasons of appearance (Fig 3.3).

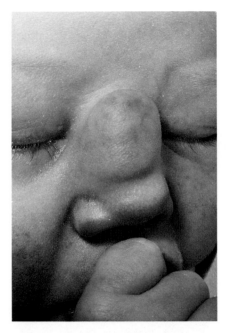

Figure 3.2 Nasal Glioma This congenital "tumor" of the nose is heterotopic neural tissue with no deep attachments.

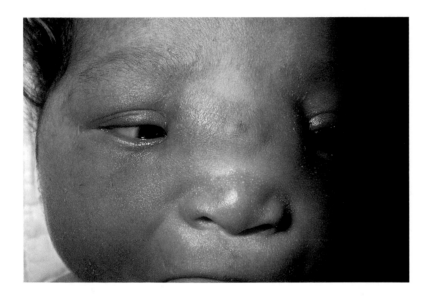

Figure 3.1 Encephalocele A soft mass of tissue, with clear margins, protrudes through a bony defect above the nose in this newborn girl.

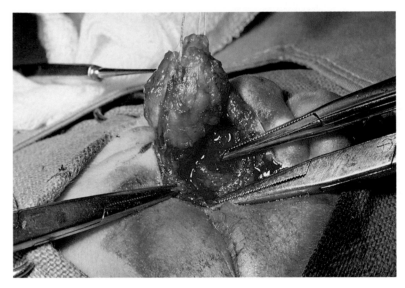

Figure 3.3 This glioma is excised. Careful plastic repair leaves a satisfactory cosmetic result.

Parotid Tumors

Hemangiomas and lymphangiomas of the parotid are handled conservatively, except in cases of rapid growth or persistent severe facial deformity. Mixed tumors of the parotid are seen most often in adolescents (Fig 3.4); very few are malignant. Superficial parotidectomy is usually adequate (Fig 3.5), although there can be local recurrence of this benign tumor. The parotid is rarely the site of several types of carcinoma, as well as lymphoma (Fig 3.6), undifferentiated sarcoma, and rhabdomyosarcoma. Identification and meticulous dissection of the facial nerve are essential in any parotid surgery.

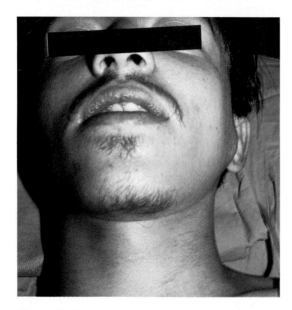

Figure 3.4 Parotid Tumor A painless mass developed in this adolescent boy's left parotid.

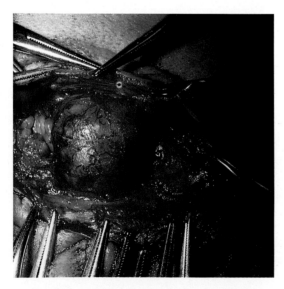

Figure 3.5 Operative dissection reveals a well-encapsulated, benign mixed tumor of the parotid.

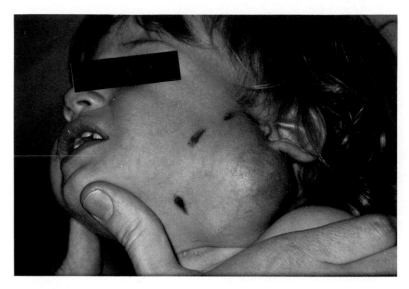

Figure 3.6 The large parotid mass of this 5-month-old girl is a lymphosarcoma. It is treated with wide excision and irradiation.

Rhabdomyosarcoma of the Head and Neck

Rhabdomyosarcoma may originate in the orbit, sinuses, nasopharynx, tongue, or scalp. Orbital and superficial lesions have the best prognosis. Management is outlined in Chapter 12.

Hodgkin's Disease

Both Hodgkin's disease and non-Hodgkin's lymphoma can first present as enlarged, firm neck lymph nodes (Fig 3.7). There is often associated mediastinal adenopathy (Fig 3.8). Biopsy of the mass, to confirm the diagnosis, and possible staging laparotomy are the only surgical procedures indicated. Radiotherapy and chemotherapy are the current treatment modalities.

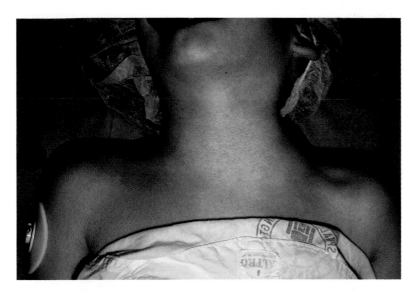

Figure 3.7 Hodgkin's Disease Enlarged, firm, fixed supraclavicular lymph nodes in this 8-year-old girl are seen prior to biopsy. The girl presented with fever, malaise, and weight loss.

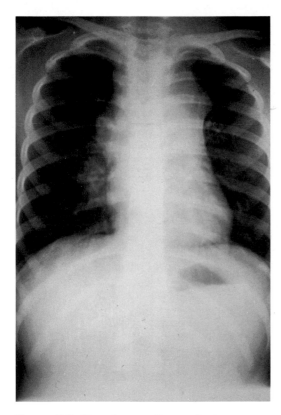

Figure 3.8 Her chest radiograph shows considerable widening of the mediastinum.

Sarcoma

Undifferentiated sarcoma can develop in any somatic tissue, including the neck (Fig 3.9). Wide excision offers the best chance for cure (Fig 3.10).

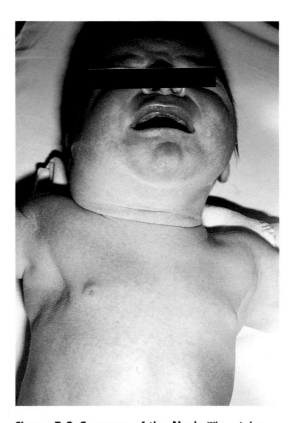

Figure 3.9 Sarcoma of the Neck The right-sided neck mass is present in this infant girl at birth. It is firm and fixed to underlying tissues.

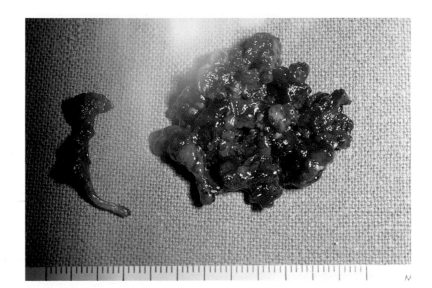

Figure 3.10 The tumor is resected, along with a segment of the attached vagus nerve on that side. It is an undifferentiated sarcoma.

Myxoma

A benign mesenchymal tumor, the myxoma frequently invades muscle and should be excised completely (Figs 3.11, 3.12).

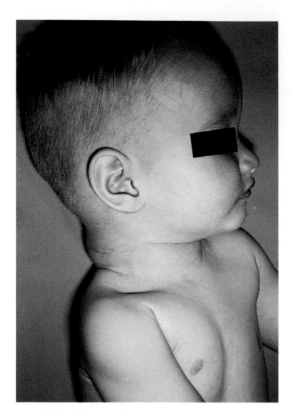

Figure 3.11 Myxoma of the Neck This 1-year-old boy has a discrete, firm mass in the posterior neck.

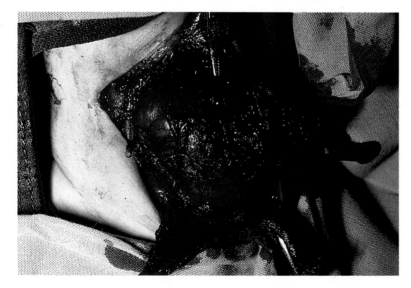

Figure 3.12 The mass involves the posterior neck muscles and must be dissected from them. It is a benign myxoma. No recurrence or disability is noted on a 26-year follow-up.

Cervical Teratoma

Teratoma presents in the infant neck as a large lateral mass with solid and cystic components (Fig 3.13). It is usually histologically benign, but may compress the airway, with serious impairment of respirations. The treatment is complete excision (Fig 3.14).

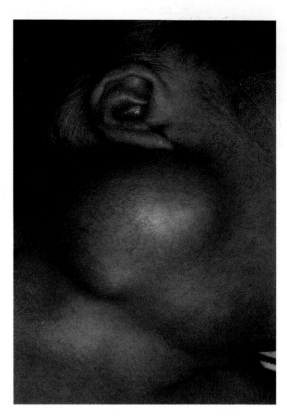

Figure 3.13 Cervical Teratoma The large mass in the neck of a newborn girl feels cystic posteriorly and more solid anteriorly. (Reprinted with permission from Connors RH: Contemporary Surgery 31(1):46–47, 1987.)

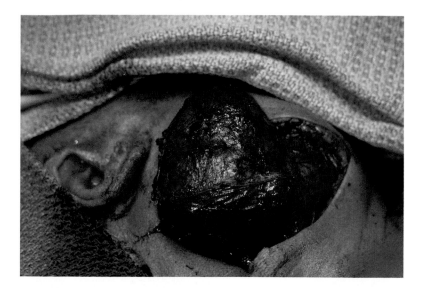

Figure 3.14 The entire tumor mass is dissected. The medial portion extends to the right thyroid lobe but is not adherent to it. All three germ layers are seen on microscopic examination and appear benign. (Reprinted with permission from Connors RH: Contemporary Surgery 31(1):46–47, 1987.)

Tongue

Tie

The short membranous lingual frenulum in infants may be sharply divided after the tissue has been crushed with a hemostat to prevent bleeding. In an older child with a demonstrable speech problem (Fig 3.15), the thick and vascular frenulum (Fig 3.16) must be divided surgically and the cut edges oversewn with absorbable suture. General anesthesia is required.

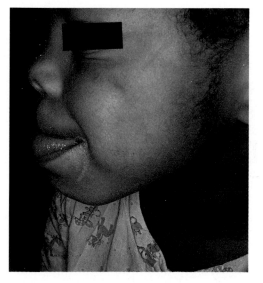

Figure 3.15 Tongue-Tie This 3-year-old cannot protrude the tip of her tongue beyond the lower teeth. She has difficulty with pronunciation, especially the "th" sound.

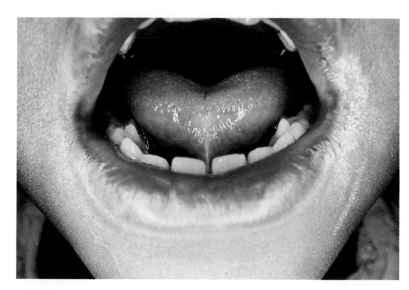

Figure 3.16 The thick, tight lingual frenulum is seen from the front.

Lymphangioma

Cystic hygroma of the neck may extend into the submandibular area, floor of the mouth, and tongue. Lymphangioma in the tongue presents on the surface as tiny vesicles (Fig 3.17) that lead to glossitis and bleeding. Electrodesiccation is used to control the vesicles. Macroglossia resulting from lymphangiomatous glossitis may require lateral tongue resection.

Hemangioma

Hemangioma of the tongue must be excised if it bleeds frequently or interferes with chewing (Fig 3.18).

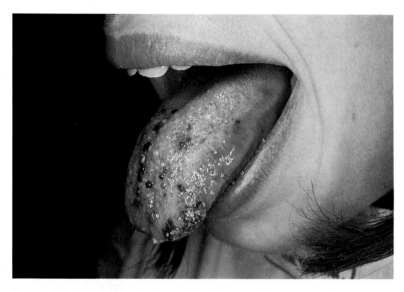

Figure 3.17 Lymphangioma of the Tongue The tongue is enlarged, and there are multiple small vesicles of dilated lymphatics on the surface.

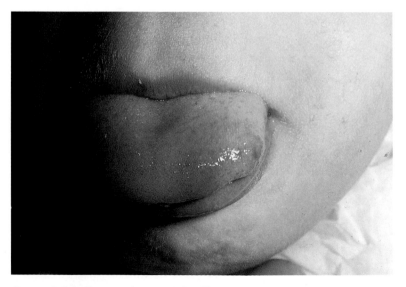

Figure 3.18 Hemangioma of the Tongue The anterolateral hemangioma of the tongue is evaluated because of a bleeding episode.

Ranula

A superficial cyst in the floor of the mouth, the ranula (Fig 3.19) is treated by incision and marsupialization to the oral mucosa using a running absorbable suture. It must be distinguished from a lymphangioma (see earlier), which is a more substantial mass in the submandibular area as well as in the mouth and should *not* be marsupialized.

Lingual Thyroid

A mass at the base of the tongue may be thyroid tissue, cyst, or tumor (see Chapter 12). Thyroid tissue can be identified by radioiodine scan or biopsy, and only obstructing lesions require thyroid suppression or surgery.

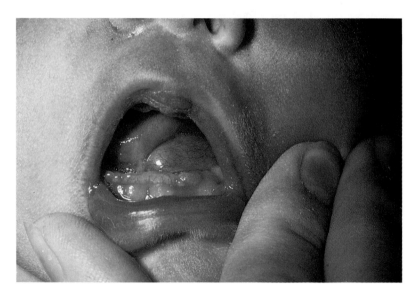

Figure 3.19 Ranula A small cyst, filled with clear fluid, is seen under the tongue of this 1-day-old infant.

Neck

Thyroglossal Duct Cyst and Sinus

The thyroglossal duct cyst presents as a round, midline mass of the anterior neck, at or below the hyoid bone; it is adherent to that bone and moves with swallowing (Figs 3.20, 3.21). It often enlarges after a respiratory infection, which stimulates mucus production in the cyst. An infected cyst may be seen initially as a midline abscess requiring drainage (Figs 3.22, 3.23). Prior infection in the cyst may have caused scarring that pulls it off the midline.

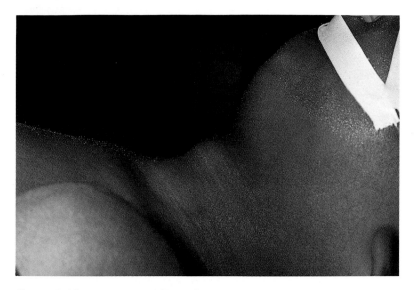

Figure 3.20 Thyroglossal Duct Cyst A round, cystic, midline mass of the neck moves with swallowing.

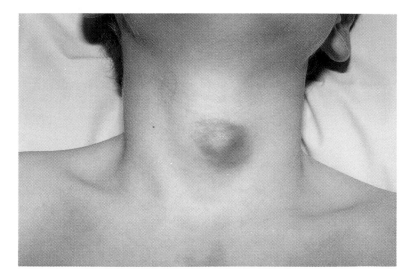

Figure 3.22 This boy presents with a round, raised, red, tender mass, slightly to the left of the midline of the neck. It is an infected thyroglossal duct cyst; the infection resolves with oral antibiotic therapy and warm compresses and does not require drainage.

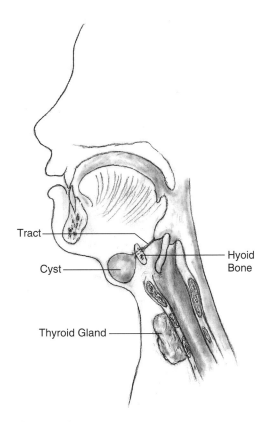

Figure 3.21 The anatomy of the cyst is shown in lateral view. It is anterior to the hyoid bone. A sinus tract extends from the cyst through the midportion of the hyoid and may continue deeper into the hypopharynx.

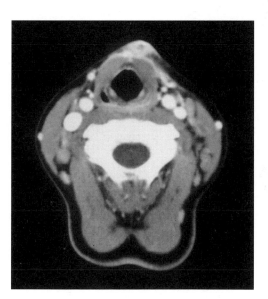

Figure 3.23 A computed tomography scan, not usually obtained, shows the protruding cystic mass, the surrounding irregular area of inflammation, and the midportion of the hyoid bone to which the cyst is adherent.

Excision of the cyst is safest in the absence of inflammation. The dissection must include the entire sinus tract attached to the cyst and the midportion of the hyoid bone through which the tract passes (Figs 3.24–3.29). Recurrent drainage is the result of incomplete removal of the tract (Figs 3.30, 3.31).

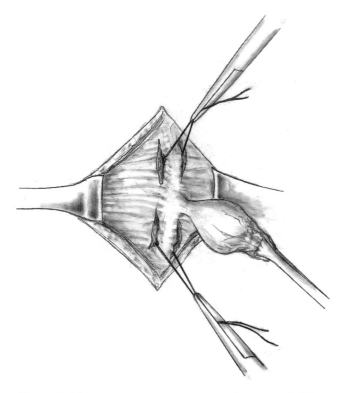

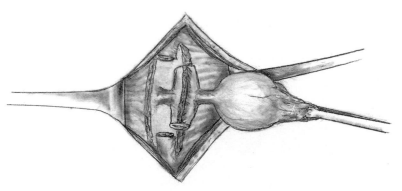

Figure 3.26 Both wings of the hyoid are divided, and a deeper extension of the thyroglossal duct sinus is visualized and dissected.

Figure 3.24 A transverse incision in the natural skin lines of the neck exposes the cyst, which is dissected from the surrounding connective tissue. Incisions into the strap muscles adherent to the palpable hyoid bone allow dissection around the thin wings of the hyoid with a right-angle clamp. A heavy silk suture is placed around each wing for traction.

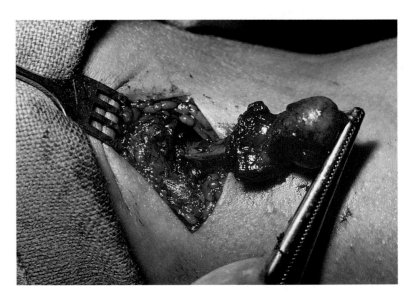

Figure 3.27 The operative dissection includes the cyst, the midportion of the hyoid bone, and a deeper sinus tract to the hypopharynx.

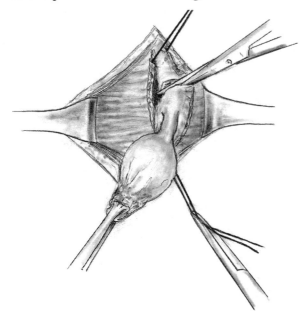

Figure 3.25 The wing of the hyoid bone is divided just lateral to its midportion.

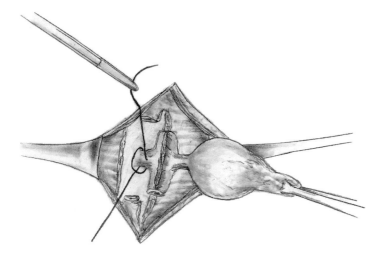

Figure 3.28 The sinus tract deep to the hyoid bone is suture-ligated prior to division.

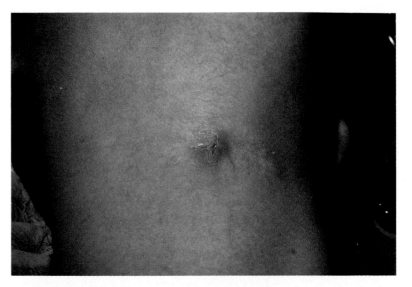

Figure 3.30 This 7-year-old boy underwent two previous attempts at surgical removal of a cyst and subsequent draining sinus. Clear mucus drains from the incisional area again, after apparent initial healing.

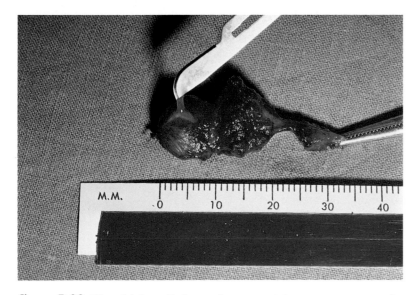

Figure 3.29 The thick-walled specimen contains mucus secreted by the respiratory epithelial lining.

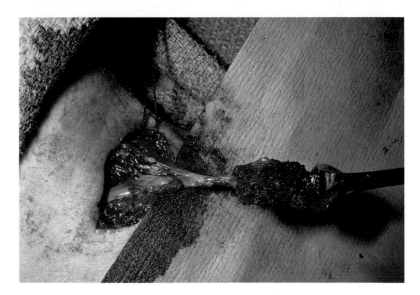

Figure 3.31 The tract is considerably scarred but extends to the middle of an intact hyoid bone. There is no recurrence after complete excision of the sinus tract *and* the midportion of the hyoid bone.

Other midline neck masses include lymph nodes, single lymphangiomatous cysts (Figs 3.32, 3.33), epidermoid cysts (see Figs 2.37–2.39), and a rare solitary midline thyroid. No experienced surgeon would mistake solid, beefy red thyroid tissue (see later) for a cyst containing mucoid material; therefore, a radioactive thyroid scan is not indicated for every child with a midline neck mass in order to prevent inadvertent removal of the child's only thyroid tissue. When found, the midline solitary thyroid should be split vertically and the halves moved laterally under each sternocleidomastoid muscle to protect the gland from future trauma.

Cystic Hygroma

Cystic hygroma is a lymphangioma of the neck, often extending onto the face, to the shoulder, and even into the mediastinum (Figs 3.34–3.37). In the newborn, it may obstruct the airway, requiring emergency excision. Magnifying loupes are recommended to help identify branches of the facial nerve during the neck dissection in infants. In the older child, the multiple cysts may coalesce into a single large cyst (Figs 3.38, 3.39). At surgery, those cysts that cannot safely be excised should be unroofed. Incomplete excision, with local regrowth, is not unusual.

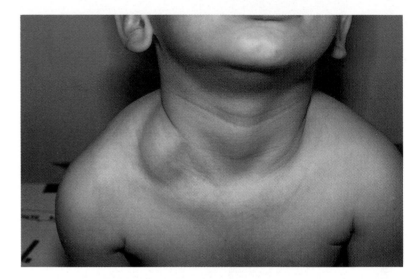

Figure 3.34 Cystic Hygroma A cystic, soft, well-circumscribed mass is seen in the right lateral neck of this child.

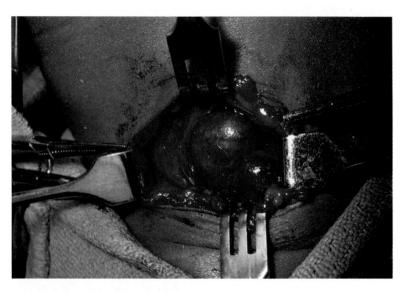

Figure 3.32 Lymphangiomatous Cyst This bilobed, single cyst, in the midline of the neck, has no deep attachments.

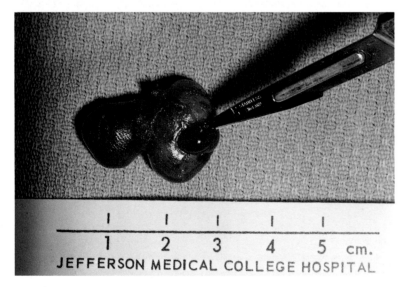

Figure 3.33 The cyst (a unilocular "cystic hygroma") contains clear fluid. Histologically it is lined with endothelium.

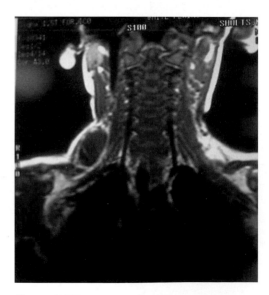

Figure 3.35 The magnetic resonance imaging scan of the neck demonstrates the mass to be an isolated cystic hygroma, without extension into surrounding tissues.

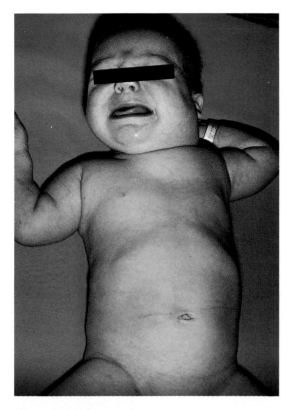

Figure 3.36 This lymphangioma of the lateral neck of an infant extends to the chest wall and into the anterior mediastinum.

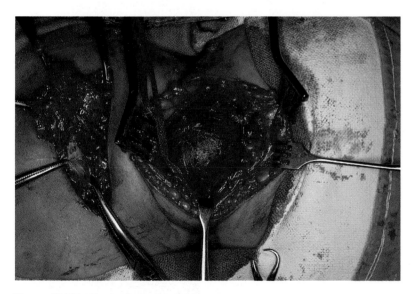

Figure 3.37 The large mass, composed of multiple cysts of varying size, is seen at the operative dissection of the neck and chest.

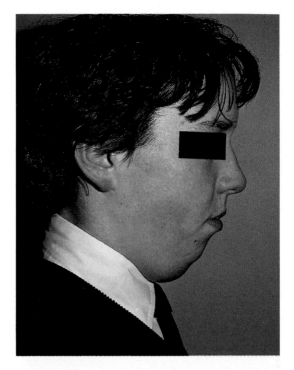

Figure 3.38 The appearance of his cystic hygroma causes great embarrassment to this teenage boy.

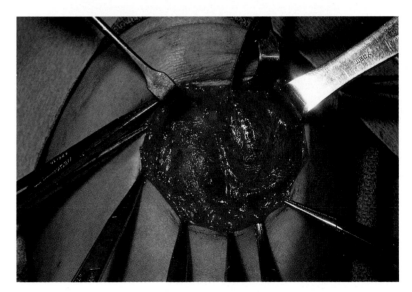

Figure 3.39 The cystic mass is of large size and extends to the sternocleidomastoid muscles on both sides and up to the floor of the mouth. The major portion of it is excised, with unroofing of several smaller cysts deep in the neck.

Thyroid

Goiter

Children, especially girls near puberty, can develop hyperthyroidism and exophthalmic goiter (Fig 3.40). Although suppressive medication, such as methimazole (Tapazole), is the first choice for therapy, some children's hyperthyroidism escapes from control and other children develop hypersensitivity to the drug. Subtotal thyroidectomy is the usual procedure of choice (Fig 3.41). Radioiodine ablation is contraindicated in childhood.

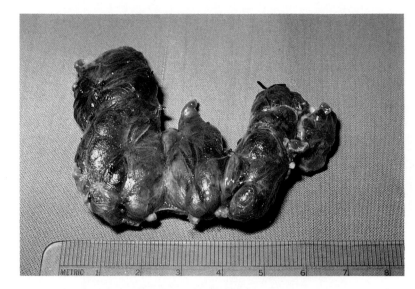

Figure 3.41 The operative specimen of a subtotal thyroidectomy is seen. Great care is taken in the dissection to identify the parathyroid glands and to preserve both recurrent and superior laryngeal nerves.

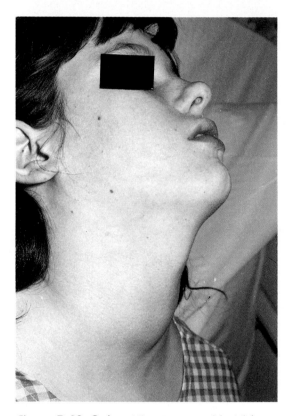

Figure 3.40 Goiter This 11-year-old girl has hyperthyroidism unresponsive to medical management.

Congenital Goiter

Congenital goiter may produce severe respiratory obstruction in the newborn (Fig 3.42). Maternal suppressive medication and rare inborn errors of infant thyroid metabolism are the principal causes. Division of the thyroid isthmus relieves the obstruction.

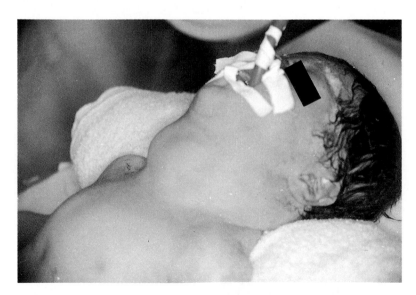

Figure 3.42 Congenital Goiter Severe respiratory distress at birth is the result of a massive goiter in this newborn. His mother was taking propylthiouracil during her pregnancy.

Thyroid Nodule

A solitary nodule in the thyroid gland of a child (Fig 3.43) is usually benign; however, it must be evaluated for the possibility of papillary carcinoma. If it is "cold" on radioiodine scan (Fig 3.44), malignancy is possible, and excision with a wide margin—usually a hemithyroidectomy—is indicated (Figs 3.45, 3.46). Benign tumors (Figs 3.47, 3.48), colloid cysts, and thyroiditis are the more frequent findings in children.

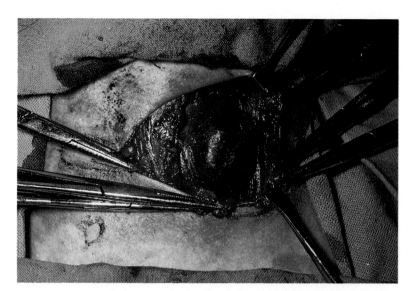

Figure 3.45 This well-defined nodule of the left thyroid lobe was present in a 6-year-old girl. A left thyroid lobectomy is performed.

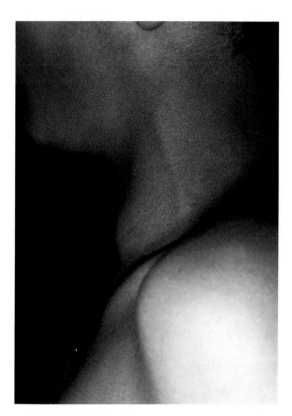

Figure 3.43 Thyroid Nodule A nodule is seen in the lower pole of the left thyroid lobe in this 12-year-old girl.

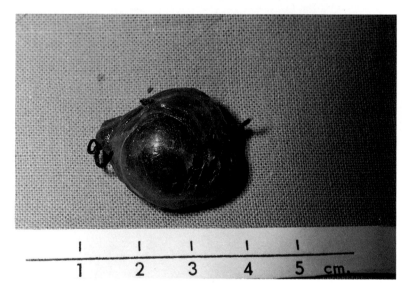

Figure 3.46 The specimen of the lobectomy is found to contain papillary carcinoma on frozen section. A wider excision is carried out. The patient, placed on suppressive thyroid medication, has no recurrence in 12 years of follow-up.

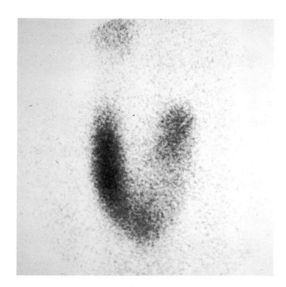

Figure 3.44 A radioiodine scan demonstrates a "cold" area in the left lobe.

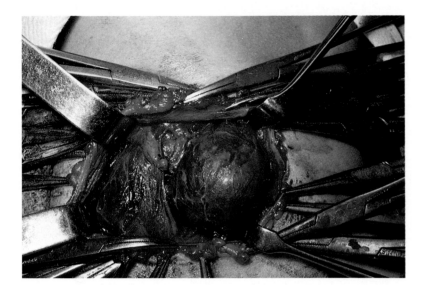

Figure 3.47 A similar thyroid nodule is seen at surgery in a 12-year-old.

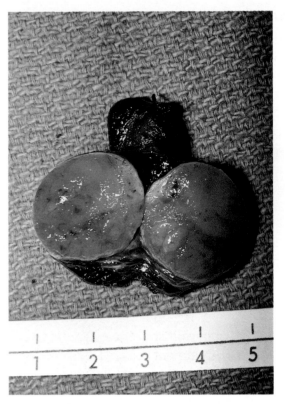

Figure 3.48 On section, it is found to be a benign follicular adenoma.

Parathyroid

Hyperparathyroidism may be seen in three forms in childhood—neonatal hyperparathyroidism, diffuse glandular hyperplasia, and adenoma.

Severe hypercalcemia secondary to hyperparathyroidism during the first week of life may be fatal if not recognized and treated by total parathyroidectomy. This rare disease may be hereditary, and screening of other family members is advised.

Familial hyperparathyroidism in children and adolescents is often associated with multiple endocrinopathies (multiple endocrine neoplasia types I and IIA). Identification of four glands and subtotal parathyroidectomy, with biopsy of apparently "normal" glands, are advised. Hyperparathyroidism is also seen in children with chronic renal failure who undergo kidney transplantation.

Single adenomas are the most frequent cause of adolescent hyperparathyroidism. Once the diagnosis has been established, the treatment consists of neck exploration with identification of all glands and excision of the adenoma.

Parathyroid cyst is an unusual cause of a visible neck mass in children (Figs 3.49, 3.50).

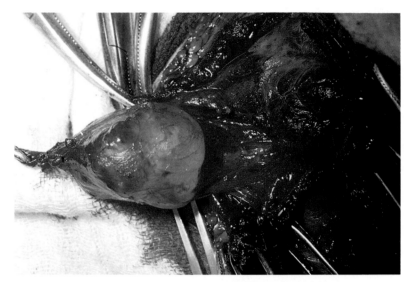

Figure 3.50 A parathyroid cyst, filled with clear fluid, is excised. There are three other parathyroid glands, which are normal.

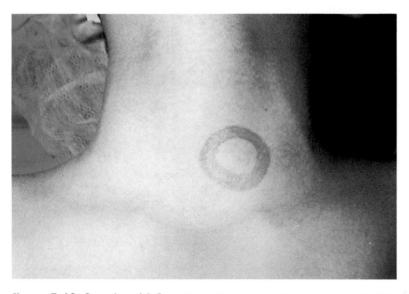

Figure 3.49 Parathyroid Cyst A cystic, nontender mass is palpable in the left lower neck, inferior to the thyroid gland.

Branchial Cleft Cysts and Sinuses

The lateral neck and preauricular face are the most frequent sites of branchial cleft cysts and sinuses (Fig 3.51). They are congenital remnants of the embryologic branchial clefts (''gill clefts''). Sinus tracts, lined with respiratory epithelium, drain clear mucus onto the skin (Fig 3.52); they often become infected (Fig 3.53) and should always be excised (Figs 3.54, 3.55). A fine lacrimal duct probe helps trace the sinus tract. Cysts in the neck accumulate secretions and may grow to significant size; excision is best performed before they become infected (Figs 3.56, 3.57).

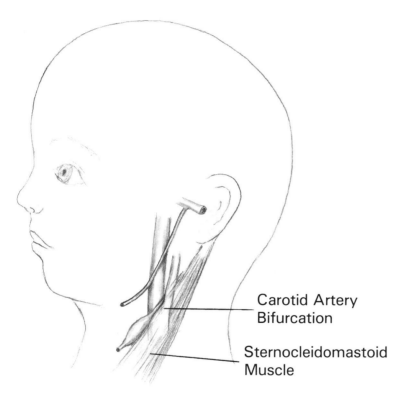

Figure 3.51 Branchial Cleft Sinus The two common sites for branchial cleft sinuses and cysts are shown in this composite drawing. Tracts from the external auditory canal drain onto the skin at the angle of the mandible. The more common sinus tract originates in the hypopharynx and exits at the anterior border of the sternocleidomastoid muscle, often passing through the bifurcation of the carotid artery.

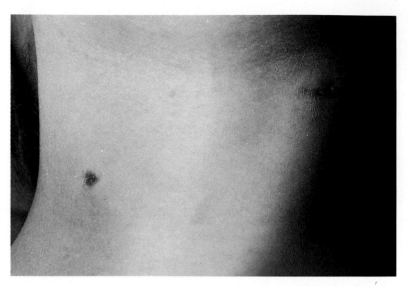

Figure 3.52 Clear mucus drains from congenital openings on both sides of this child's neck.

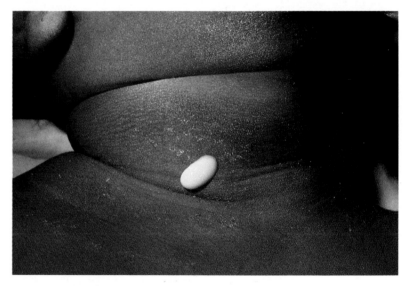

Figure 3.53 Purulent drainage is seen from the infected branchial cleft sinus in this 2-year-old.

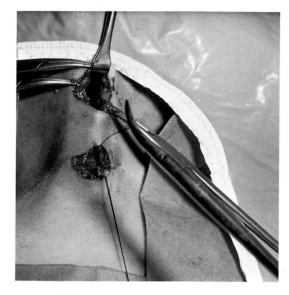

Figure 3.54 A branchial sinus tract is dissected from the lower neck to the level of the hypopharynx. "Stepladder" transverse incisions are used to expose the entire tract.

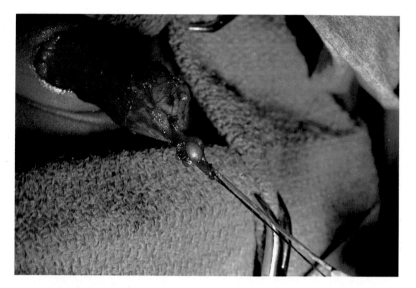

Figure 3.56 Branchial Cleft Cyst The palpable cyst drained mucus and occasionally pus onto the skin. A lacrimal duct probe enters the tract for identification and ease in dissection.

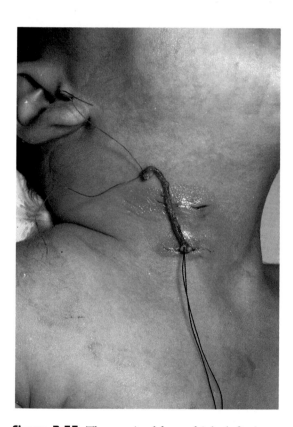

Figure 3.55 The excised branchial cleft sinus tract is seen next to the neck. Subcuticular closure of the skin-crease incisions gives a very satisfactory cosmetic result.

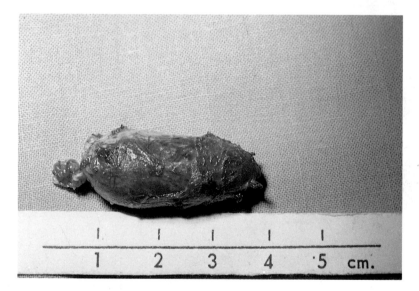

Figure 3.57 The 4-cm cyst and draining sinus are excised.

The preauricular branchial cyst is excised only after it presents with infection or enlargement (Figs 3.58–3.60). Care must be taken in dissection, because the tract is adherent to the tragal cartilage. The procedure should always be done under general anesthesia in children.

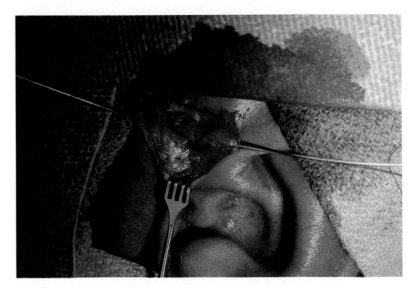

Figure 3.60 The dissection shows the sinus and cyst. Care is taken to avoid damage to branches of the facial nerve and the temporal artery.

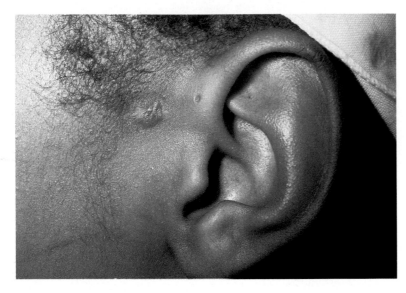

Figure 3.58 Preauricular Cyst and Sinus The preauricular cyst shows signs of previous infection and scarring. The entrance of the sinus tract is in the anterior pinna of the ear.

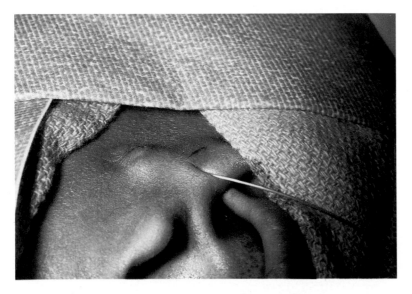

Figure 3.59 A probe in the sinus tract demonstrates its extent.

Torticollis

The infant who presents at 3–6 weeks of age with a tilt of the head to one side, limitation of neck rotation to the opposite side, and a mass in the sternocleidomastoid muscle has torticollis, or wryneck (Fig 3.61). Occasionally, the muscle mass is seen without neck distortion; it should not be mistaken for a neoplasm. The firm, discrete, nontender mass is a hematoma in an injured muscle, probably from intrauterine malposition. Local massage and simple stretching exercises for several weeks in early infancy prevent permanent muscle scarring and shortening in the majority of infants.

In older children with fixed torticollis, there may be marked facial asymmetry and visual problems from a nonhorizontal relationship of the eyes. The scarred muscle must be completely divided (Figs 3.62, 3.63) and subsequent exercise undertaken to maintain correction.

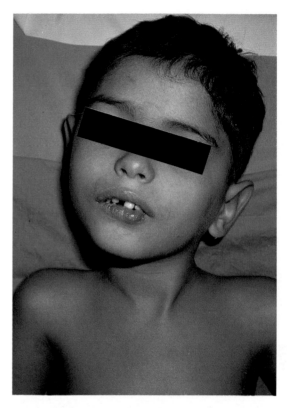

Figure 3.62 This 5-year-old boy has a fixed torticollis and facial asymmetry.

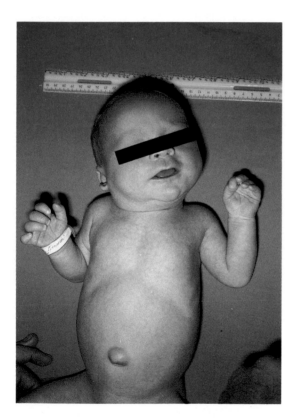

Figure 3.61 Torticollis This newborn with a firm mass in the right sternocleidomastoid muscle tilts his head to that side and lacks full neck rotation to the opposite side.

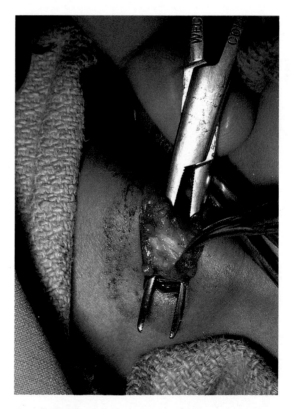

Figure 3.63 The thick, tight scar of the muscle is exposed and will be completely divided.

Chapter 4

Chest

Wall Deformities

Pectus Excavatum

Overgrowth of the lower costal cartilages is thought to be the cause of this concave lower sternal deformity (Fig 4.1); it is often familial. Some children have associated scoliosis, especially those with Marfan's syndrome. Many children are asymptomatic and are referred for cosmetic correction because of a poor body image and self-consciousness. A common story is that of a boy who will not take off his shirt in public, even to swim. In other children, cardiac displacement and narrowing of the anteroposterior diameter of the chest are felt to cause symptoms of decreased exercise tolerance and increased pulmonary infections. Radiographs of the chest (Figs 4.2, 4.3), with barium paste in the sternal concavity, are helpful in assessing the depth of the deformity, the degree of

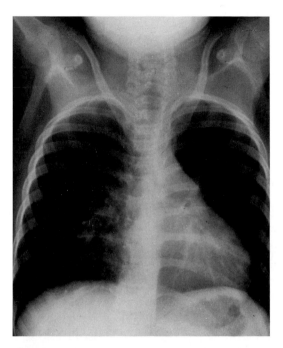

Figure 4.2 The heart is only slightly displaced to the left in this asymptomatic 10-year-old girl with pectus excavatum.

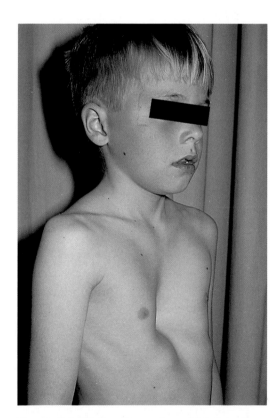

Figure 4.1 Pectus Excavatum This boy has a deep depression in the lower sternum, causing him great embarrassment. He is normally active.

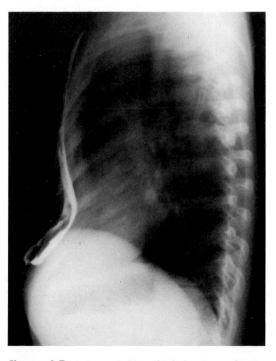

Figure 4.3 A lateral film with barium shows the depth of the sternal depression.

cardiac displacement, and the existence of scoliosis. Other, noninvasive, cardiopulmonary studies may be performed for postoperative comparison. Several studies have reported improvement in maximal ventilatory capacity, cardiac output, and exercise performance after repair.

Correction is recommended before puberty, some suggest as early as the age of 2 years. Repair may be performed through a vertical or a transverse incision; most pediatric surgeons prefer the transverse incision, which leaves a more cosmetically acceptable scar. The procedure involves complete bilateral excision of the third to sixth costal cartilages and the medial portion of the seventh, leaving the perichondrium in place (Figs 4.4–4.6). The sternum is wedged and elevated (Fig 4.7), and a supporting stainless steel strut is placed over the sternum and sutured to the ribs (Fig 4.8). Subcutaneous suction drainage is maintained for 24–48 hours. The strut is removed in 6–12 months. Good results are the rule (Fig 4.9).

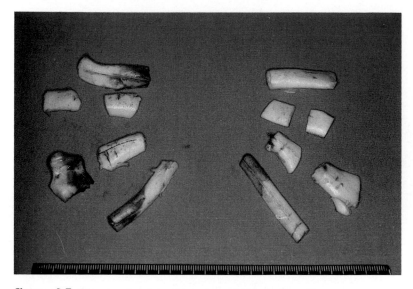

Figure 4.5 The excised cartilages are arranged as they were removed.

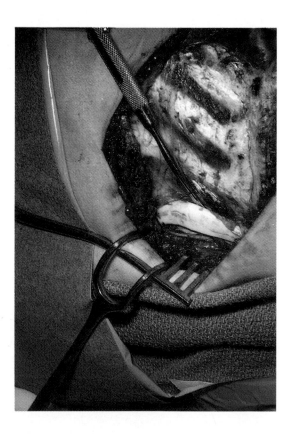

Figure 4.4 The costal cartilages are exposed, the perichondrium is incised over the length of the cartilage, and a periosteal elevator is used to separate the cartilage from the perichondrium.

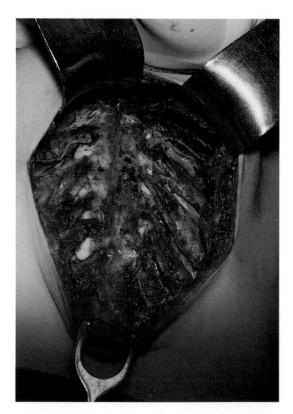

Figure 4.6 The intact perichondrium is seen after removal of all resected cartilage.

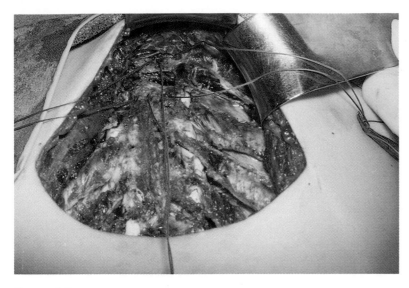

Figure 4.7 A transverse wedge of bone is taken from the anterior sternum at the angle of Louis, and the lower sternum is elevated. Sutures of heavy nonabsorbable material are placed through the bone at the wedge site, to maintain the elevation.

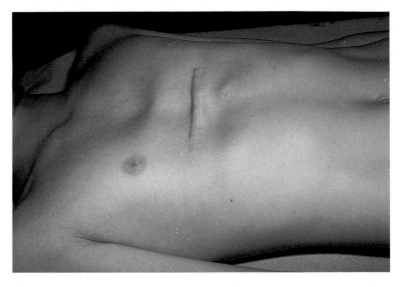

Figure 4.9 A healed repair is seen at the time of removal of the steel strut.

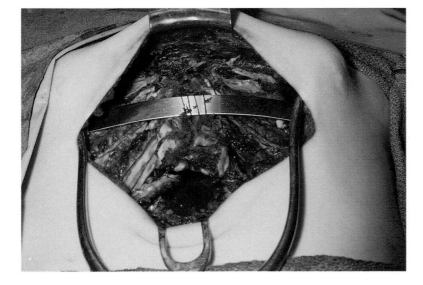

Figure 4.8 A single steel strut supports the repair. It is sutured to the ribs laterally—usually the fourth ribs—and to the periosteum of the sternum in the midline.

Pectus Carinatum

Anterior protrusion of the sternum, sometimes called *pigeon breast,* is also postulated to be a result of overgrowth of the costal cartilages. It is associated primarily with emphysematous lung changes. The deformity is corrected by cartilaginous resection, similar to that for pectus excavatum, and double transverse osteotomies to align the sternum properly; the pectoral fascia is approximated anteriorly, and no internal support is needed.

Sternal Cleft

Sternal clefts may be partial—upper or lower—or complete midline defects. Cardiac and pericardial abnormalities, as well as anterior diaphragmatic hernia and epigastric omphalocele, may accompany some sternal clefts (Cantrell's pentalogy). Ectopia cordis is the most dramatic associated abnormality and is almost invariably fatal.

Upper defects present with a bulge in the midline (Fig 4.10). They are best repaired in infancy, when the cartilaginous structures are easily approximated (Figs 4.11–4.13). A total cleft may also be repaired primarily if there are no major cardiac, pericardial, or diaphragmatic defects.

Repair of a lower sternal cleft and associated defects of abdominal wall, diaphragm, pericardium, and heart frequently requires several stages.

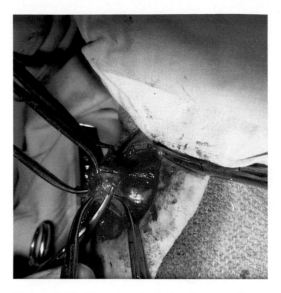

Figure 4.11 The skin is incised vertically. Great care is taken in dissecting the subcutaneous tissues from the adherent pericardium.

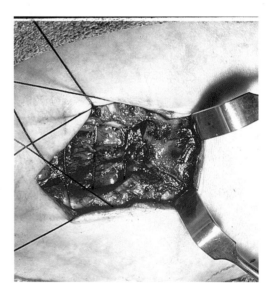

Figure 4.12 A medial wedge of cartilage is taken from the junction of the intact sternum and the cleft sternum on each side. Heavy nonabsorbable sutures are passed around both sides of the cleft sternum.

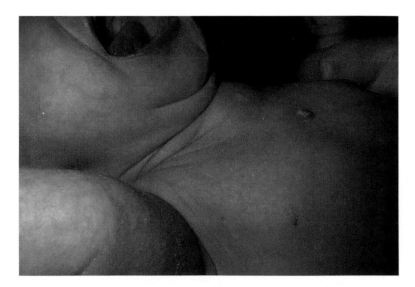

Figure 4.10 Sternal Cleft The bulge through a defect in the upper sternum is seen in this crying infant.

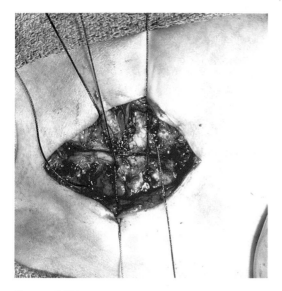

Figure 4.13 The sutures are tied, closing the cleft.

Breast

Neonatal Enlargement

The breast of the newborn may be enlarged and may produce a colostrumlike fluid (Fig 4.14) in response to the stimulation of maternal hormones during pregnancy. The enlargement regresses in several weeks, and the fluid secretion stops.

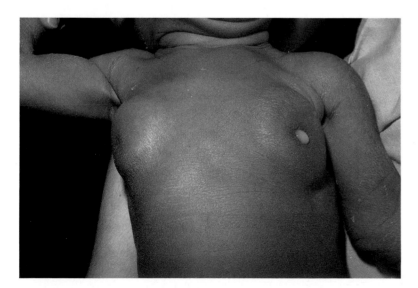

Figure 4.14 Neonatal Breast Hypertrophy Both breasts are enlarged and secrete colostrumlike fluid in this newborn.

Abscess

Mastitis in the sensitive hormone-stimulated neonatal breast can lead to an abscess, which requires surgical drainage (Fig 4.15). *Staphylococcus aureus* is the commonest pathogen, although *Escherichia coli* also may infect the newborn breast. A subareolar drainage incision minimizes injury to the breast tissue; however, the parents should be informed that the infection itself may interfere with future breast development.

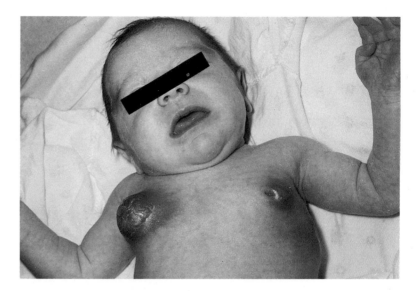

Figure 4.15 Neonatal Breast Abscess *Mastitis neonatorum* is another name for breast abscesses like the ones seen in this 10-day-old girl.

Gynecomastia

Persistence or exaggeration of the normally transient enlargement of the male breast just after puberty may lead to considerable embarrassment. Boys with liver and endocrine abnormalities associated with elevated estrogen levels also may have significant breast enlargement (Fig 4.16). Subcutaneous mastectomy, preferably through a lower circumareolar incision, is recommended (Fig 4.17).

Cysts and Fibrocystic Disease

Simple cysts of the breast may occur at any age (Fig 4.18). Surgical excision is not recommended, especially in the prepubertal girl, in whom damage to normal breast tissue may impede future breast development.

Fibrocystic disease is found, uncommonly, in adolescent girls. Poorly circumscribed areas of cordlike fibrous thickening, with one or more small cysts, are palpable. They characteristically become more tender and enlarged just prior to menses. Persistence or enlargement of the mass may lead to excisional biopsy for diagnosis. Cancer is rare.

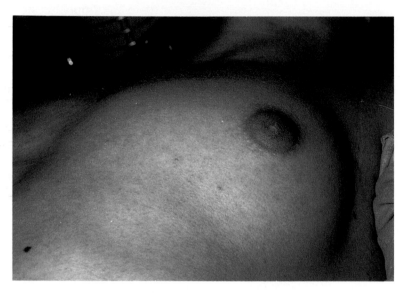

Figure 4.16 Gynecomastia Enlargement of normal breast tissue in this adolescent boy is secondary to liver disease with a defect in estrogen breakdown.

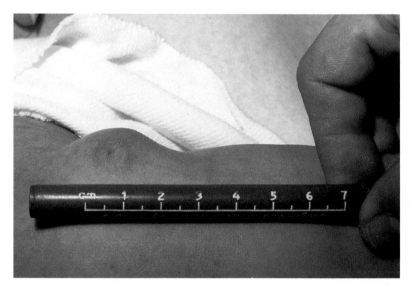

Figure 4.18 Simple Breast Cyst A 1.5-cm cyst of the breast is seen in this 7-week-old girl. It is neither excised nor aspirated.

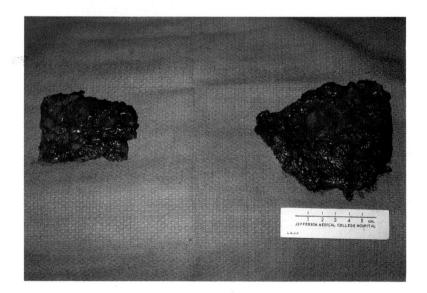

Figure 4.17 The specimens are from bilateral subcutaneous mastectomy.

Fibroadenomas

The most common solitary breast masses in children, fibroadenomas are benign fibrous tumors that may slowly enlarge. On palpation, they are firm, discrete, mobile, and nontender. Excision is indicated for diagnosis.

Juvenile Hypertrophy of the Breast

Massive breast enlargement with firm, nodular tissue is seen in some adolescent girls (Fig 4.19). There is no associated endocrine abnormality. Reduction mammoplasty, with nipple transplantation, is the usual procedure (Fig 4.20).

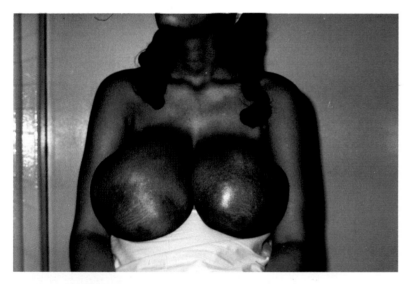

Figure 4.19 Juvenile Breast Hypertrophy There is huge, firm, irregular enlargement of both breasts in this adolescent girl.

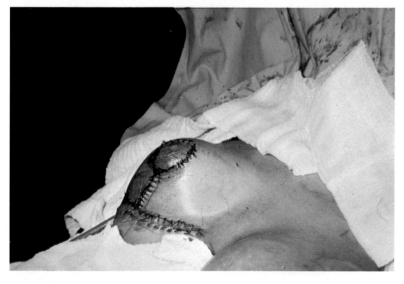

Figure 4.20 Reduction mammoplasty, with transplantation of the nipple, leaves a normal-appearing breast.

Lungs and Pleura

Pneumothorax

Spontaneous pneumothorax is seen most often in the neonate with respiratory distress and in the active teenager who ruptures a pleural bleb. Trauma is the third most common cause of pneumothorax in children (see Chapter 13).

In the newborn, sudden deterioration of cardiopulmonary status is accompanied by loss of breath sounds on the affected side and mediastinal shift to the opposite side (Fig 4.21). For immediate relief, air should be evacuated through a small needle or plastic needle-catheter placed in the anterolateral chest. Definitive treatment is placement of a chest tube through the third or fourth intercostal space; in infants, a lateral, rather than midclavicular, insertion avoids damage to the structures of the mediastinum (Fig 4.22). The author uses a sterile hemostat to spread the intercostal muscle and to enter the pleura; the tube is then inserted between the open jaws of the hemostat. A sharp stylet is never used to puncture the chest wall for introduction of the tube.

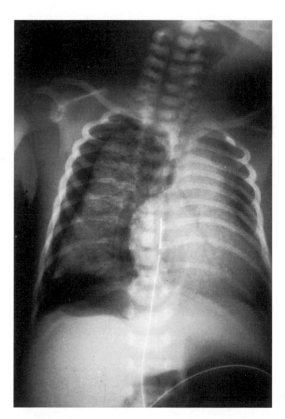

Figure 4.21 Pneumothorax A large spontaneous right pneumothorax displaces the mediastinal structures to the left in this neonate.

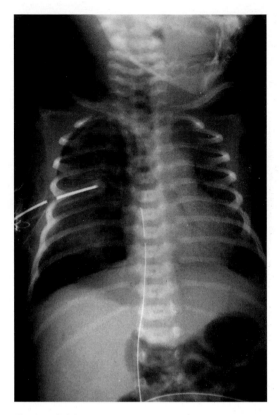

Figure 4.22 A thoracostomy tube is placed in the fourth intercostal space through a lateral incision. Note that the last hole of the tube, seen as a lucent defect in the radiopaque marker, is outside the chest wall; the tube must be advanced so that all drainage holes lie within the chest cavity.

Sudden chest pain is the first symptom in most adolescents (Fig 4.23). Unless a progressive tension pneumothorax develops, there may be respiratory symptoms only on exertion. For any pneumothorax more than 20% of the lung volume, a chest tube should be placed and put on water-seal suction. With the lung fully expanded, the tube is left in place for 48–72 hours to promote pleural adhesion. Recurrent episodes of pneumothorax indicate probable rupture of pulmonary pleural blebs (Fig 4.24). In the past, the author performed an open thoracotomy and pleurodesis, with excision of the blebs. Thoracoscopic excision is now the preferred treatment of the apical blebs, and pleurodesis or talc poudrage under thoracoscopic control are ways of preventing recurrent pneumothorax (see Chapter 8).

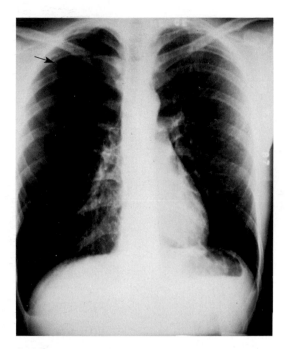

Figure 4.23 There is a moderate-sized right apical pneumothorax in this thin teenage boy who noted the sudden onset of chest pain. At the left apex can be seen a row of surgical staples where pleural blebs were excised after recurrent episodes of pneumothorax.

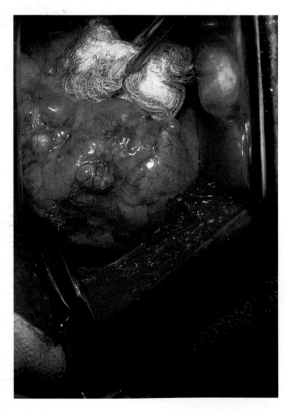

Figure 4.24 Pleural blebs are seen in the right upper lobe at thoracotomy. They, too, will be excised and a pleurodesis will be performed, as on the opposite side.

Lobar Emphysema

Congenital lobar emphysema presents in early infancy with progressive respiratory distress secondary to impingement of an overinflated lobe on the rest of the thoracic contents—ipsilateral lung, mediastinum, and even the contralateral lung (Fig 4.25). The left upper lobe is most commonly involved, followed in frequency by the right upper and middle lobes. Lobectomy is the treatment of choice when there are progressive symptoms (Figs 4.26, 4.27). Surgery may be withheld in some older infants with lobar emphysema who have no increasing respiratory distress.

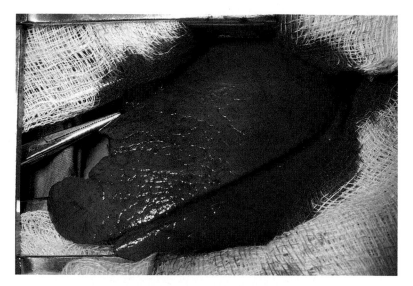

Figure 4.26 The involved upper lobe is seen at thoracotomy. It does not collapse, even without positive airway pressure.

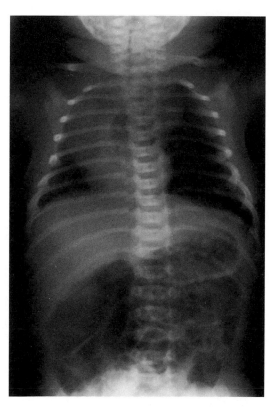

Figure 4.25 Congenital Lobar Emphysema A hyperinflated left upper lobe displaces the mediastinum and protrudes to the right of the midline.

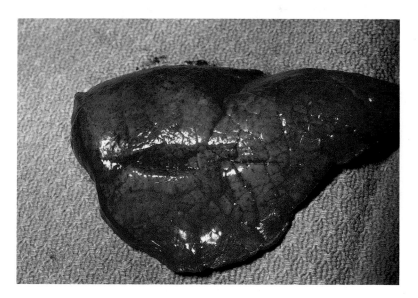

Figure 4.27 The abnormal lobe does not decompress after removal. A honeycomb appearance is visible on cut section.

Cystic Adenomatoid Malformation

Cystic adenomatoid malformation is thought to be the result of an overgrowth of terminal bronchial structures. There is a bulky pulmonary lobe with multiple cysts of varying sizes, lined by cuboidal or columnar bronchial epithelium; a single lobe is involved more often than multiple lobes. The clinical presentation is that of either progressive respiratory distress in the newborn or recurring pulmonary infections in later infancy. Radiographs and computed tomography of the chest indicate the diagnosis (Figs 4.28–4.30). The treatment is resection of the involved lobe or lobes (Fig 4.31).

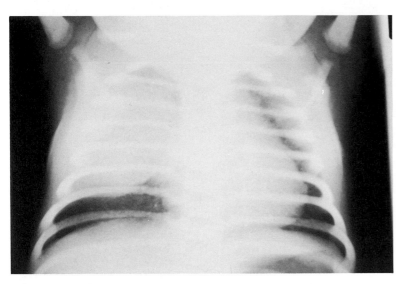

Figure 4.28 Cystic Adenomatoid Malformation of the Lung A rounded density is seen in the right upper lobe of this neonate with mild respiratory distress.

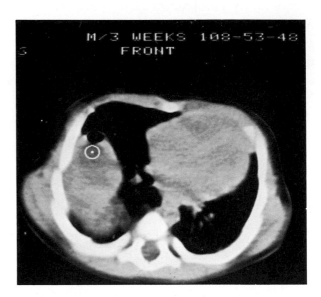

Figure 4.30 Computed tomography also demonstrates the multiple cysts in this lung malformation.

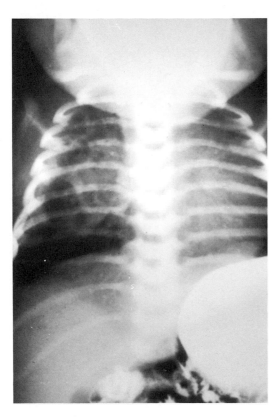

Figure 4.29 Three weeks later, the pulmonary density contains scattered radiolucent cysts and displaces the mediastinum to the opposite side.

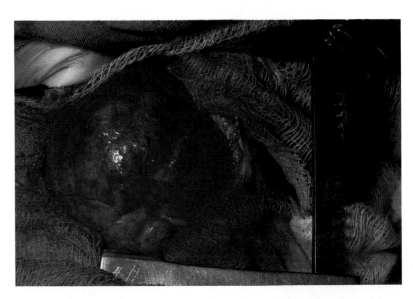

Figure 4.31 The cystic right upper lobe is seen at surgery and will be excised.

Pulmonary Sequestration

A sequestration is a mass of nonfunctioning lung tissue, lacking bronchial connection and having an anomalous systemic arterial supply. It may be intralobar or extralobar. The left lower chest is the most common location, and the systemic blood supply may originate below the diaphragm. Failure to locate and control the systemic arterial blood supply at surgery can lead to significant bleeding from vessels that may retract below the diaphragm. Intralobar sequestrations, with the abnormal tissue contained within normal lung, are detected as incidental findings on chest radiographs or may become infected (Fig 4.32). Computed tomography is sometimes helpful in confirming the diagnosis, as is angiography. Lobectomy or segmental resection is the treatment of choice (Figs 4.33, 4.34).

Extralobar sequestrations lie outside the lung and the visceral pleura. They may be seen on chest radiographs, appearing as paraspinal "tumors" (Fig 4.35). Computed tomography (CT) may help clarify the diagnosis (Fig 4.36). Sometimes they are seen as incidental findings at surgery. Most are excised (Figs 4.37, 4.38).

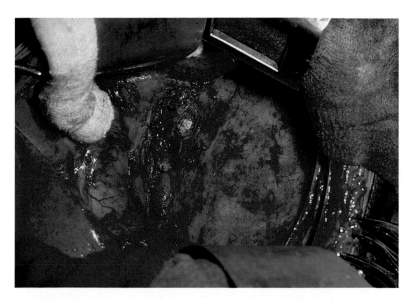

Figure 4.33 The systemic blood supply to the right-lower-lobe sequestration comes through the diaphragm from the abdomen. The vessels are seen ligated and divided.

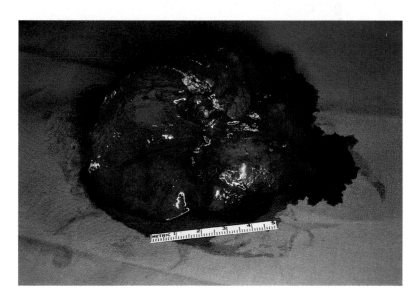

Figure 4.34 The sequestration is resected.

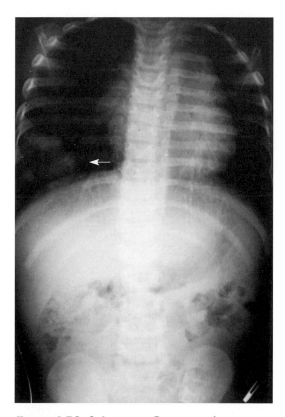

Figure 4.32 Pulmonary Sequestration A right-lower-lobe sequestration is seen in this boy with recurrent infections.

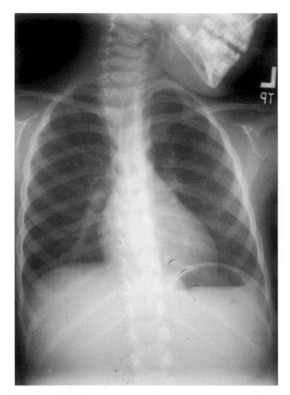

Figure 4.35 A left posterior mediastinal mass is discovered on this chest radiograph.

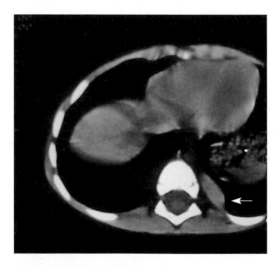

Figure 4.36 The CT scan shows the mass to be an oval, intrapleural lesion.

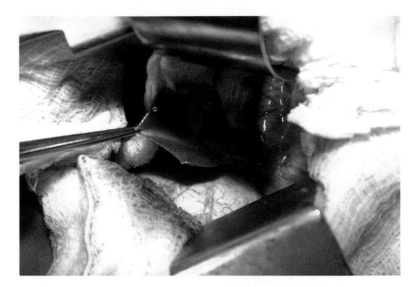

Figure 4.37 At thoracotomy, a small segment of pulmonary tissue, separate from the lung, is seen to have a systemic blood supply directly from the aorta.

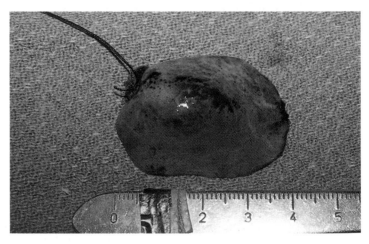

Figure 4.38 The extralobar sequestration is excised. A silk ligature is tied around the specimen side of the systemic artery.

Systemic Lobar Artery

Rarely, one sees a systemic artery from the aorta supplying the circulation to an entire pulmonary lobe with a normal bronchial attachment and normal pulmonary venous return. The left lower lobe is the most common site. Although some consider this anomaly a form of sequestration, the normal bronchial supply puts it into a separate catagory. The children present with tachycardia and a cardiac murmur; unlike children with pulmonary arteriovenous malformations with right-to-left shunting, there is no cyanosis or clubbing. The diagnosis is made by angiography (Fig 4.39). For those children in whom the lobe is abnormal or does not ventilate properly, lobectomy is indicated. In the others, the systemic artery may be detached from the aorta and anastomosed to the ipsilateral pulmonary artery (Figs 4.40–4.42).

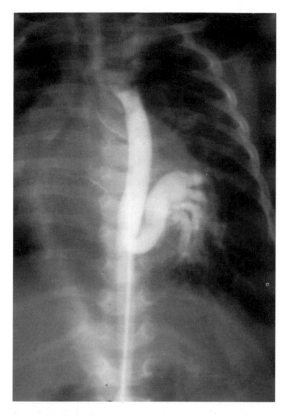

Figure 4.39 Systemic Lobar Artery A 5-month-old boy presents with tachycardia and a systolic murmur. This aortogram shows the entire left lower lobe supplied by a single artery from the aorta. The venous phase of the arteriogram demonstrates venous return through normal, but dilated, pulmonary veins.

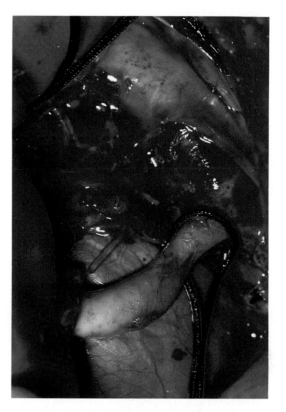

Figure 4.41 The entire length of the artery is dissected free. The silk tie is around the aortic origin.

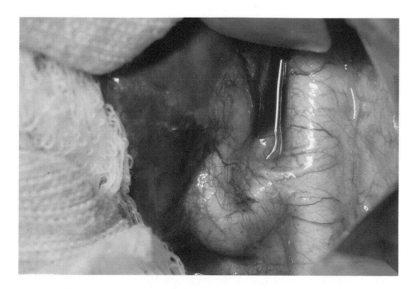

Figure 4.40 Through a left thoracotomy, the systemic artery is visualized from the aorta to the anteriorly retracted left lower lobe.

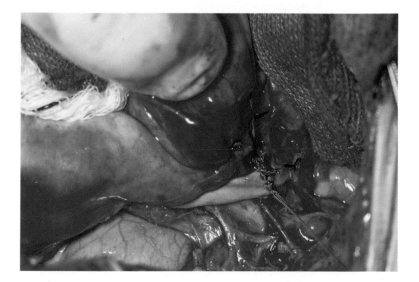

Figure 4.42 The artery is divided, the aortic origin is closed, and the end of the artery is anastomosed to the left pulmonary artery.

Bronchogenic Cyst

The bronchogenic cyst, lined with respiratory epithelium, may be found in the lung or adherent to the trachea or bronchi. Symptoms are those of airway compression. Many cysts cannot be detected on plain radiographs. A few have been missed at surgical exploration, only to be found at autopsy (Figs 4.43, 4.44).

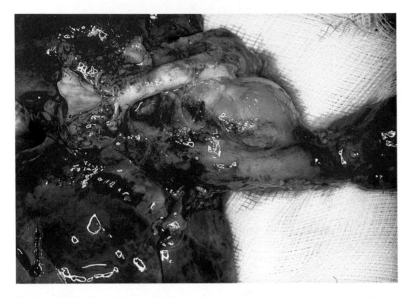

Figure 4.43 Bronchogenic Cyst A large bronchogenic cyst, which caused respiratory obstruction from posterior tracheal compression, is seen at autopsy of this unfortunate 15-month-old.

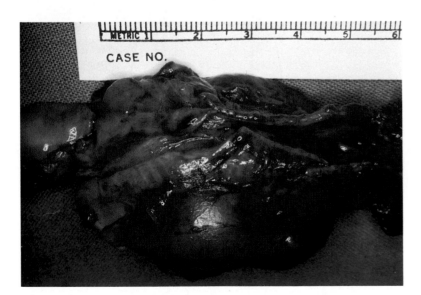

Figure 4.44 The relationship of the cyst to the trachea is seen more clearly in the dissected specimen.

Lung Abscess

Chronic aspiration, especially in brain-damaged children, and staphylococcal pneumonia in any child may produce a lung abscess (Fig 4.45). Failure to control the infection, despite adequate antibiotic therapy, is the indication for drainage. Most surgeons prefer external tube or open drainage. Lobectomy is reserved for chronic abscess formation with lobar destruction.

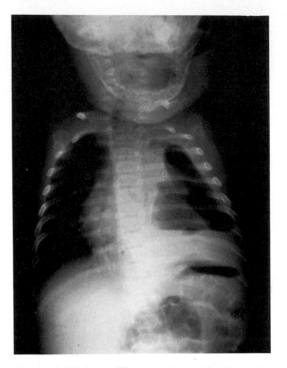

Figure 4.45 Lung Abscess An air-fluid (pus) level is seen in a staphylococcal abscess of this infant. Tube drainage and antibiotic therapy resolve the infection.

Tracheobronchial Foreign Bodies

Children aspirate a variety of foreign materials, from peanuts to toy parts (Fig 4.46) to pointed metallic objects (Figs 4.47, 4.48). Laryngeal or tracheal obstruction may be a life-threatening emergency, requiring immediate Heimlich maneuver or cricothyroidotomy. The presence of a foreign body in the bronchial tree is suggested by a history of sudden coughing or dyspnea, especially in a child who has been eating nuts or holding a small object in the mouth; by continuing wheezing or whistling breaths; or by the development of localized air trapping or atelectasis. Modern pediatric bronchoscopes, with excellent optics and fiberoptic illumination, facilitate foreign body visualization; fine forceps can be placed through the bronchoscope to grasp irregular objects; and a thin balloon catheter can be threaded past some bronchial foreign bodies, which are removed when the balloon is inflated and the catheter is withdrawn.

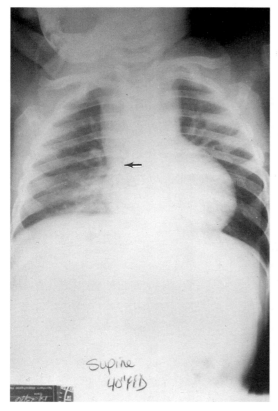

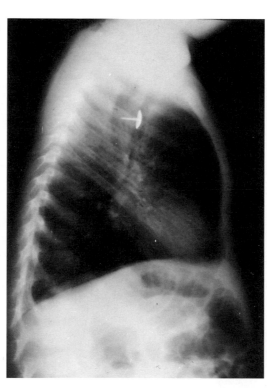

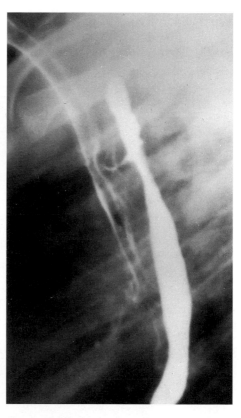

Figure 4.46 Tracheobronchial Foreign Bodies A small, round, plastic bead *(arrow)* is seen on this chest radiography of a 13-month-old boy who suddenly began to cough and wheeze after playing with a toy.

Figure 4.47 An aspirated tack points directly into the esophagus from the trachea.

Figure 4.48 An acquired tracheo-esophageal fistula is the result, demonstrated on barium swallow. Surgical closure is required in this child.

Diaphragm

Diaphragmatic Hernia

Congenital diaphragmatic hernia results from a failure of closure of the embryologic opening between the abdominal and thoracic cavities—the pleuroperitoneal canal. Abdominal contents herniate into the chest and compress the ipsilateral lung, preventing it from growing and developing normally during fetal life. In some infants, both lungs are hypoplastic. Bochdalek defects, in the posterolateral diaphragm, are the most common. Less common is absence of the entire lateral diaphragm. Seventy-five percent of diaphragmatic hernias occur on the left side. Some infants have small hernia defects of the right diaphragm that are occluded by the liver until birth, when increased intraabdominal pressure pushes intestine or liver into the chest for the first time; these infants have normal lungs.

The infant born with this anomaly develops progressive respiratory distress with his or her first breaths, as swallowed air distends the intrathoracic intestine, further compressing the mediastinal structures and the contralateral lung. There may be prominence of the chest on the involved side and a scaphoid abdomen (Fig 4.49). Breath sounds are absent on the side of the hernia, and the heart is displaced toward the opposite chest wall. A chest radiograph confirms the diagnosis (Fig 4.50).

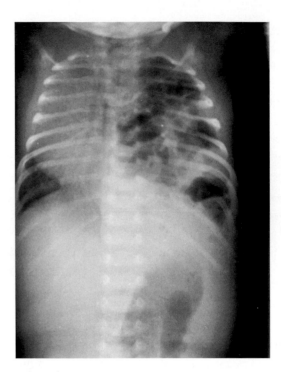

Figure 4.50 Bowel loops fill the left hemithorax, displacing the heart and mediastinum to the right side.

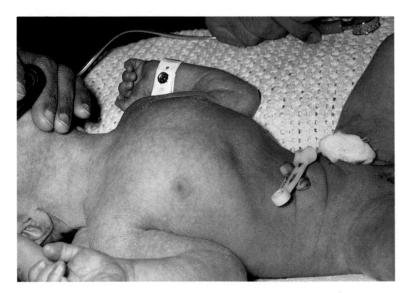

Figure 4.49 Congenital Diaphragmatic Hernia This newborn with respiratory distress and a prominent left hemithorax has a scaphoid abdomen. Most of the abdominal contents are in the left side of the chest.

Therapy must be initiated rapidly to reverse hypoxia, treat acidosis, and prevent further respiratory embarrassment prior to surgical repair. Nasogastric decompression with a catheter of adequate size (#8 or #10 Fr) prevents further intestinal distention. Oxygen is administered. Endotracheal intubation is almost always indicated by the infant's respiratory status or the need to transport him or her to another hospital for definitive care. The baby's lungs are ventilated rapidly—60 or more breaths per minute—and gently; a tension pneumothorax, especially of the uninvolved lung, might prove fatal. To correct the expected respiratory and metabolic acidosis, sodium bicarbonate, 2 mEq/kg, may be given empirically before the results of arterial blood gas measurements are known. Further corrective measures are determined by laboratory data.

A small number of children with congenital diaphragmatic hernias present after the newborn period with respiratory or gastrointestinal symptoms (Fig 4.51). The repair is the same.

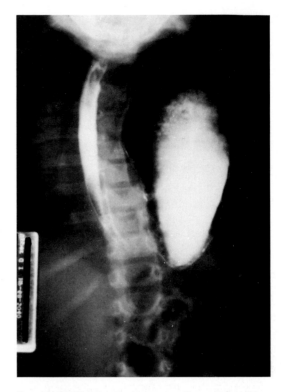

Figure 4.51 This barium swallow, in a 10-month-old with feeding problems, shows the entire stomach protruding through the diaphragm into the left side of the chest.

Surgical Approach

In the past, the repair of a diaphragmatic hernia was always an immediate surgical emergency. The infant was rushed to the operating room, being ventilated with high concentrations of oxygen and receiving intravenous bicarbonate to correct respiratory and metabolic acidosis. It was felt that relief of intrathoracic pressure on the lungs and closure of the diaphragm were the most important steps leading to survival. More recently, the focus has shifted to stabilization of the infant's pulmonary and metabolic status prior to surgical correction. In some centers, infants with severe, but potentially reversible, lung problems may be placed on extracorporeal membrane oxygenation (ECMO) even prior to repair of the hernia and may undergo surgery while on partial bypass.

The surgical repair may be approached via the abdomen or the chest. The author prefers a rapid thoracotomy to give relief from mediastinal and pulmonary compression and for ease of diaphragmatic repair (Figs 4.52, 4.53). Bochdalek defects, with a residual rim of diaphragm, are amenable to primary suture repair (Figs 4.54, 4.55). Large lateral defects may require patch closure (Fig 4.56). Following repair, a chest catheter is connected to water-seal drainage, with suction of no more than 5 cm of water, to allow slow expansion of the underdeveloped lung. The majority of infants do well after surgery. The very high mortality rate for those with severe lung hypoplasia and pulmonary artery hypertension (persistent fetal circulation) has been lowered by the use of ECMO, which gives time for spontaneous recovery of the lungs.

Maternal sonography has enabled physicians to diagnose diaphragmatic hernia antenatally and to have the baby delivered in a setting where full supportive and surgical care can be given. Fetal intervention, with reduction of the viscera into the abdomen and repair of the defect with the fetus in utero, has been carried out in very few specialized medical centers. The determination of which infants will not survive without fetal intervention is difficult, and the ethical issues of subjecting both mother and child to surgery are still controversial.

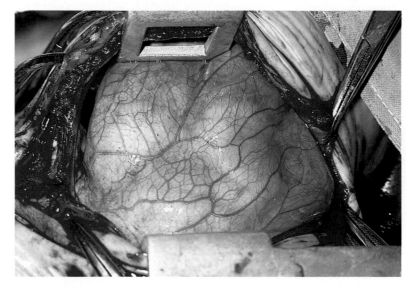

Figure 4.52 A persistent membrane covers the intestine in the left side of the chest. Some diaphragmatic hernias have no sac, and the intestine lies free in the pleural cavity.

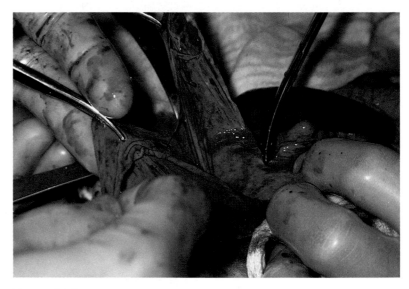

Figure 4.53 After the contents are reduced into the abdomen, the hernia sac is excised at the rim of the diaphragmatic defect. Failure to do so may lead to recurrence of the hernia.

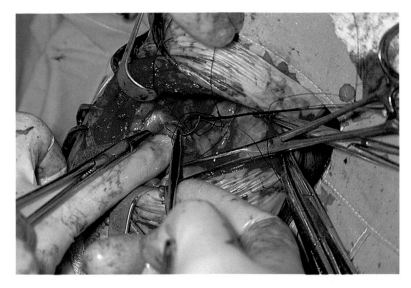

Figure 4.54 Nonabsorbable sutures are placed in the rim of the Bochdalek defect.

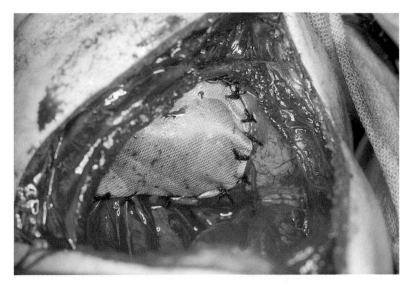

Figure 4.56 The diaphragmatic defect in this child is too large for primary closure. A patch of Silastic material is used.

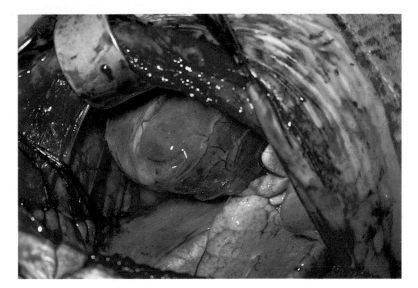

Figure 4.55 The diaphragmatic hernia is closed. This child also has congenital absence of the pericardium.

Eventration

Eventration is the flaccid protrusion of the diaphragm into the thorax; its passive and paradoxical motion with respirations is visualized on fluoroscopy. Birth injury to the phrenic nerve is one cause. Others are congenital, with a variable absence of normal diaphragmatic muscle. Respiratory difficulty in the neonate and frequent pulmonary infections in the older infant are the common presenting symptoms. Repair consists of diaphragmatic plication via thoracotomy. Ventilation-perfusion studies may be helpful in determining the need for surgery in questionable cases.

Hiatus Hernia

Repeated vomiting is the common symptom of paraesophageal hiatus hernia in children. Incarceration of the stomach is possible, but rare. The diagnosis is made on barium swallow (Fig 4.57). Repair involves closure of the defect and fundoplication (Figs 4.58, 4.59).

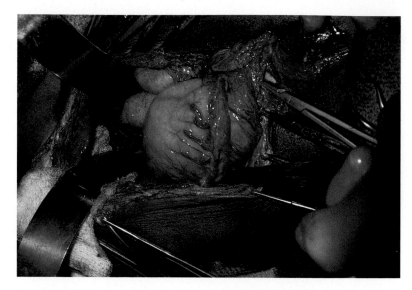

Figure 4.58 The stomach is reduced from the hiatus.

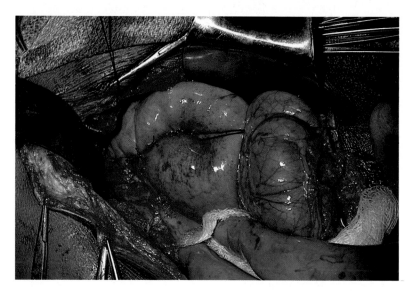

Figure 4.59 A fundoplication and closure of the hiatus are completed.

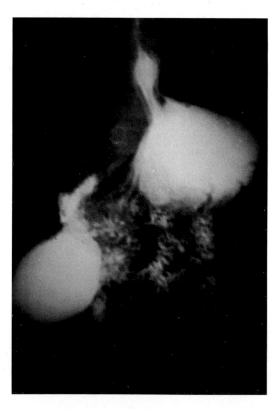

Figure 4.57 Hiatus Hernia A paraesophageal hiatus hernia is demonstrated on this barium study of an 11-year-old with recurrent vomiting episodes.

Morgagni Hernia

This anteromedial diaphragmatic opening is often discovered as an incidental finding, with only rare incarceration of intestine (Figs 4.60, 4.61). Repair is accomplished from the abdomen, with excision of the hernia sac and suturing of the edge of the defect to the posterior rectus sheath at the costal margin (Fig 4.62).

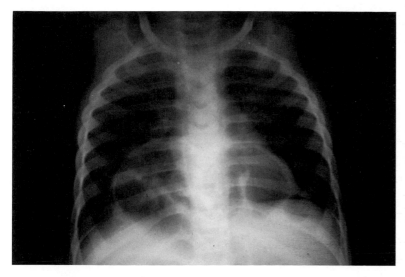

Figure 4.60 Foramen of Morgagni Hernia Air-filled bowel loops are seen in the lower mediastinum on this chest radiograph. (Reprinted with permission from Kimmelstiel FM, Holgersen LO, Hilfer C: Retrosternal [Morgagni] hernia with small bowel obstruction secondary to a Richter's incarceration. Journal of Pediatric Surgery 22:998–1000, 1987.)

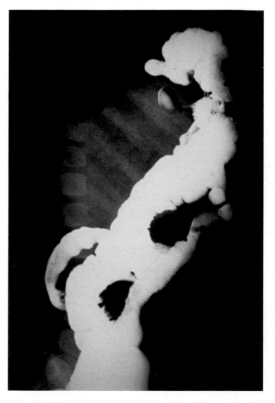

Figure 4.61 A barium study shows intestine protruding through the anterior diaphragmatic defect. (Reproduced with permission from Kimmelstiel FM, Holgersen LO, Hilfer C: Retrosternal [Morgagni] hernia with small bowel obstruction secondary to a Richter's incarceration. Journal of Pediatric Surgery 22:998–1000, 1987.)

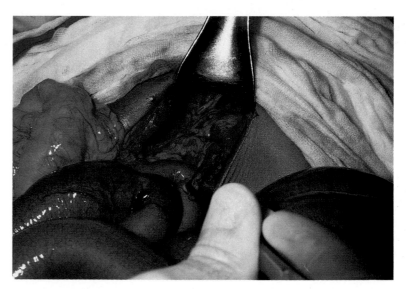

Figure 4.62 The hernia defect is seen, just below the retractor, after intestine is reduced from the hernia.

Esophagus

Atresia

Congenital absence of continuity of the esophagus—esophageal atresia—may be an isolated malformation; more commonly, it is associated with one or more abnormal fistulas to the trachea or bronchi (Fig 4.63). In 80%–85% of cases, there is a single fistula from the trachea to the distal esophagus. Atresia without fistula occurs in 10%–12%. Fistulas to the trachea from the proximal esophagus, with or without a distal fistula, are present in only 5%.

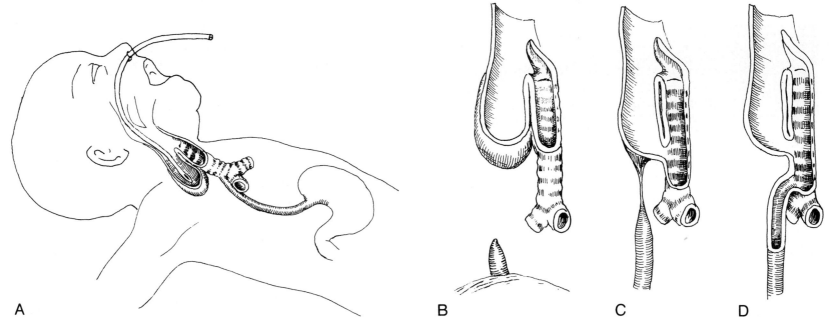

A   B   C   D

Figure 4.63 Esophageal Atresia A. The most common type of esophageal atresia, with a blind upper pouch and a tracheal or bronchial fistula to the lower esophagus. Suction through a double-lumen sump catheter keeps secretions from pooling in the upper pouch. **B.** An atresia without fistula, with the usual wide separation of upper and lower esophagus. **C** and **D.** The two rarest types, a single proximal tracheoesophageal fistula and a double fistula.

The presenting symptom in the newborn infant is excessive salivation or immediate regurgitation of feedings. Attempted passage of a nasogastric tube, which stops or coils in the midesophagus (Figs 4.64–4.66), confirms the diagnosis. This simple maneuver, if performed routinely in the delivery room, would always establish the diagnosis at birth.

The infant with esophageal atresia and distal fistula should be kept with the head elevated to prevent gastric acid regurgitation and aspiration—the most frequent and serious complication (Fig 4.66). A double-lumen sump catheter is placed in the blind-ending upper esophageal pouch; constant suction keeps secretions from pooling and being aspirated. Oxygen is given as needed.

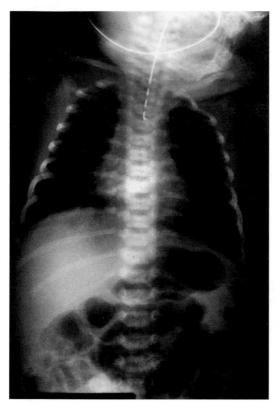

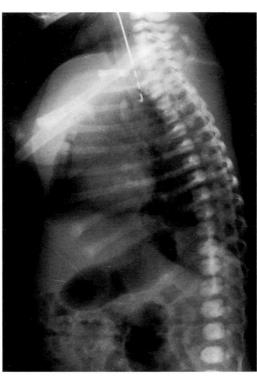

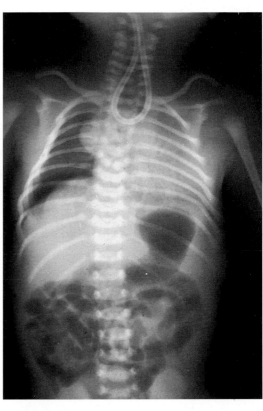

Figure 4.64 The radiopaque sump catheter stops in the upper esophagus. Air in the intestine confirms the presence of a distal tracheal fistula.

Figure 4.65 A lateral radiograph shows the catheter to be in the esophagus, posterior to the air-filled trachea.

Figure 4.66 The tube is coiled in the upper esophagus, confirming the diagnosis of esophageal atresia; there is a distal tracheoesophageal fistula. Before these diagnoses were made, the baby, who also had an imperforate anus, was turned head-down for radiographs of the bowel in the pelvis. Gastric acid flooded the lungs, producing a fatal aspiration pneumonia.

Surgical Repair

Prompt repair is indicated if the baby has no other major contraindications to general anesthesia and thoracotomy (Figs 4.67–4.70). The severely premature infant (less than 1500 g) or one with serious cardiac or pulmonary disease may benefit from a staged approach: a preliminary gastrostomy is performed to decompress the stomach, with a sump catheter on constant suction to remove saliva from the upper pouch; when the infant is of suitable size and health, he or she will undergo thoracotomy, division of the fistula, and esophageal anastomosis.

The approach to isolated esophageal atresia depends on the distance between the upper and lower ends. After preliminary gastrostomy, an attempt is made to stretch the esophagus with bougies from above and dilators from below (Figs 4.71, 4.72). These maneuvers may then permit a subsequent primary anastomosis (Figs 4.73, 4.74). The alternative is a form of intestinal interposition—substernal colon (Figs 4.75–4.77), intrathoracic colon (Fig 4.78), or gastric tube.

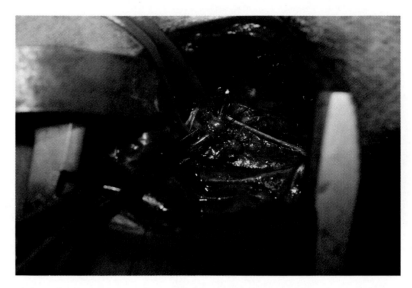

Figure 4.67 Repair is accomplished through a right thoracotomy, unless there is a right aortic arch and right descending aorta. The pleura is not entered, but is gently dissected from the chest wall and mediastinum. The azygos vein is divided to expose the dilated upper esophagus. The lower esophagus and tracheal fistula are identified, as shown. The esophagus is to the left and the trachea to the right. Fine silk traction sutures are placed at the edges of the fistula, 2–3 mm from the trachea.

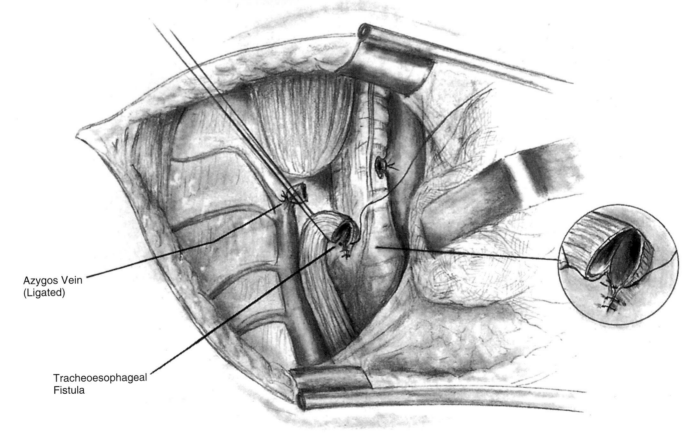

Azygos Vein
(Ligated)

Tracheoesophageal
Fistula

Figure 4.68 The fistula is divided, leaving a 3-mm cuff on the tracheal side to avoid narrowing the trachea. Interrupted 5-0 silk sutures close the fistula, which should be airtight. With warm saline in the infant's chest, the anesthesiologist inflates the lungs; if there is no bubbling of air, the tracheal closure is adequate.

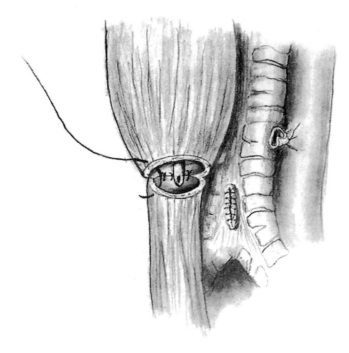

Figure 4.69 An anastomosis is performed between the upper and lower esophagus, using fine interrupted silk sutures.

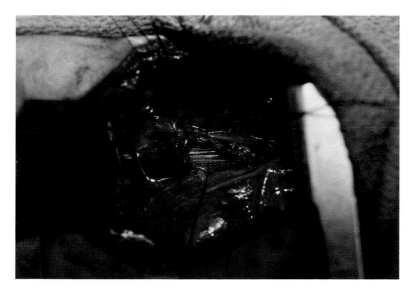

Figure 4.70 A single-layer esophageal anastomosis is performed, with the nasogastric tube in the esophagus to aid in the placement of the lateral sutures. When the anastomosis is complete, the tube is advanced into the stomach for postoperative decompression.

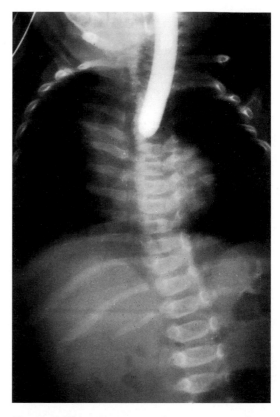

Figure 4.71 A bougie in the upper esophagus of this infant with isolated atresia demonstrates the level to which it can be stretched—not enough for a primary anastomosis.

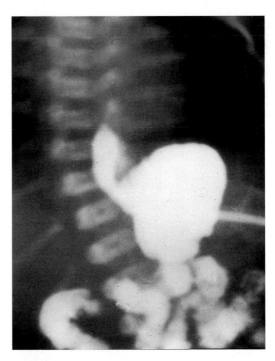

Figure 4.72 Barium through a gastrostomy tube shows the level of the distal esophagus.

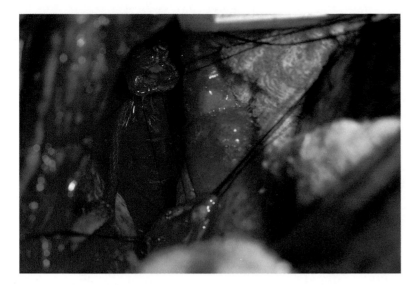

Figure 4.73 In this delayed primary anastomosis, several sutures are placed through the upper and lower esophagus before they are brought together.

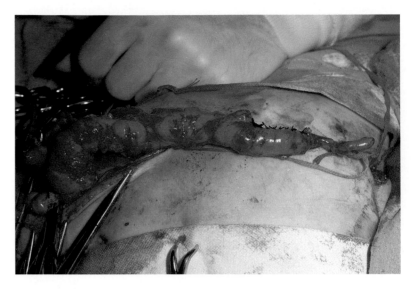

Figure 4.75 The right colon is mobilized to reach the neck in this child with isolated esophageal atresia and a wide gap between ends.

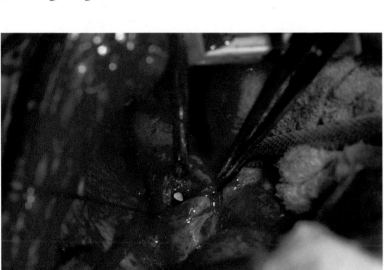

Figure 4.74 The posterior row of sutures has been tied. A nasogastric tube in the esophagus facilitates placement of the remaining sutures.

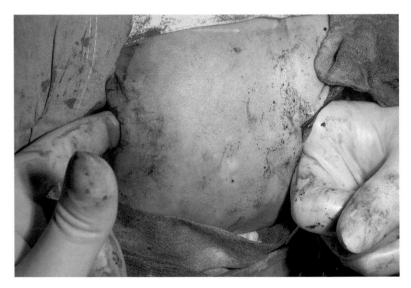

Figure 4.76 A substernal tunnel is created by the surgeon's fingers.

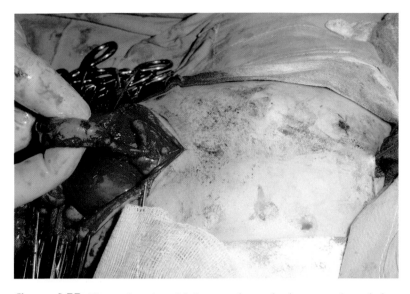

Figure 4.77 The colon is withdrawn through the tunnel, and the cecum is anastomosed to the esophagus in the neck and to the stomach in the abdomen.

Tracheoesophageal (H-Type) Fistula

The isolated fistula between intact trachea and esophagus (H-type fistula) is a rare anomaly that usually is not apparent in the neonate. Coughing with feeding or recurrent episodes of pneumonia in infancy raise the possibility of this diagnosis. Radiographic studies of the esophagus with dilute contrast media will demonstrate some fistulas, which run diagonally from the esophagus to a higher level of the membranous trachea (Figs 4.79, 4.80). Other fistulas not seen radiographically may sometimes be visualized with an infant bronchoscope or esophagoscope. Some surgeons pass a fine ureteral catheter through the fistula during preoperative bronchoscopy, as an aid to identifying the tract for surgical division. The majority of H-type fistulas are high and can be approached and divided through a supraclavicular cervical incision (Figs 4.81–4.83).

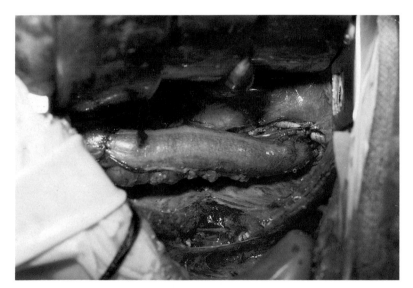

Figure 4.78 A vascularized colon segment is brought through the diaphragm into the chest to bridge the gap between the upper and lower esophagus.

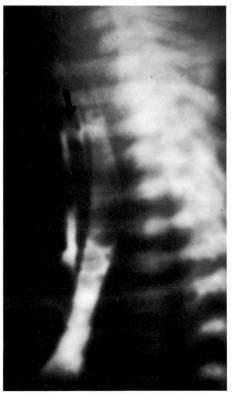

Figure 4.79 A proximal H-type tracheoesophageal fistula is outlined on this barium study.

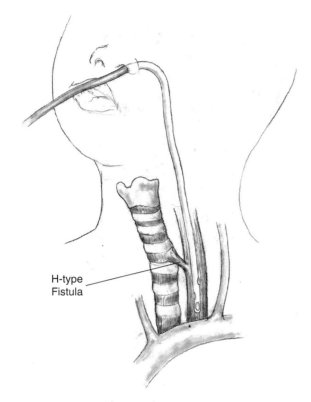

H-type
Fistula

Figure 4.80 The oblique fistula tract
between the trachea and esophagus
is illustrated.

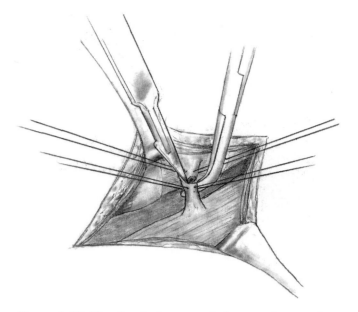

Figure 4.82 The fistula is severed close to the esophagus and sutured closed at both ends. Placement of
traction sutures on both sides of the fistula, as shown,
facilitates fistula closure.

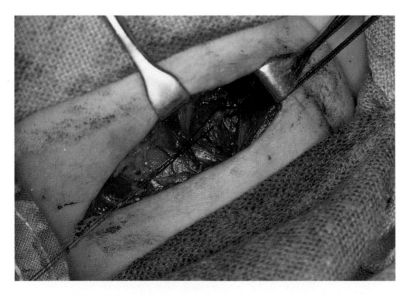

Figure 4.81 The H-type tracheoesophageal fistula is approached
through a left low cervical incision. Some advocate a right-sided
incision to avoid damage to the thoracic duct. The fistula is seen
isolated and dissected.

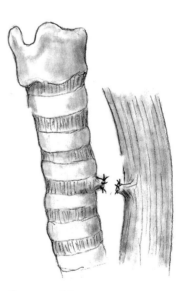

Figure 4.83 Fine interrupted
sutures close the tracheal and
esophageal sides of the fistula.

Esophageal Web

A congenital web or membrane across the esophagus,
usually in the middle or lower third, most often has a
central or eccentric perforation (Fig 4.84). It is a form of
esophageal stenosis, which becomes apparent at an age
when solid food obstructs the lumen. Some respond to
simple dilatation. The thicker ones must be resected (Figs
4.85–4.87).

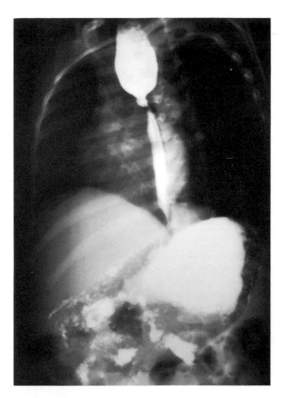

Figure 4.84 Esophageal Web Marked narrowing of the upper esophagus, with proximal dilatation, is seen on this barium swallow.

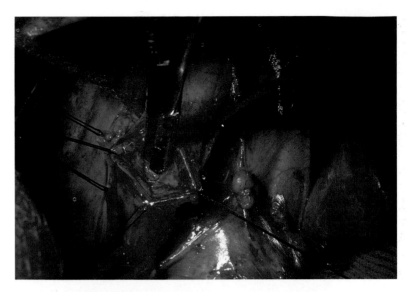

Figure 4.86 A hemostat demonstrates the small opening in the esophageal web.

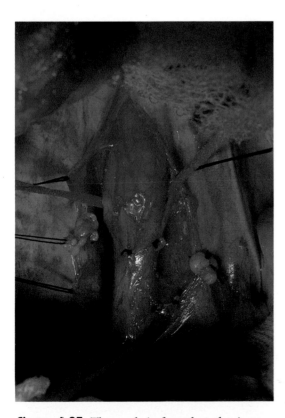

Figure 4.85 The web is found at the junction between dilated proximal and normal-caliber distal esophagus.

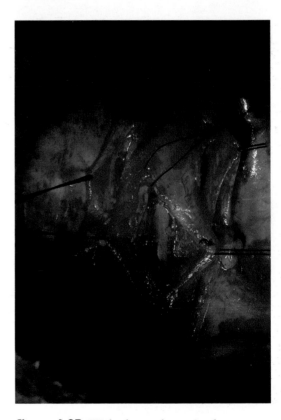

Figure 4.87 With the web excised, a nasogastric tube passes easily through the esophageal lumen. The vertical incision is closed transversely to prevent narrowing.

Duplication

Duplications of the esophagus and of the trachea may form cysts in the wall of the esophagus. They may present with dysphagia or may be incidental radiographic findings (Figs 4.88, 4.89). Excision of the cyst is always advised (Figs 4.90–4.92).

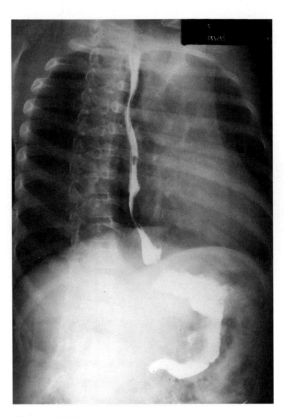

Figure 4.89 Indentation on the lower esophagus is demonstrated by this barium swallow.

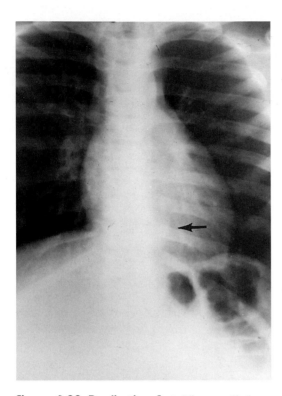

Figure 4.88 Duplication Cyst The small density behind the heart is seen on this plain radiograph.

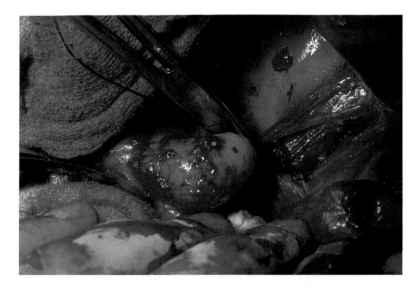

Figure 4.90 At thoracotomy, a cyst is dissected from the wall of the esophagus.

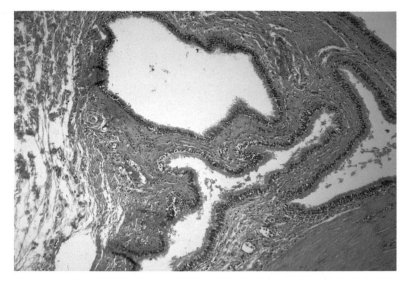

Figure 4.92 A columnar epithelial lining, characteristic of bronchial origin, is seen in this photomicrograph of the specimen.

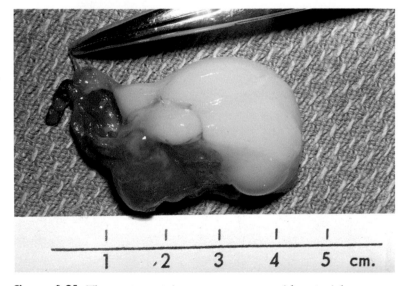

Figure 4.91 The cyst contains a creamy mucoid material.

Foreign Bodies

Ingested foreign bodies can lodge in the esophagus (Fig 4.93). Sharp or pointed ones may perforate. The two common sites of hold-up are the hypopharynx and the gastroesophageal junction. A lateral radiograph will reveal the presence of overlapping objects, such as multiple coins. Round objects, such as coins, that are stuck in the hypopharynx may be dislodged with a balloon catheter without anesthesia (Fig 4.94). Others, especially of odd shape, may require endoscopic removal (Figs 4.95, 4.96).

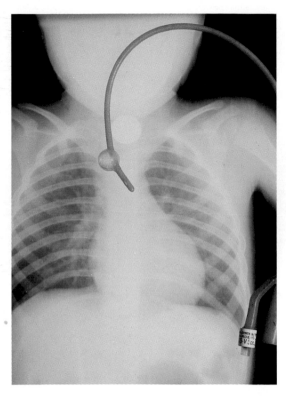

Figure 4.94 Round objects, such as the coin in this child's hypopharynx, can often be dislodged by passage of a balloon catheter beyond the object and withdrawal of the catheter with the balloon inflated.

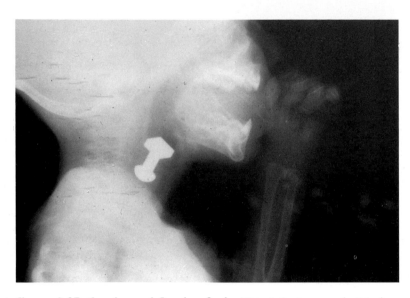

Figure 4.93 Esophageal Foreign Body This infant was admitted for evaluation of dysphagia and weight loss. The cause is seen on the lateral neck radiograph.

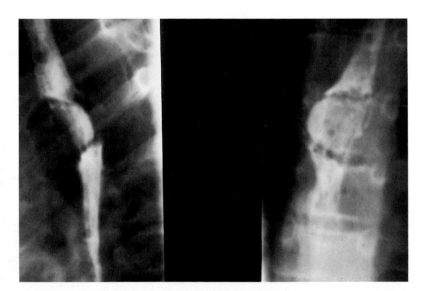

Figure 4.95 An unusual-shaped object is outlined by barium in the esophagus of this 10-year-old girl.

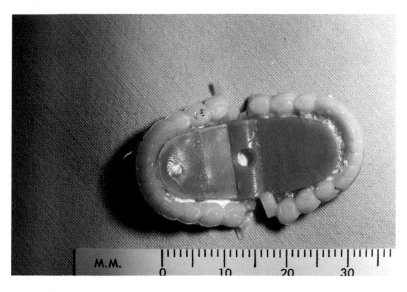

Figure 4.96 Esophagoscopy under general anesthesia was necessary to remove this set of plastic "false teeth."

Caustic Injury

The unsupervised toddler who has access to caustic household products, such as drain cleaners, may find and swallow one, resulting in lye burns of the mouth, pharynx, and esophagus. Children in whom caustic ingestion is suspected should be examined at once by direct and endoscopic means to determine the extent and location of the burns. Systemic steroids and antibiotics are administered if caustic injury is demonstrated. No attempt is made at dilatation for at least 2 weeks, and then only after demonstration of a stricture (Fig 4.97). Short-segment strictures respond better than long ones to dilatation. Esophageal substitution, similar to that for isolated esophageal atresia, using colon or small intestine, has been performed for severe or extensive scarring.

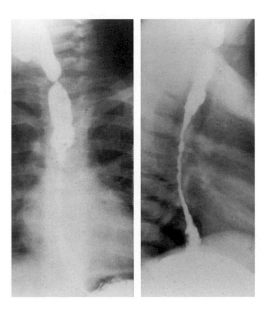

Figure 4.97 Caustic Esophageal Stricture
Stricture following lye ingestion is seen on the anteroposterior and lateral views of the barium-filled esophagus of a 2-year-old.

Achalasia

Lack of relaxation of the lower esophageal sphincter presents with dysphagia and retention and regurgitation of food. The barium swallow shows a dilated proximal esophagus, with poor contractions and a tapered narrowing distally. A Heller esophagomyotomy is required, as balloon dilatation is considered dangerous in children. The Heller procedure has been performed under video-assisted thoracotomy (thoracoscopy), with good reported results.

Mediastinum

Teratoma

The classic location of mediastinal teratomas is anterior, although some may originate posteriorly (Figs 4.98, 4.99) or within the pericardium. The tumors may be cystic or solid, and they produce symptoms by compression of lung and mediastinum. Malignant degeneration is found in 20%. Others may become infected or may erode into mediastinal structures. The diagnosis of mediastinal teratoma, by radiography or computed tomography, is an indication for excision (Figs 4.100–4.102).

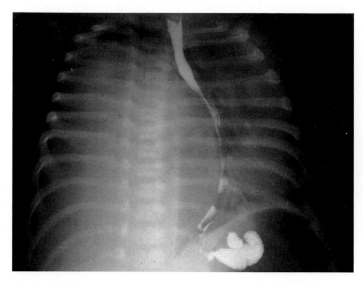

Figure 4.99 The mass fills the right chest and displaces the barium-filled esophagus to the left.

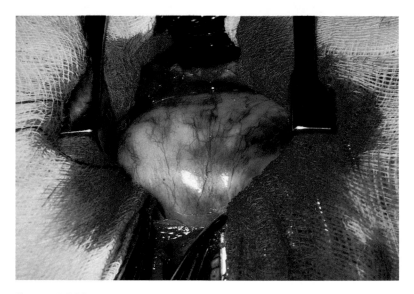

Figure 4.100 The large cystic and solid mass is seen at thoracotomy.

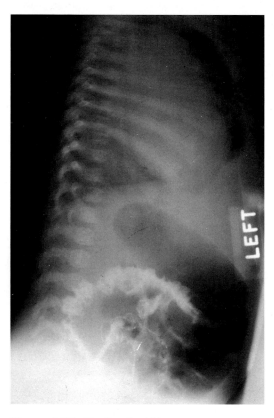

Figure 4.98 Mediastinal Teratoma A posterior mediastinal mass compresses the lung, producing respiratory distress in this 2-month-old girl.

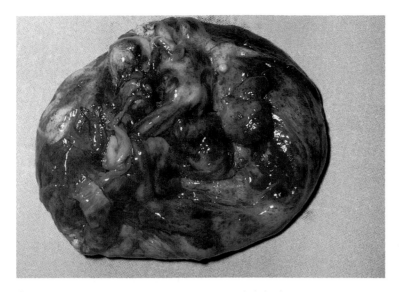

Figure 4.101 The open specimen has an irregular lining and some nodules of firm tissue.

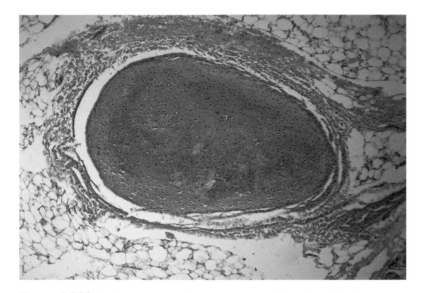

Figure 4.102 All three germ layers are found and are benign. This photomicrograph demonstrates one of the firm areas to be cartilage.

Lymphoma

The anterior mediastinum is a common site for the appearance of lymphoma. With the introduction of thoracoscopic biopsy, thoracotomy is no longer needed for those lesions that cannot be diagnosed by cervical node biopsy or needle biopsy of the mediastinal mass (Fig 4.103).

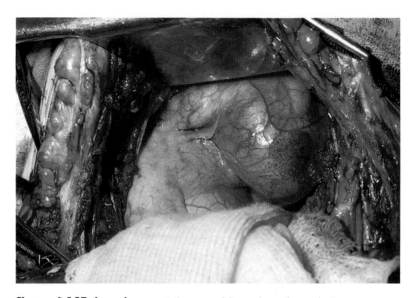

Figure 4.103 Lymphoma A large rubbery lymph node is seen at thoracotomy in this 12-year-old girl with fever and a widened mediastinum on chest radiograph. A supraclavicular node had been excised and was found to be normal.

Ganglioneuroma

Ganglioneuroma is a benign, well-encapsulated tumor of sympathetic-chain origin that is seen in the posterior mediastinum (Figs 4.104, 4.105). Excision is indicated for diagnosis (Figs 4.106–4.108) to distinguish it from neuroblastoma.

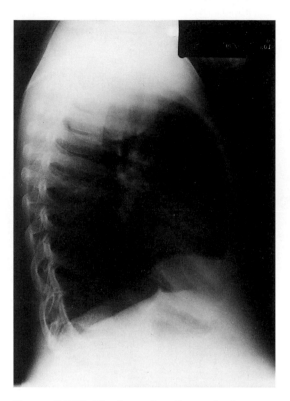

Figure 4.105 The lateral radiograph shows the mass to be in the posterior mediastinum.

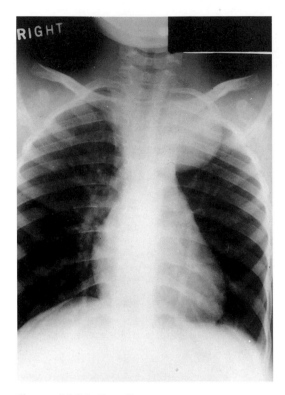

Figure 4.104 Ganglioneuroma A discrete round mediastinal mass is found on the chest radiograph of an asymptomatic 7-year-old.

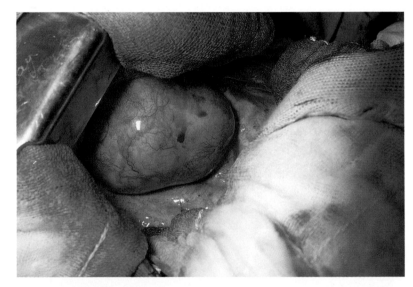

Figure 4.106 The smooth, encapsulated mass is dissected at thoracotomy.

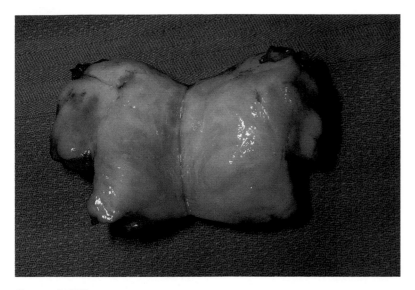

Figure 4.107 The sectioned specimen has a uniform consistency and appearance.

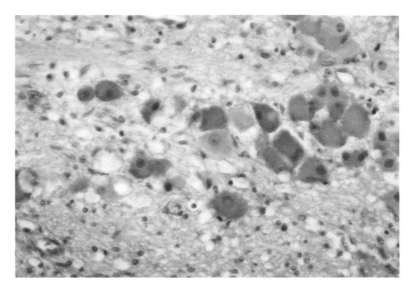

Figure 4.108 The ganglion cells of a benign ganglioneuroma are seen in this photomicrograph.

Thymoma

Thymic enlargement in childhood rarely represents a malignant tumor. The thymus is normally large in children to the age of 18 months; it shrinks rapidly with stress or after a short course of steroids.

Thymoma (Figs 4.109, 4.110), thymic cyst, and thymolipoma are the most common thymic lesions. Thymectomy is achieved through a cervical or sternum-splitting approach (Figs 4.111, 4.112), depending on the location of the bulk of the mass.

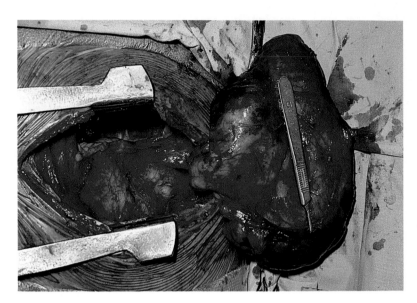

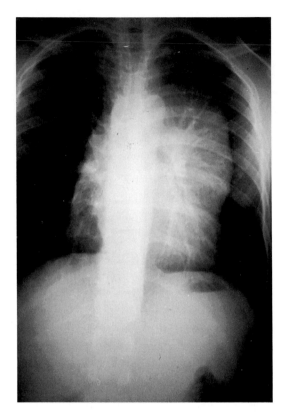

Figure 4.109 Thymoma A chest radiograph, taken of a 14-year-old boy for wheezing, discloses this huge anterior mediastinal mass.

Figure 4.111 The huge mass is seen dissected from the underlying mediastinal structures. Exposure is through a median sternotomy.

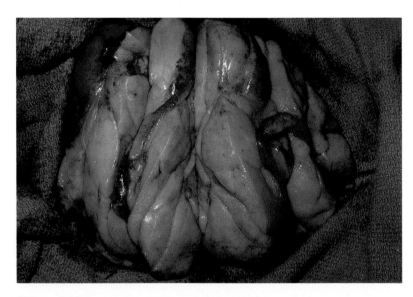

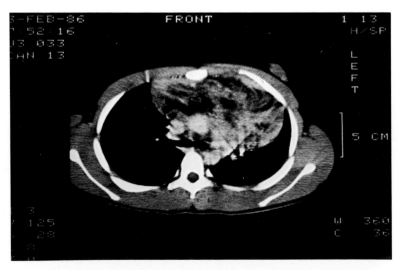

Figure 4.110 A computed tomogram of the chest shows the location and extent of this mass of variable density.

Figure 4.112 A soft, uniform consistency is found in the mass, which proves to be a benign thymoma.

Vascular Ring

Abnormal embryologic development of the aortic arch often leads to a vascular ring around the trachea and esophagus. The double aortic arch arises from the ascending aorta and encircles the trachea and esophagus; the narrower arch is usually divided. A ring may also be formed by the combination of a right aortic arch, a retro-esophageal left subclavian artery, a ductus arteriosus, and the pulmonary artery anteriorly (Fig 4.113). The diagnosis is made by barium swallow (Fig 4.114) and aortography. Relief of the constriction is achieved by division of the ductus arteriosus (or ligamentum arteriosum); the aberrant left subclavian artery may also be divided, if necessary (Figs 4.115, 4.116).

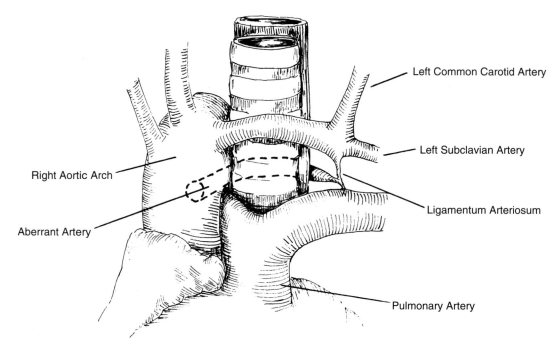

Figure 4.113 Congenital Vascular Ring The illustration is of an aortovascular ring formed by the following structures: (1) an aberrant left innominate artery, which arises from a right descending aorta and passes posterior to the trachea and esophagus; (2) a rudimentary, blind-ending, anterior left aortic arch, which has a fibrous adherence to the left innominate and to (3) the pulmonary artery and ligamentum arteriosum anterior to the trachea and esophagus.

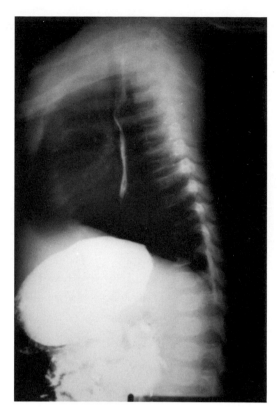

Figure 4.114 A barium swallow shows the indentation of the vascular ring on the posterior esophagus of a 4-month-old boy whose mother revived him from a sudden apneic episode.

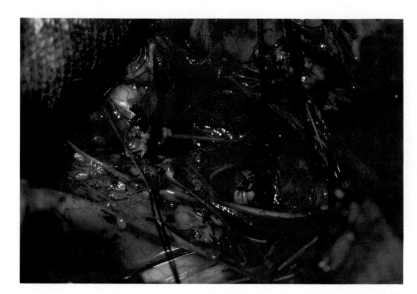

Figure 4.116 Division of the ligamentum frees the trachea and esophagus from circular compression.

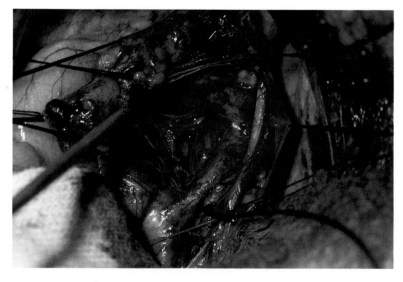

Figure 4.115 At surgery, the pulmonary artery is seen at the lower left and gives rise to the ligamentum arteriosum, which is isolated by a large black suture. It attaches to the left innominate artery and rudimentary left aortic arch.

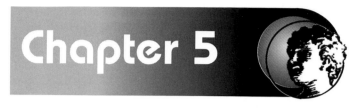

Chapter 5

Hernias and Defects of the Abdominal Wall

Congenital defects of the abdominal wall are all visible or palpable. Hernias may be found at the umbilicus, in the epigastrium, in the lumbar area, in the groin, and in the femoral space. Omphalocele and gastroschisis present dramatically, as abdominal contents protrude either into the umbilical cord or out of the abdomen through a paraumbilical defect. The patent urachus or omphalomesenteric duct drains urine or intestinal contents at the umbilicus. Absence of the abdominal musculature is called ''prune-belly'' because of the lax abdominal wall and wrinkled skin.

Inguinal Hernia

Indirect inguinal hernia, present in 1%–3% of all children, is the most common congenital problem requiring surgery. The processus vaginalis, a protrusion of peritoneum through the internal ring into the inguinal canal, normally obliterates by the 8th or 9th intrauterine month (Fig 5.1). Failure of closure by the time of birth leaves a patent processus vaginalis, or hernia sac, which peritoneal fluid or an abdominal viscus may enter. The left side generally closes first; therefore, right inguinal hernias are more common. Premature infants are more likely to have hernias, and have a higher proportion of bilateral hernias, than do full-term babies. Although hernias occur primarily in boys, the female proportion is a significant 12%–14%.

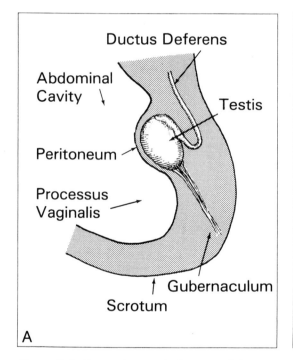
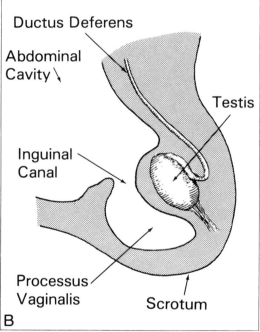
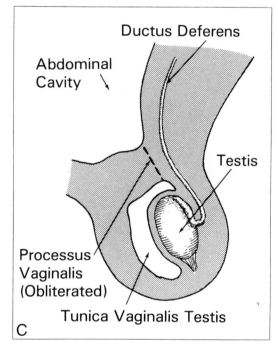

Figure 5.1 Formation and closure of the processus vaginalis: **A.** A protrusion of peritoneum accompanies the testis (or round ligament in the female) into the inguinal area to form the processus vaginalis. **B.** The processus vaginalis descends into the scrotum (or labium). **C.** The proximal processus obliterates, leaving only a potential space in the scrotum, the tunica vaginalis testis.

The diagnosis of a large hernia is made on the observation of a mass protruding through the internal inguinal ring into the inguinal canal, and sometimes extending into the labium or scrotum (Fig 5.2). With a smaller hernia, an inguinal bulge appears only when the child cries or strains (Fig 5.3). Hernias in children produce pain only when incarcerated.

A very narrow opening may present as a communicating hydrocele, which fluctuates in size as peritoneal fluid passes into and out of the patent sac (Figs 5.4–5.7). It must be distinguished from the noncommunicating hydrocele of infancy, in which fluid is trapped in the tunica vaginalis testis or the processus vaginalis at the time of normal closure (Fig 5.8); the trapped peritoneal fluid slowly resorbs by the age of 6–7 months in most cases.

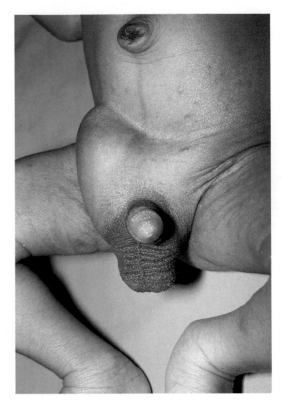

Figure 5.3 A hernia mass containing intestine appears in the groin when this 2-month-old cries and reduces spontaneously when he relaxes.

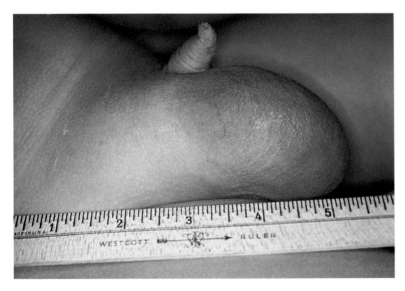

Figure 5.2 This right inguinal hernia, in a 3½-year-old, fills the scrotum. It is found at surgery to contain the cecum and appendix.

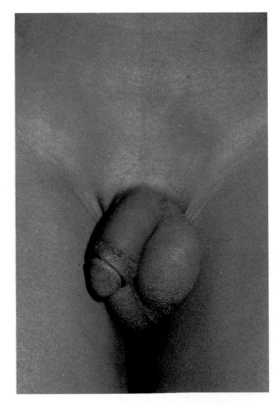

Figure 5.4 Soft fluid swelling is noted in the left side of the scrotum.

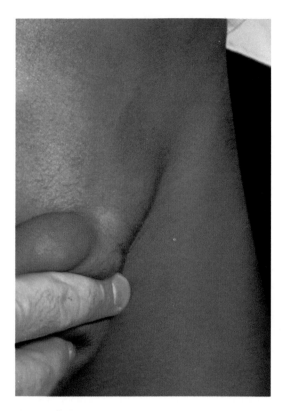

Figure 5.5 Gentle, steady pressure forces the fluid back into the peritoneal cavity through a patent processus vaginalis. Most communicating hydroceles do *not* empty this easily.

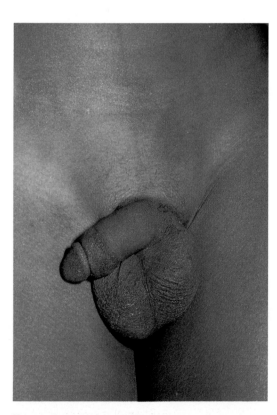

Figure 5.6 The left side of the scrotum is empty of fluid but refills after the boy has been up and active.

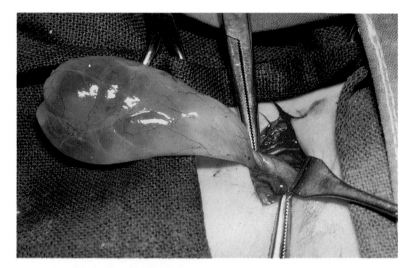

Figure 5.7 In this 19-month-old boy, the entire hernia sac can be seen as a communicating hydrocele containing peritoneal fluid. The neck of the sac has been twisted prior to suture ligation.

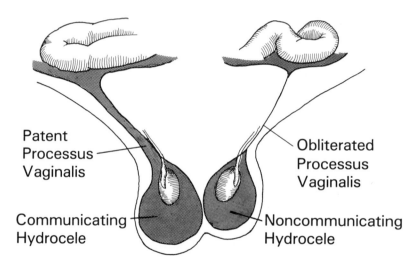

Patent Processus Vaginalis

Obliterated Processus Vaginalis

Communicating Hydrocele

Noncommunicating Hydrocele

Figure 5.8 The left side of the illustration shows a communicating hydrocele with a narrow patent sac; it is the equivalent of an inguinal hernia. On the right is depicted a noncommunicating hydrocele, the result of fluid trapped in the tunica vaginalis testis at the time of normal obliteration of the sac.

When there is a clinical history of a hernia but no visible or palpable mass at the time of examination, the finding of a palpable thickening of cord structures or round ligament—or an inguinal "impulse" with crying or coughing—helps confirm the presence of a suspected hernia (Fig 5.9). A cooperative child may be asked to "blow up your finger like a balloon" to increase intraabdominal pressure. If there is a question about the diagnosis, the child is reexamined in a few weeks, and the parents alerted to watch for inguinal or scrotolabial swelling.

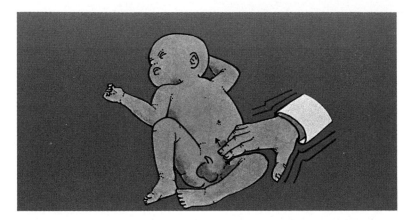

Figure 5.9 Gentle palpation perpendicular to the cord structures in the inguinal canal reveals the thickening of a patent sac. Inversion of the scrotum to palpate the inguinal canal in a child gives no useful information and frequently produces pain. (Reprinted with permission from Liebert PS: Inguinal Hernias in Children [a teaching slide/sound series]. Teaching Dynamics, Philadelphia, 1972.)

Treatment of Inguinal Hernias

An inguinal hernia or communicating hydrocele should be repaired electively soon after the diagnosis is confirmed, consistent with the child's state of health and the anesthetic and surgical expertise available. The recommendation for repair is based on the possibility of incarceration and subsequent strangulation of a viscus. Incarceration of intestine in a hernia is a problem requiring urgent attention. A rapidly appearing hydrocele of the cord or the scrotum may be mistaken for an incarcerated hernia; with a hydrocele alone, there are no palpable intestinal contents protruding through the internal ring. Transillumination of the scrotum does not always distinguish intestine from hydrocele fluid, especially in infants.

An incarcerated hernia (Figs 5.10, 5.11) should be reduced manually if there are no signs of strangulation of the contents. Attempts at reduction may include one or more of the following: (1) barbiturate sedation (pentobarbital, 1.5–2 mg/kg), (2) elevation of the foot of the bed or crib (Trendelenburg position), (3) ice pack to the groin to minimize soft tissue swelling, and (4) gentle persistent pressure over the internal inguinal ring (Fig 5.12). After successful reduction, the author routinely admits the child to the hospital and performs a herniorrhaphy in a day or two, after the local edema subsides. Parents should be informed that testicular atrophy sometimes follows prolonged cord compression from an incarcerated hernia.

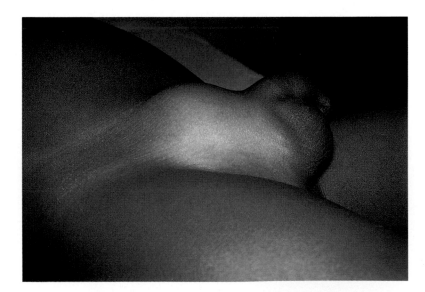

Figure 5.10 This right-sided inguinal hernia in a 3-year-old boy is incarcerated for only a short time and can be reduced manually.

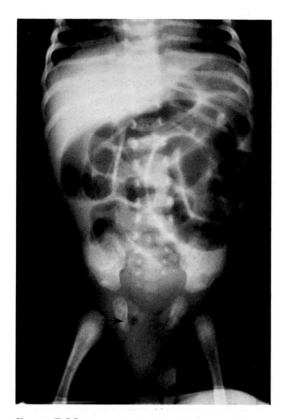

Figure 5.11 The diagnosis of incarcerated hernia was made on the basis of air in the right inguinal canal, seen on an abdominal radiograph of a 3-week-old evaluated for intestinal obstruction. Direct observation is the usual method of making the diagnosis.

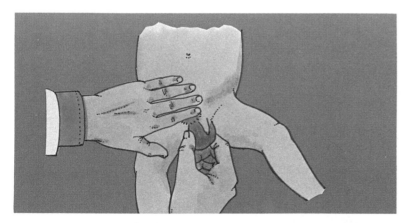

Figure 5.12 The technique for reduction of an incarcerated inguinal hernia requires displacement of the hernia contents toward the internal inguinal ring with one hand, with exertion of steady, continuous pressure over the internal ring with the other. It may take up to 5–10 minutes of pressure to achieve reduction. (Reproduced with permission from Liebert PS: Inguinal Hernias in Children [a teaching slide/sound series]. Teaching Dynamics, Philadelphia, 1972.)

Edema and erythema of the overlying skin, fever, leukocytosis, and toxic appearance of the child are signs of possible strangulation of the hernia contents and require prompt surgery (Figs 5.13, 5.14).

Because of the high incidence of unrecognized bilateral hernias, the author routinely explores both sides at elective repair in children younger than 10 years of age. Unless there is a clinically apparent contralateral hernia, only the involved side is repaired at emergency surgery for an incarcerated hernia or for the hernia found in association with an undescended testis.

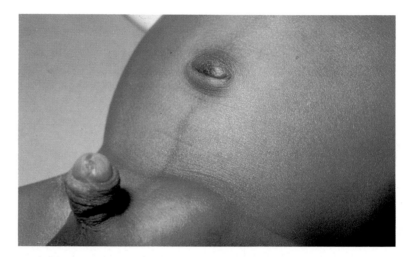

Figure 5.13 This 3-week-old presents with a 1-day history of irritability, followed by fever and vomiting. His abdomen is distended, and there are edema and erythema over the obvious left-sided inguinal bulge. No attempt is made to reduce the hernia preoperatively.

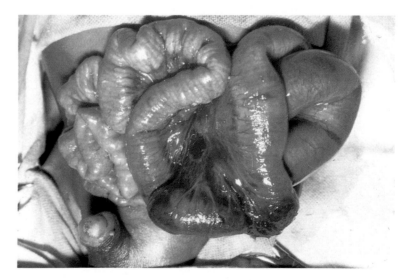

Figure 5.14 At surgery, performed through a low transverse abdominal incision, the strangulated hernia is reduced with great difficulty. The gangrenous ileum seen here is resected, and the child recovers without incident.

Surgical Repair

Inguinal hernia repair in a child consists of suture ligation of the hernia sac at the internal inguinal ring after reduction of the sac contents (Figs 5.15–5.23). When the entire contents cannot be reduced, as determined by careful palpation of the neck of the sac, the sac must be opened to determine the possibility of a sliding hernia—one with an abdominal viscus adherent to the peritoneal lining of the hernia sac. In the female (Fig 5.24), the hernia sac should always be opened and inspected for a fallopian tube or ovary as a sliding component (Figs 5.25, 5.26). The author repairs a sliding hernia by placing a purse-string suture at the neck of the sac from the outside and then inverting the sac and its contents into the abdomen before tying the suture (Figs 5.27–5.30). In all patients the transverse, skin-crease incision is closed in layers, using absorbable suture material. A subcuticular skin closure gives optimal healing and appearance.

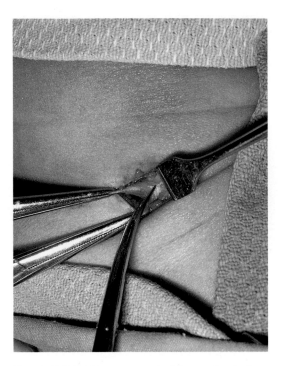

Figure 5.16 The external oblique fascia is opened in the direction of its fibers to expose the hernia sac and cord structures. The external inguinal ring is left intact, except when a large incarcerated hernia must be reduced.

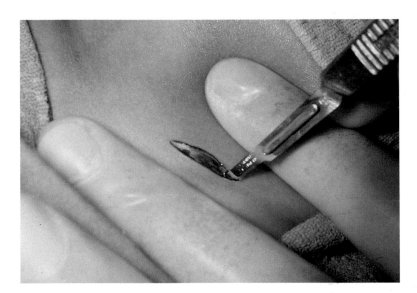

Figure 5.15 A transverse incision in the low abdominal skin crease, just lateral to the pubic tubercle, gives the best exposure of the internal inguinal ring and leaves the best cosmetic result.

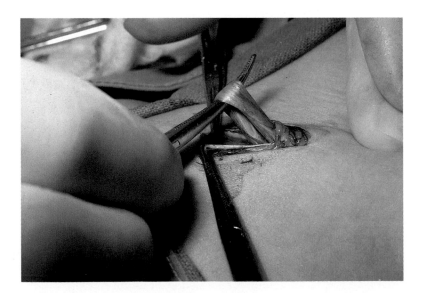

Figure 5.17 The cord structures and hernia sac are gently elevated together from the inguinal canal in this male patient.

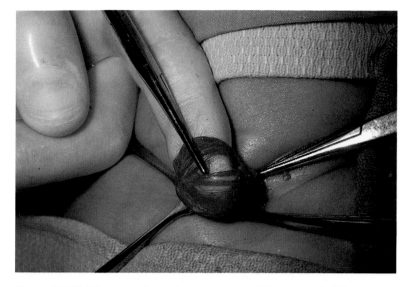

Figure 5.18 The vessels and vas are carefully separated from the hernia sac under direct vision. The vas and vessels are never clamped or pinched between forceps, but are teased from the sac.

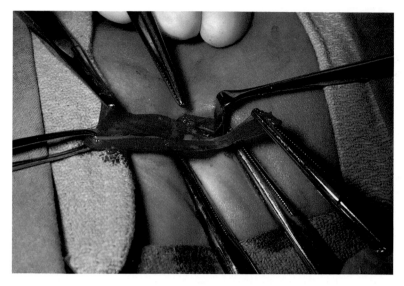

Figure 5.20 The vessels and vas are carefully separated from the sac to the level of the internal inguinal ring.

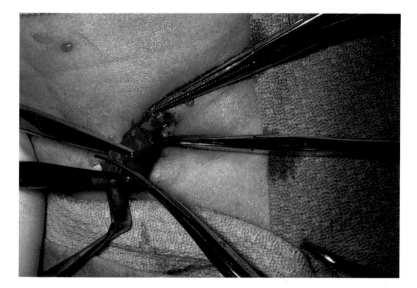

Figure 5.19 The sac is divided between hemostats. No attempt is made to excise the entire distal sac, which is emptied of fluid and left in place. There may be a transient accumulation of fluid, which is then absorbed spontaneously and causes no subsequent problem.

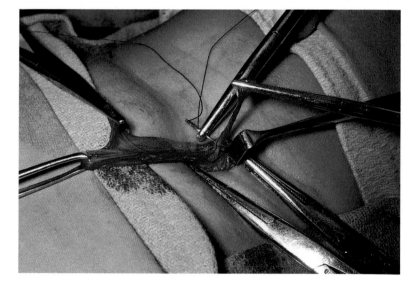

Figure 5.21 After palpation confirms the absence of a contained viscus, the proximal sac is twisted to consolidate it and is doubly suture-ligated. The silk suture shown here is no longer used and has been replaced by absorbable suture material.

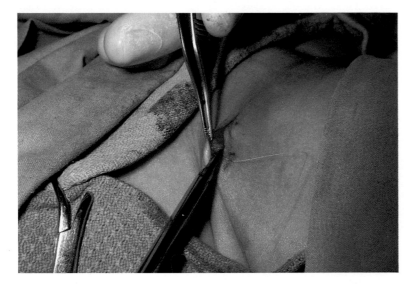

Figure 5.22 The cord structures are straightened in the inguinal canal; the external oblique fascia and Scarpa's fascia are approximated with simple sutures; and the skin is closed with interrupted, absorbable subcuticular sutures.

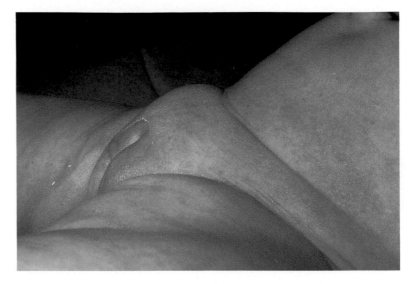

Figure 5.24 This 7-week-old girl has a visible inguinal bulge, representing a right inguinal hernia containing an ovary.

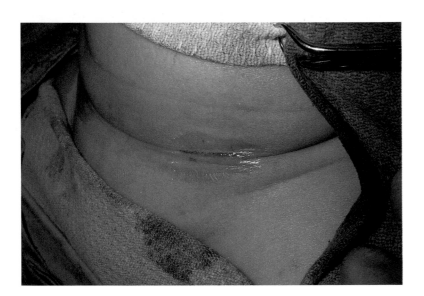

Figure 5.23 A simple layer of collodion dressing protects the incision and obviates dressing changes postoperatively.

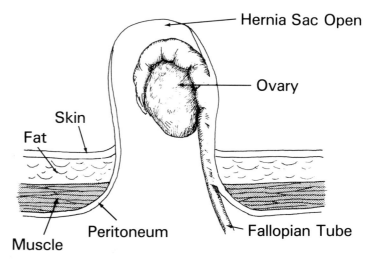

Figure 5.25 A sliding hernia containing fallopian tube and ovary is seen in cross-section.

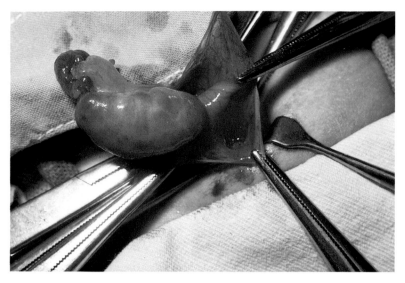

Figure 5.26 The opened sac reveals a sliding hernia containing the ovary and fimbriated end of the fallopian tube. The finding of a normal tube rules out the possibility of testicular feminization syndrome; no buccal smear or chromosome studies are indicated.

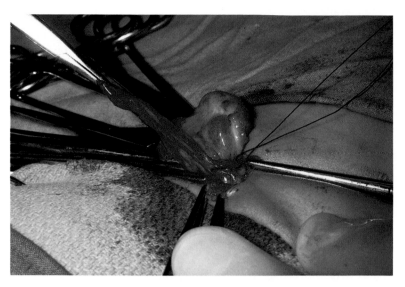

Figure 5.28 A pursestring suture is placed at the neck of the sac from the outside. Small superficial bites are used to avoid damage to the hernia contents. The author no longer uses silk suture material.

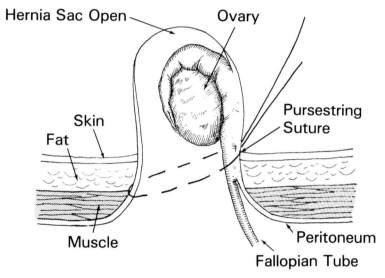

Figure 5.27 The level of placement of the pursestring suture just below the internal ring is illustrated.

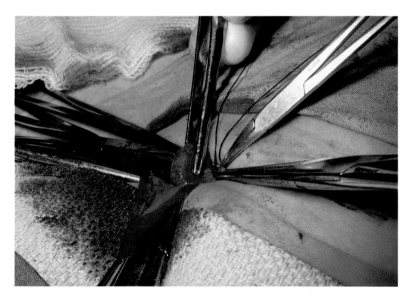

Figure 5.29 The ovary is then reduced as the hernia sac is inverted into the abdomen.

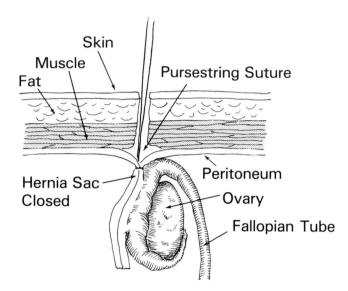

Figure 5.30 This diagram of the repair shows the tube and ovary reduced into the abdomen and the hernia sac closed with the pursestring suture.

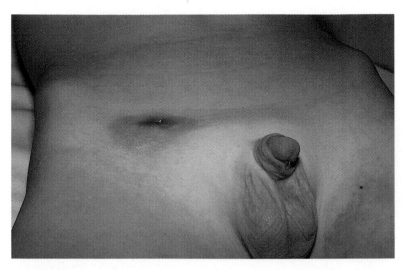

Figure 5.31 In this 5-year-old, erythema, swelling, and mild tenderness are found at the site of a right inguinal herniorrhaphy performed 2½ years previously.

The author has specifically stopped using nonabsorbable suture material (silk) for the closure of the inguinal hernia sac and external oblique fascia, as depicted in Figs 5.21 and 5.28. He has operated on five children with deep silk suture granulomas that appeared from 1½–7 years after herniorrhaphy (Figs 5.31, 5.32). In addition, polyglycolic acid sutures are no longer used for the subcuticular skin closure because of occasional reactions to the chemical breakdown products of that suture material 3–8 weeks after complete incisional healing; 4-0 or 5-0 plain gut has been used for the subcuticular closure since the mid-1980s, with no postoperative suture reactions.

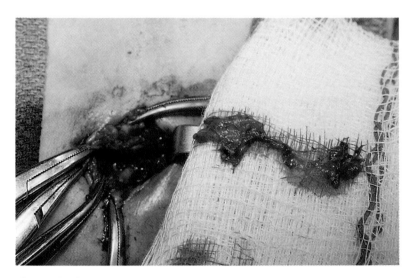

Figure 5.32 At surgery, a large granuloma extends to the internal inguinal ring, where a black silk suture remnant is found, seen in the center of the photograph.

Femoral Hernia

Femoral hernias are unusual in childhood. They are frequently missed or are mistaken for inguinal hernias. As in the adult, they occur more often in females. The hernia bulge presents *inferior* to the inguinal ligament and never extends into the scrotum or labium (Fig 5.33). Isolation and ligation of the sac and a Cooper's ligament fascial repair are performed through a low inguinal incision (Figs 5.34, 5.35).

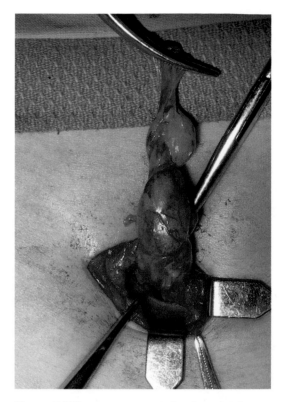

Figure 5.34 Dissection of the femoral hernia is shown. The sac and its contents (omentum) are reduced through the femoral hernia defect.

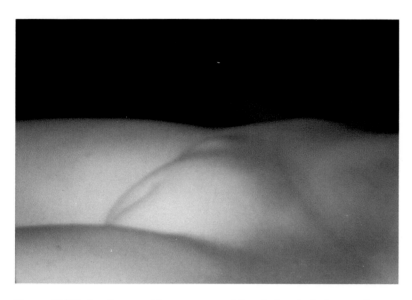

Figure 5.33 An 8-year-old presents with a bulge inferior to the inguinal ligament. Compare the appearance with that of Figure 5.24.

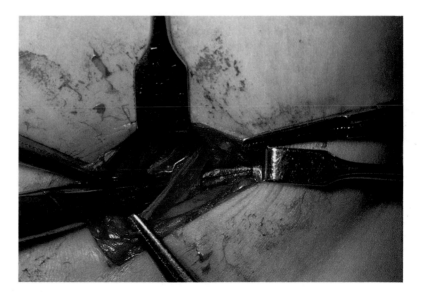

Figure 5.35 A hemostat clearly demonstrates the femoral defect. It is closed with nonabsorbable sutures from the anterior edge of the fascial defect to Cooper's ligament.

Umbilical Hernia

Although more numerous at birth than inguinal hernias, umbilical hernias have a high rate of spontaneous closure and, therefore, less commonly require surgical repair. They result from a defect in the fascia at the umbilical ring. Two thirds close by 1 year of age. Fascial defects less than 1.0 cm in diameter generally close by the age of 3 years and almost always by the age of 5 years (Fig 5.36). Fascial defects more than 2.0 cm in size (Fig 5.37)

rarely close spontaneously and may be repaired electively at any time, preferably between the ages of 2 and 5 years. Rarely, a hernia has so large a protrusion that repair is indicated because of size alone (Figs 5.38, 5.39). Any umbilical hernia in a child older than 6 years old should be repaired. Although incarceration is unusual in childhood, the likelihood of this complication increases with age. Incarceration of an umbilical hernia at any age is a clear indication for surgical repair.

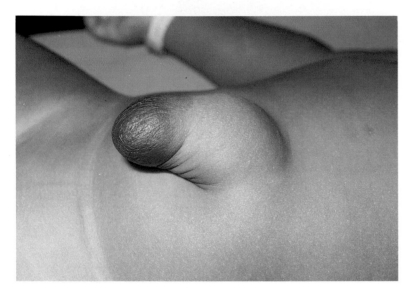

Figure 5.36 The ''proboscis'' seen here is a long umbilical hernia in a 14-month-old girl. The diameter of the abdominal wall defect is only 1.5 cm, allowing the possibility of spontaneous closure.

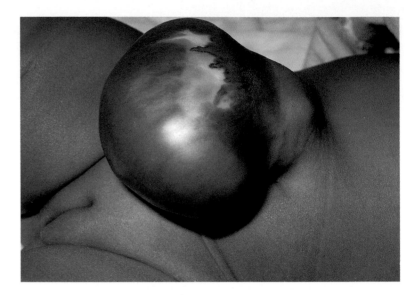

Figure 5.38 This ''giant'' umbilical hernia measures 10 cm across, with an abdominal wall opening of 2.5 cm. Surgery is performed at the age of 7 months because of erosion of the umbilical skin by the diaper.

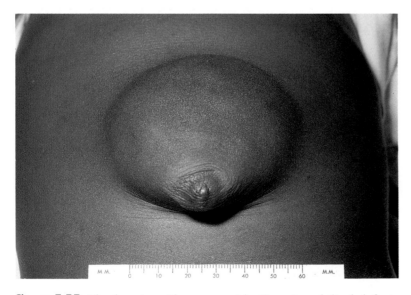

Figure 5.37 The hernia with a very wide (3 cm) umbilical defect is repaired, as there is no expectation of spontaneous closure.

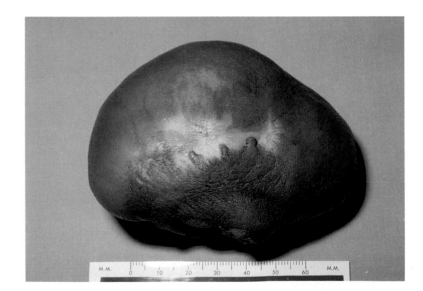

Figure 5.39 The skin and sac of the ''giant'' hernia are excised. In umbilical hernia repairs in children, skin is rarely removed.

Umbilical herniorrhaphy consists of dissection and closure of the hernia sac and repair of the fascial defect (Figs 5.40–5.43). The author prefers vertical approximation of the medial edges of the anterior rectus fascia, restoring the linea alba, with simple nonabsorbable sutures. One of the fascial sutures is placed through the undersurface of the umbilical skin to tack it down and ensure flattening of the redundant skin (Fig 5.44). A pressure dressing obliterates dead space and minimizes subcutaneous edema and hematoma formation postoperatively. It is removed in 24 hours.

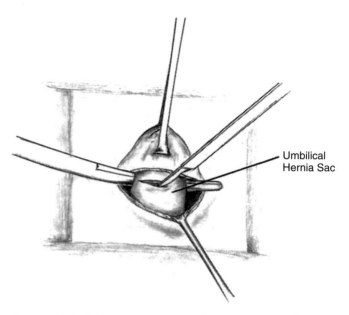

Figure 5.41 The sac is transected, leaving a small portion adherent to the umbilical skin; the residual sac causes no problem.

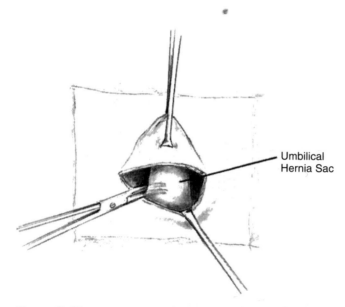

Figure 5.40 A transverse infraumbilical incision is made in the natural skin lines. The hernia sac is separated from the skin circumferentially by blunt scissor dissection.

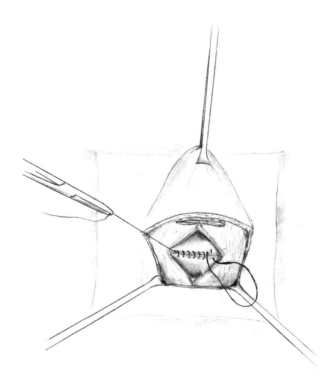

Figure 5.42 After the medial portions of rectus fascia are cleaned of subcutaneous tissue, the peritoneum is closed transversely with a running absorbable suture (chromic catgut). In large defects, the ends of the suture are tied together to consolidate the sac in the midline, which facilitates vertical fascial closure.

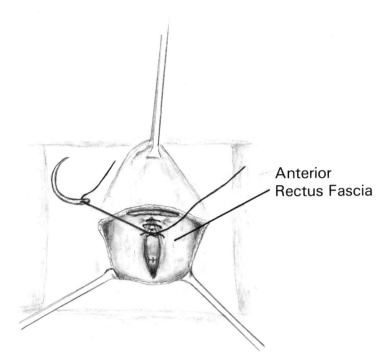

Anterior
Rectus Fascia

Figure 5.43 Vertical closure of the rectus fascia in the midline is performed with interrupted sutures of nonabsorbable material, with buried knots.

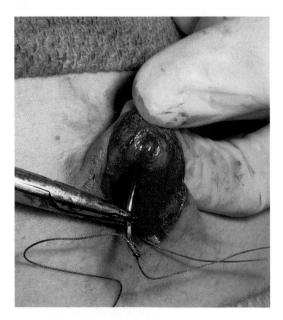

Figure 5.44 A central fascial suture is used to tack down the loose umbilical skin. Collodion seals the incision, and a pressure dressing minimizes swelling during the first day after surgery.

Lumbar Hernia

Lumbar hernia is rare in children, usually presenting in the neonate as a bulge in the flank. The defect in the triangle of Petit inferiorly or in the triangle of Grynfeltt superiorly is thought to result from a failure of development of the somite in the lumbar area. Associated with other somatic defects, such as rib and vertebral anomalies, congenital lumbar hernias are frequently bilateral (Figs 5.45, 5.46). Repair is advised in infancy, when tissues can be mobilized more easily for careful fascial closure. Approximation of the external oblique muscle to the latissimus dorsi, or the two muscles to the iliac crest, forms the basis of the repair (Figs 5.47, 5.48). Rarely, prosthetic materials, such as Marlex or sheet Silastic, are required for closure.

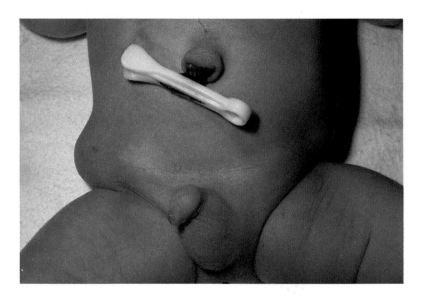

Figure 5.45 This infant boy is born with bilateral lumbar hernias.

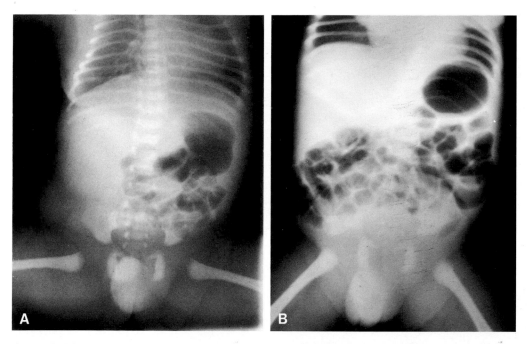

Figure 5.46 A. A radiograph at birth shows only the soft-tissue bulge at the right flank. **B.** Two days later, air-filled intestine protrudes into the hernia.

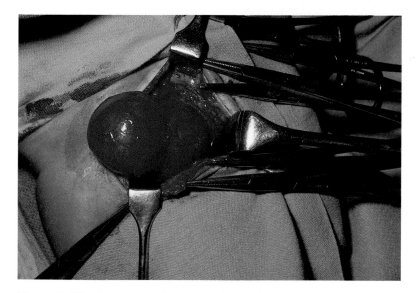

Figure 5.47 The hernia defect on the right is dissected.

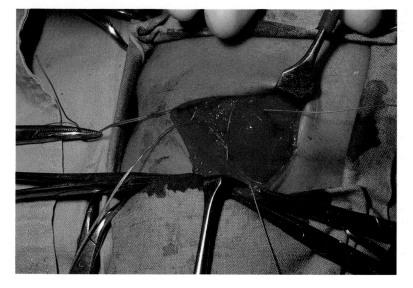

Figure 5.48 Repair of the defect is performed with local musculofascial approximation. The internal and external oblique fasciae and latissimus dorsi are sutured to the fascia and periosteum overlying the iliac crest.

Epigastric Hernia

A small fascial defect in the midline of the upper abdomen, the epigastric hernia presents as a visible or palpable mass of protruding properitoneal fat (Fig 5.49). It is symptomatic, with pain and tenderness, when a wad of fat incarcerates. Most epigastric hernias require repair; the defect rarely closes spontaneously. Because the fat contents may become reduced from the defect on induction of anesthesia, making localization difficult, it has been recommended that the skin over the hernia be marked just prior to surgery. Closure can be effected by simple fascial approximation with nonabsorbable sutures (Fig 5.50).

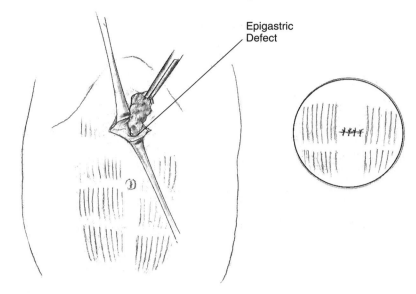

Figure 5.50 This drawing shows the epigastric fascial defect and the sutured closure.

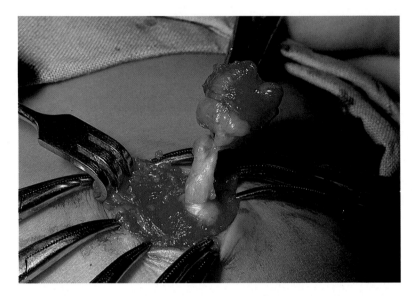

Figure 5.49 A symptomatic epigastric hernia in a 12-year-old boy is dissected. Properitoneal fat is seen protruding through the defect; the fat is excised, and the defect is closed with simple interrupted sutures.

Omphalocele and Gastroschisis

An omphalocele is a hernia into the umbilical cord (Fig 5.51). A small one may contain only fluid or a single loop of intestine (Fig 5.52). The thin sac of a large omphalocele may contain large and small bowel, stomach, liver, and spleen (Fig 5.53). Other anomalies are commonly associated with omphalocele; these include intestinal atresias, duplications, and enteric remnants (Figs 5.54–5.56), and cardiac, urinary (see Fig 10.28), skeletal, and chromosomal abnormalities. With the increasing use of maternal ultrasonography, the diagnosis is often made prenatally (Fig 5.57).

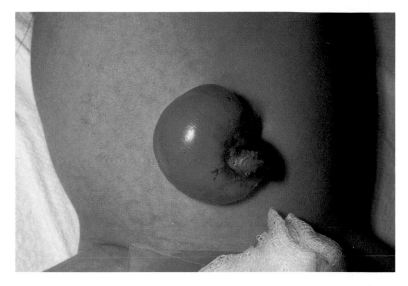

Figure 5.52 This tiny omphalocele contains only fluid and no viscus. It is the type of omphalocele that can be caught in an umbilical clamp or tie at delivery, with a leak of peritoneal fluid or evisceration of the intestine when the cord falls off.

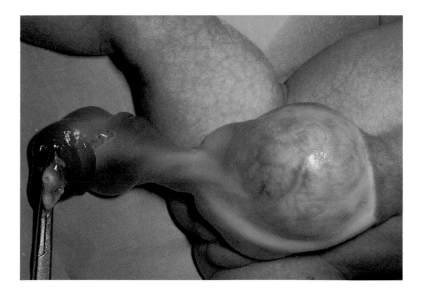

Figure 5.51 A moderate-sized omphalocele, with intestine herniating into the umbilical cord, is present in a newborn girl.

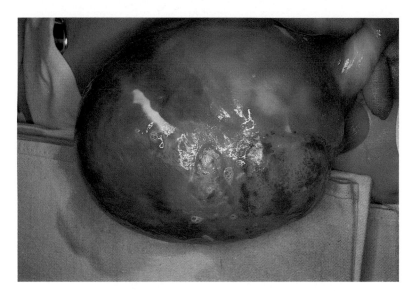

Figure 5.53 A large omphalocele contains most of the abdominal viscera. The liver and small intestine are clearly visible.

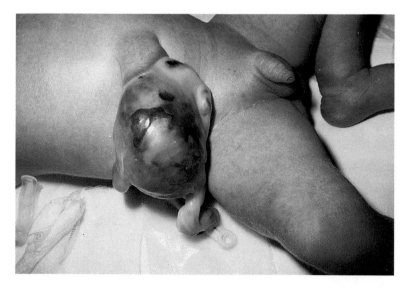

Figure 5.54 The moderate-sized omphalocele in this boy contains atretic ileum.

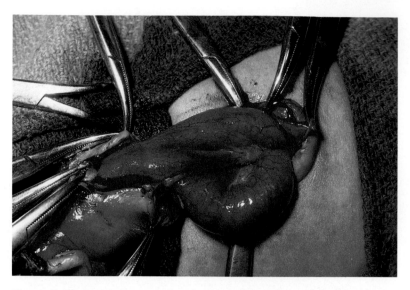

Figure 5.56 An omphalomesenteric duct remnant (Meckel's diverticulum) is adherent to the sac of this omphalocele.

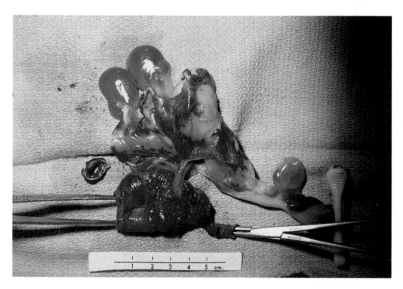

Figure 5.55 The atretic ileal segment is adherent to the wall of the omphalocele. A forceps is placed in the dilated proximal ileum, and a hemostat in the narrow distal end. The omphalocele is closed primarily after ileal resection and anastomosis.

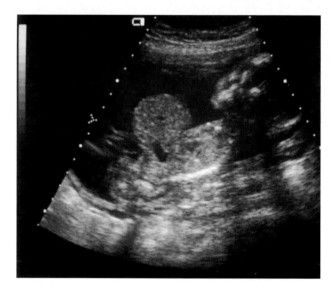

Figure 5.57 The maternal sonogram at 20 weeks' gestation shows a large omphalocele. At birth, the baby is found to have a cardiac defect as well.

Gastroschisis is the herniation of abdominal contents, usually intestine alone, through an extraumbilical defect in the abdominal wall. It does not have a sac. The intestine, when exposed to amniotic fluid before birth, has a thick edematous wall and lacks pliability (Fig 5.58); it may have a "peel" of adherent exudate. These factors make reduction and primary repair more difficult (Fig 5.59).

Initial therapy for newborns with omphalocele or gastroschisis is aimed at preventing infection, heat loss, fluid loss, and intestinal distention. With the baby in a temperature-controlled incubator, the omphalocele membrane—or the exposed intestine in gastroschisis—is covered with warm sterile saline dressings under an impermeable plastic wrap. A #8 or #10 Fr nasogastric tube is placed for continuous intestinal decompression, and an intravenous line is placed for administration of fluids, electrolytes, glucose, and antibiotics. These maneuvers are especially important if the infant must be transported to another hospital for definitive care.

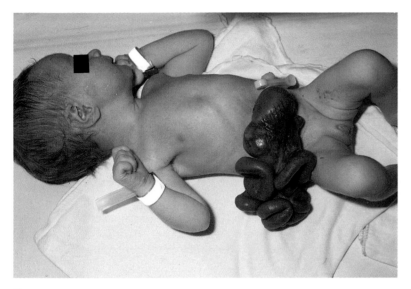

Figure 5.58 This newborn girl has a gastroschisis. The intestine protrudes from a defect in the abdominal wall to the right of the intact umbilical cord, and there is no covering membrane.

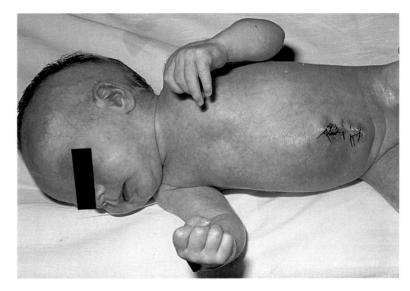

Figure 5.59 Despite the considerable amount of thick-walled edematous intestine and stomach that protrudes, they are completely reduced into the abdomen, and the defect is closed primarily.

Primary Repair

Primary repair may be attempted for all but the largest defects, if there is adequate space in the abdominal cavity (Fig 5.60) or if the abdominal wall can be stretched manually to accommodate the viscera. With too tight a closure, pressure of the reduced viscera elevates the diaphragms and obstructs caval venous return. The sac is excised (Fig 5.61), associated anomalies are corrected when possible, and the peritoneum and fascia are closed in layers. A subcuticular pursestring suture of absorbable material may be used to pucker the skin at the appropriate part of the incision to give the appearance of an umbilicus (Fig 5.62).

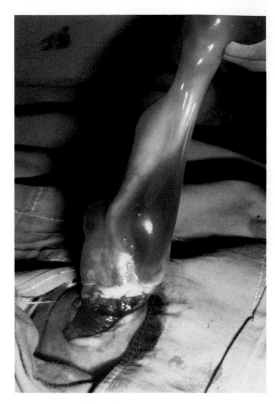

Figure 5.61 The cord and hernia sac are excised, with ligation of the vessels. In this case, there is a normal number of vessels, two arteries and one vein. A single umbilical artery is often associated with other congenital anomalies.

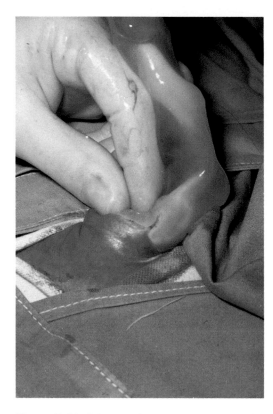

Figure 5.60 Primary Omphalocele Repair The contents of the omphalocele seen in Figure 5.51 are reduced manually in the operating room with the baby under general anesthesia.

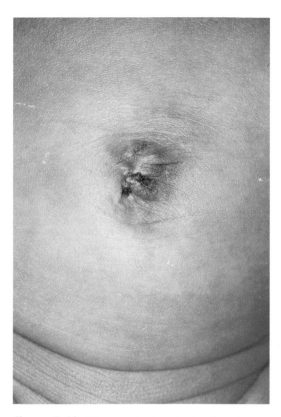

Figure 5.62 The omphalocele is closed primarily with interrupted sutures through the fascia and peritoneum. The skin is closed with an absorbable subcuticular pursestring suture to give a slight dimpling effect and to save the child from the stigma of lacking a "belly button."

"Silo" Repair

When the size of the defect or the disparity between visceral volume and abdominal cavity prevents primary closure (Fig 5.63), a sheet of Silastic is sewn to the peritoneal and fascial edges of the opening to create a pouch or "silo" (Fig 5.64). Dressings of antibacterial solution (silver nitrate or povidone-iodine) or cream (sulfadiazine silver) are applied regularly over the pouch to prevent infection. The pouch is then slowly reduced in size until it can be removed and primary fascial and skin closure can be achieved—usually within a week, but occasionally longer (Figs 5.65, 5.66). Central venous alimentation is advisable, because normal intestinal function may not return for 3–5 weeks, especially in babies with gastroschisis.

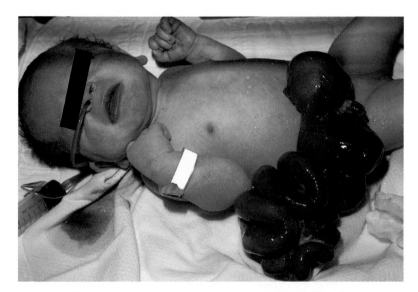

Figure 5.63 The intestine of this newborn girl cannot be reduced into the existing space of the small abdominal cavity without markedly displacing the diaphragms and severely compromising respiration. Note the #10 Fr nasogastric tube draining bile from the stomach.

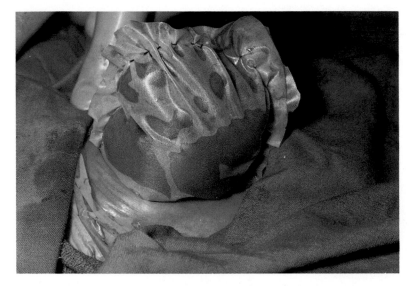

Figure 5.64 A sac is created from Silastic-impregnated fabric, which is sewn to the fascial edges of the defect. The sac is then closed over the protruding intestine.

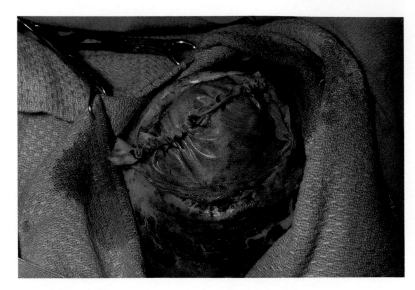

Figure 5.66 The omphalocele contents are completely reduced, in this case after 6 days, and the sac will be excised. Primary closure of the peritoneum and fascia in one layer, followed by approximation of the skin, completes the repair.

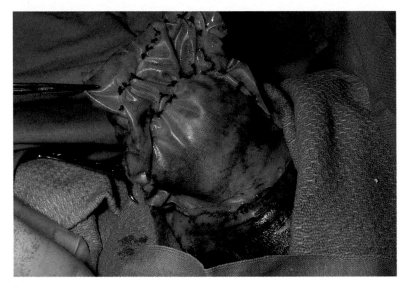

Figure 5.65 The Silastic sac is narrowed daily, forcing the contents into the abdomen, which slowly stretches to accommodate them. The antibacterial dressing is reapplied each time.

Patent Urachus

A remnant of the embryologic connection between the dome of the bladder and the umbilical cord, the patent urachus presents as a mucosa-lined opening in the umbilicus, discharging urine (Fig 5.67). The diagnosis is confirmed with a cystogram or sinogram, and resection of the tract to the bladder is advised (see Chapter 10). The remaining umbilical defect is closed primarily, as with a small omphalocele, and an umbilicoplasty is performed for normal appearance.

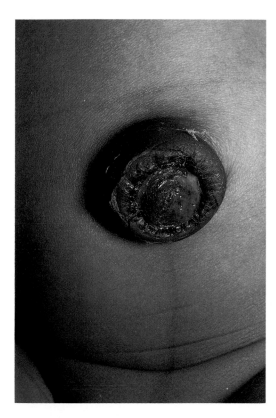

Figure 5.67 Urine has been seen coming from the pink opening in the center of the umbilicus of this 5-day-old boy.

Patent Omphalomesenteric Duct

The omphalomesenteric (vitelline) duct, an intestinal communication between the midileum and the umbilical stalk in the embryo, can fail to resorb before birth. If the entire duct remains, there is a congenital enterocutaneous fistula, lined with ileal mucosa. When the umbilical cord separates, intestinal contents may discharge from the umbilicus, and vigorous crying may even lead to prolapse of the limbs of the adjacent ileum (Figs 5.68, 5.69). Surgical repair consists of dissection of the omphalomesenteric duct (Fig 5.70), excision of the duct at the ileum—as for a Meckel's diverticulum (see Chapter 6)—and closure of the umbilical defect.

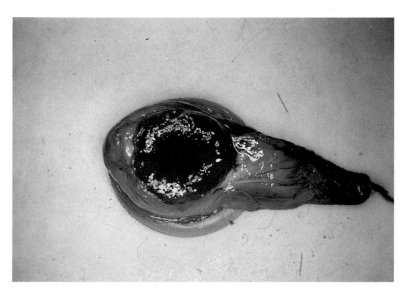

Figure 5.68 Following the sloughing of the cord in this 5-day-old, a mucosa-lined structure fills the umbilicus.

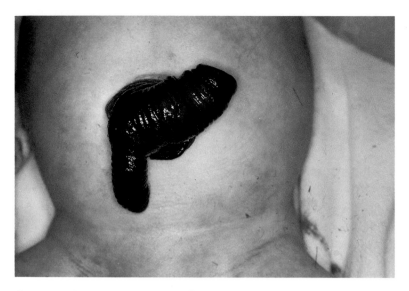

Figure 5.69 A vigorous cry produces a prolapse of proximal and distal ileum through this patent omphalomesenteric duct. The prolapsed intestine cannot be reduced, and immediate surgery is necessary.

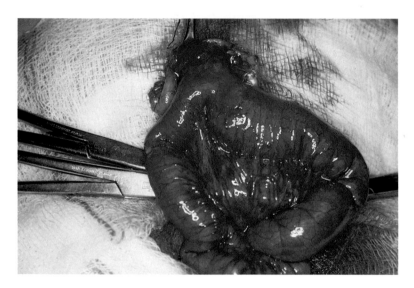

Figure 5.70 The two limbs of prolapsed ileum are reduced, and the opening of the duct is dissected from the umbilicus. The duct originates at the antimesenteric side of the midileum. It is excised.

Umbilicoenteric Remnant

A remnant of the urachal tract without bladder communication—or the omphalomesenteric duct without intestinal connection—may drain through the umbilicus. The tract is lined with bladder or intestinal mucosa and generally has a small amount of clear drainage; if it is infected, purulent material will drain. A contrast sinogram (Fig 5.71) may demonstrate the blind-ending tract. Surgical excision is advised (Fig 5.72).

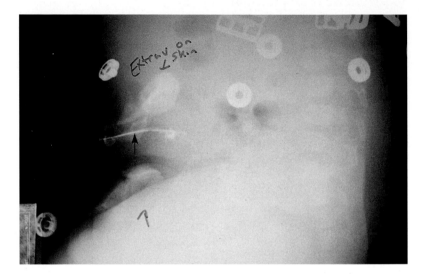

Figure 5.71 Water-soluble contrast material is injected into the tract that drains through this infant's umbilicus. No communication with an abdominal viscus is demonstrated.

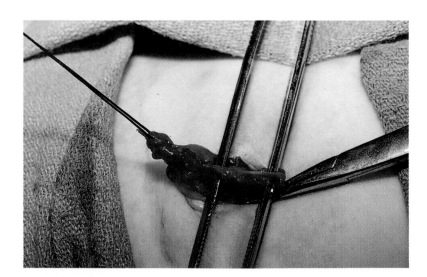

Figure 5.72 Exploration at the umbilicus reveals this tract, which ends blindly in the peritoneal cavity. The excised tract is lined with intestinal epithelium.

Absent Abdominal Musculature

Congenital absence of the abdominal musculature ("prune belly") occurs almost exclusively in males and is associated with a variety of genitourinary abnormalities. Examination of the neonate reveals the absence of musculature, especially in the lower abdomen; resultant wrinkling of the skin over minimal subcutaneous fat (Fig 5.73); undescended testes; and occasionally an associated patent urachus (Fig 5.74). Imaging studies are necessary to delineate the potential abnormalities of the kidneys, ureters, bladder, and urethra (see Figs 10.17–10.19), and care must be taken to avoid introduction of infection into the urinary tract. Surgical drainage or repair of the urinary tract abnormalities should be aimed at preservation of renal function. Randolph* has described reconstruction of the abdomen, with excision of the full thickness of the lower abdominal wall; excellent cosmetic and improved functional results are reported (Figs 5.75–5.81).

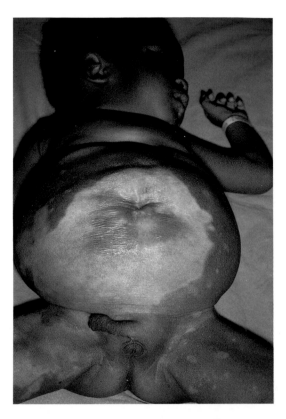

Figure 5.74 This 17-month-old boy has undescended testes and a patent urachus associated with absent abdominal musculature.

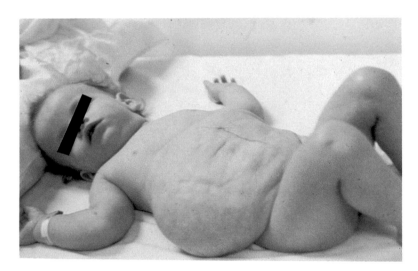

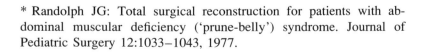

Figure 5.73 This infant demonstrates the lax abdominal musculature and wrinkled skin of the "prune-belly" syndrome.

---

* Randolph JG: Total surgical reconstruction for patients with abdominal muscular deficiency ('prune-belly') syndrome. Journal of Pediatric Surgery 12:1033–1043, 1977.

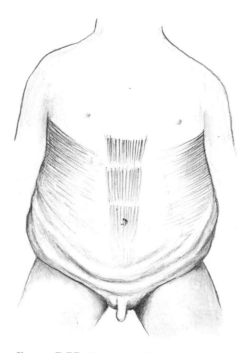

Figure 5.75 Absence of the lower abdominal musculature, typical of ''prune-belly'' syndrome, is illustrated graphically.

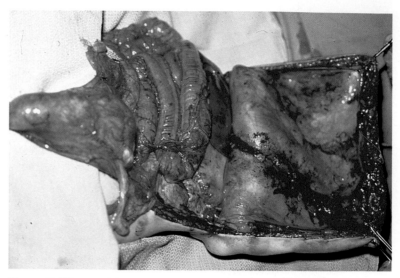

Figure 5.77 The U-shaped flap of abdominal wall is elevated to show its size and the extent of dissection. (Courtesy of Judson Randolph, M.D.)

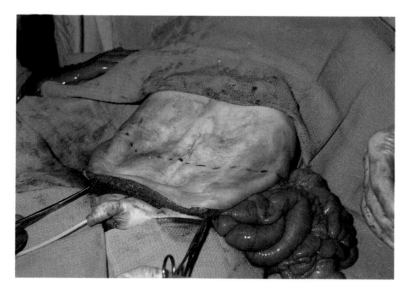

Figure 5.76 A large U-shaped incision is made from both flanks down to the suprapubic area and includes the full thickness of the anterior abdominal wall. Intestine is seen in the open peritoneal cavity. (Courtesy of Judson Randolph, M.D.)

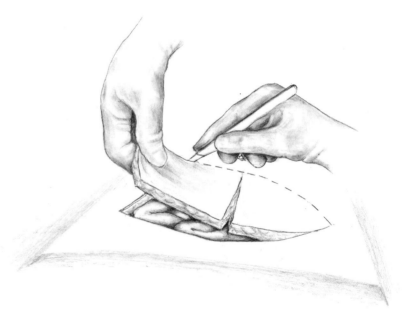

Figure 5.78 The technique for excision of a full-thickness segment of the lower portion of the abdominal flap is illustrated.

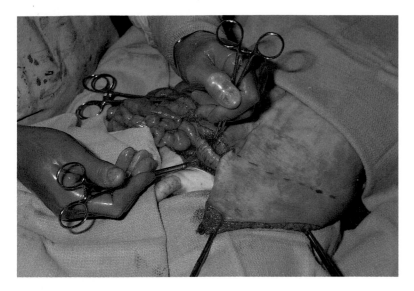

Figure 5.79 Half of the abdominal wall resection is completed. (Courtesy of Judson Randolph, M.D.)

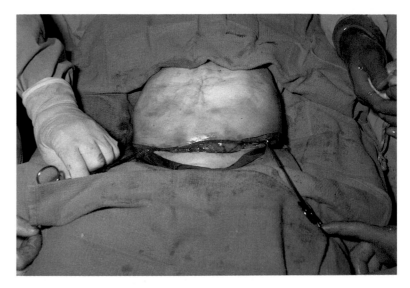

Figure 5.81 Traction on the fascia and peritoneum aids the final closure of the layers of the abdominal wall. (Courtesy of Judson Randolph, M.D.)

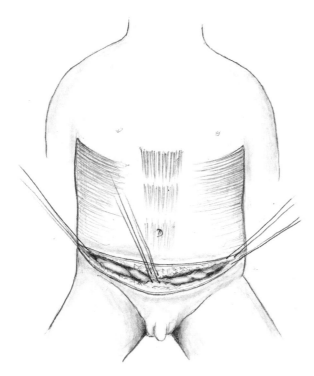

Figure 5.80 The final repair is illustrated.

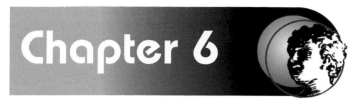

Chapter 6

Upper Gastrointestinal Tract

Congenital and acquired obstructions, inflammation, perforation, and ulceration are the major—and sometimes life-threatening—upper gastrointestinal problems of infants and children.

Pyloric Stenosis

One of the most common pediatric surgical problems, pyloric stenosis results from progressive thickening of the muscle at the gastric outlet during the first 2–6 weeks of life—it is not present at birth except in the rarest cases. Although the stimulus to hypertrophy of the muscle is not known, it has a definite genetic predisposition and occurs more frequently in boys.

Vomiting after feeding, with no loss of appetite, often progresses to projectile vomiting—the classic symptom of pyloric stenosis. Gastric peristalsis, when present, can be seen as a visible wave moving from the left upper to the right middle abdomen (Fig 6.1). Palpation of the rubbery,

oval, hypertrophied pyloric muscle ("olive") confirms the diagnosis. The thickened pylorus may lie behind the liver or in another location where it cannot be palpated. Sonography has become the first diagnostic imaging study used to detect a nonpalpable pyloric "olive" (Figs 6.2, 6.3). The accuracy of the study is dependent on the sonographer's experience (operator dependent) and the position of the pylorus; it is only 75%–80% reliable. Contrast radiographs are indicated only if the diagnosis cannot be confirmed by palpation or sonography or if other causes of partial gastric outlet obstruction are being

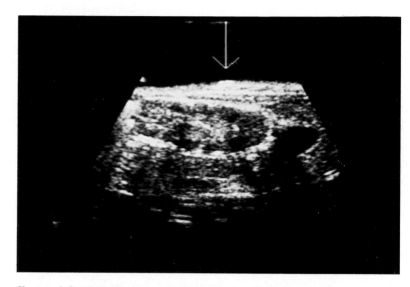

Figure 6.2 This ultrasound study shows thickening of the pyloric muscle and narrowing of the lumen.

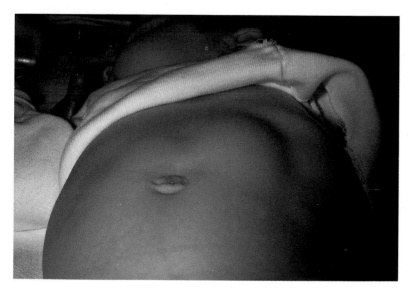

Figure 6.1 Pyloric Stenosis There are visible gastric waves (peristalsis) in a girl of 4 weeks. Although gastric waves are not seen in every infant with pyloric stenosis, when present they are indicative of partial gastric-outlet obstruction.

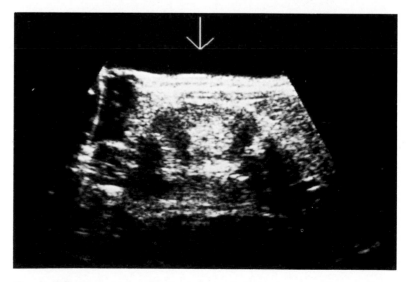

Figure 6.3 The same infant's pylorus is seen in ultrasonographic cross-section.

considered (Figs 6.4, 6.5). The differential diagnosis of nonbilious vomiting in the infant includes overfeeding, gastroesophageal reflux, and gastric antral web; other causes, such as sepsis and metabolic derangements, generally produce a sick infant without appetite.

For an examiner to be successful in palpating the pyloric "olive," both the examiner and the baby must be relaxed. Sitting allows the examiner to relax; a nipple in the baby's mouth and rolled towel under the baby's thighs relax the abdominal muscles to permit palpation. Gentle palpation in the right epigastrium, deep to the border of the right rectus muscle, identifies the firm pylorus in most cases. The pyloric mass is most prominent when the baby's stomach is full or immediately after the baby vomits.

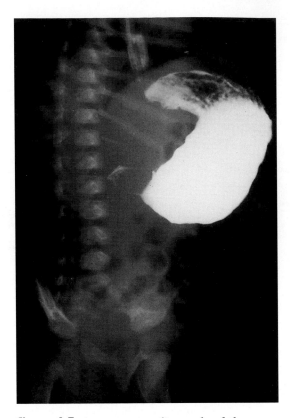

Figure 6.5 A contrast radiograph of the same infant clearly shows a narrow pyloric channel ("string sign") and widening at the duodenal cap. One can also see the negative shadow of the thick pyloric muscle at the outlet of the distended stomach.

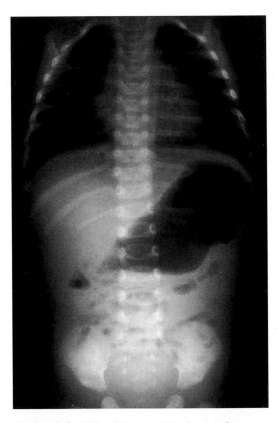

Figure 6.4 This abdominal radiograph shows air distending the stomach, with visible narrowing at the pylorus and a paucity of air in the distal intestine. The problem is not usually seen so easily without contrast material in the stomach.

The infant with prolonged vomiting of gastric contents may develop metabolic alkalosis, dehydration, and weight loss. The electrolyte and fluid abnormalities must be corrected prior to surgery (see Chapter 1 under ''Fluids and Electrolytes''). Feeding after pyloromyotomy will correct the nutritional deficit. Jaundice, seen in a small number of infants with pyloric stenosis and thought to be caused by bile stasis, also resolves after surgery.

The technique for pyloromyotomy is illustrated in detail (Figs 6.6–6.16). Within 8–12 hours of surgery, the baby may start a slowly progressive feeding regimen, from glucose water to dilute, and then full-strength, formula or breast milk. Vomiting of some feedings during the first postoperative day or two is common and should not be cause for concern. Following an adequate pyloromyotomy, vomiting eventually stops, and most infants may be discharged within 3 days after surgery. Once corrected, pyloric stenosis does not recur. In time, the muscle reverts to normal thickness, and the myotomy closes, leaving a normal-appearing and functioning pylorus. There is no known predisposition to future gastric problems.

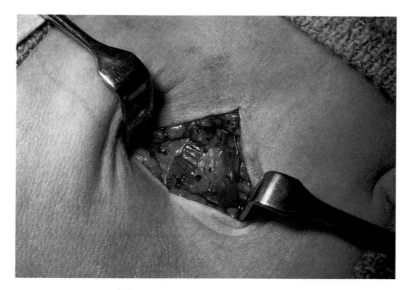

Figure 6.7 The transverse skin incision is deepened to the anterior rectus fascia, which is incised transversely.

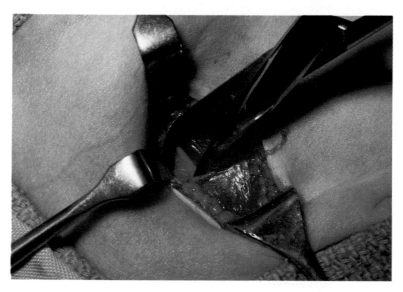

Figure 6.8 The rectus muscle is split longitudinally, in the direction of its fibers, to the level of the posterior fascia and peritoneum.

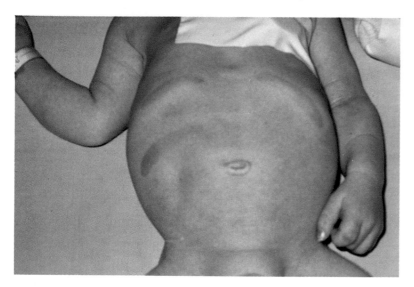

Figure 6.6 Pyloromyotomy The yellow lines painted on this infant's abdomen represent the following: both costal margins superiorly, the liver edge inferiorly, and the incision line over the right rectus muscle—one third of the distance from the xiphoid to the umbilicus.

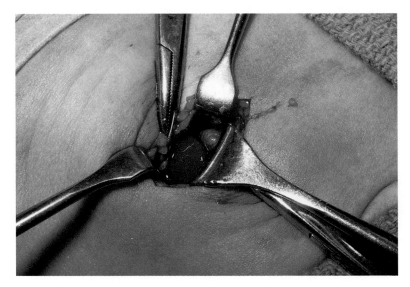

Figure 6.9 The transverse peritoneal incision reveals the liver edge and transverse colon; the liver will buttress the peritoneal closure and help prevent intestinal adhesion to it.

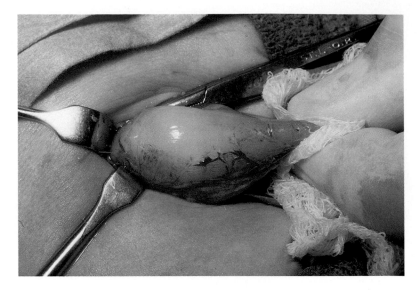

Figure 6.11 The pylorus is delivered by gentle traction on the stomach; a rocking or rotary motion of the surgeon's right hand is used.

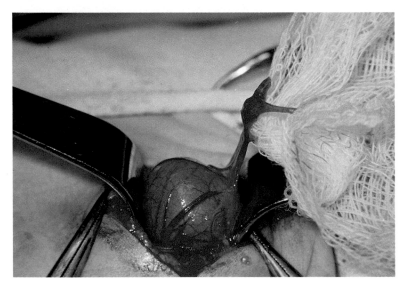

Figure 6.10 A moist gauze withdraws the omentum and transverse colon from the abdomen. Further traction on the colon will deliver the stomach.

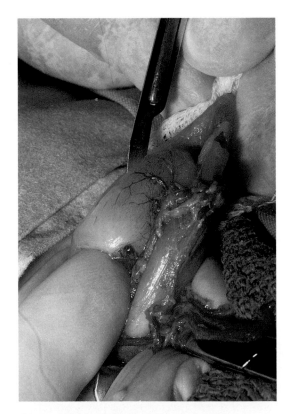

Figure 6.12 With the surgeon's index finger on the distal end of the pylorus to protect the thin-walled duodenum, a longitudinal incision is made along the least vascular portion of pyloric muscle and is extended proximally onto the antrum.

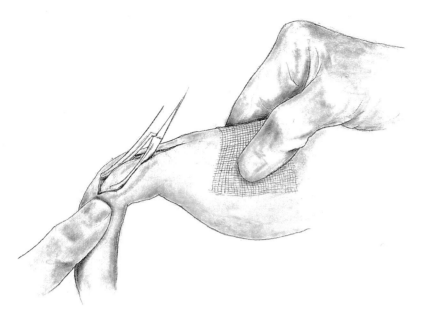

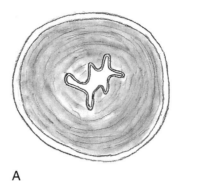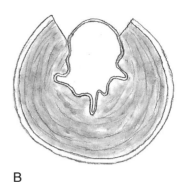

A   B

Figure 6.15 The cross-sectional view of the pylorus in pyloric stenosis is shown (**A**) before myotomy, with the hypertrophied thick muscle compressing the mucosa and narrowing the lumen, and (**B**) after myotomy, with release of some of the luminal compression.

Figure 6.13 This drawing shows the technique for spreading of the pyloric muscle. Traction on the antrum of the stomach keeps the pylorus prominent, as the surgeon gently spreads the incision to the depth of the muscularis mucosae.

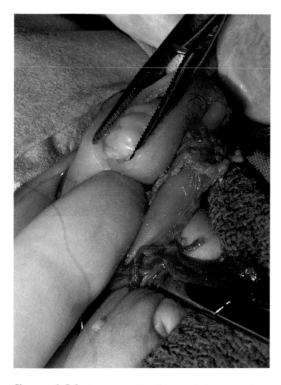

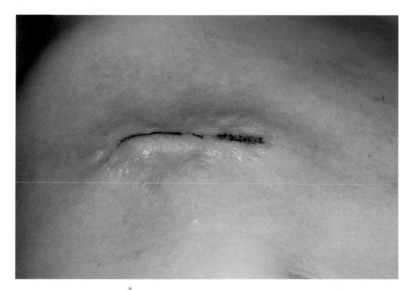

Figure 6.16 The incision is closed in layers. The subcuticular skin closure and transparent, waterproof collodion dressing require no special care. The result is a thin scar, which eventually lies at the costal margin of the fully grown child.

Figure 6.14 A mosquito hemostat spreads the muscle to the underlying muscularis mucosae for the length of the incision. Before the stomach is replaced in the abdomen, it is compressed to ensure that there is no mucosal leak. If a leak is discovered, a two-layer closure of mucosa and muscle is performed, and a pyloromyotomy is done on the opposite side.

Neonatal Gastric Perforation

During the first 5 days of life, an infant who has experienced some neonatal stress may suddenly develop massive abdominal distention (Fig 6.17). Spontaneous gastric perforation is the presumptive diagnosis when an abdominal radiograph shows a large pneumoperitoneum (Fig 6.18). At the time of emergency laparotomy, the surgeon will find a ragged-edged defect of variable size in the gastric wall; it almost always involves the greater curvature (Fig 6.19). Surgical closure, in two layers, follows freshening or debridement of any necrotic edges (Fig 6.20). Gastrostomy decompression is advised. The etiology of spontaneous gastric perforation is not clear; local ischemia and gastric overdistention have been suggested as possibilities.

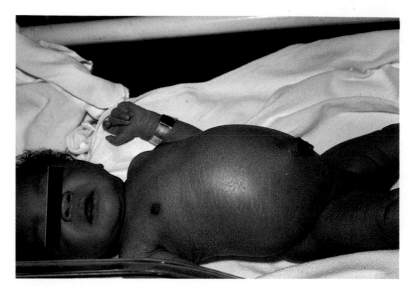

Figure 6.17 This 3-day-old girl had been taking formula for a day when she began vomiting and developed sudden, massive abdominal distention.

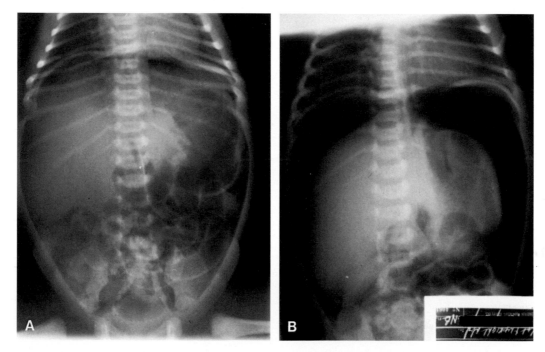

Figure 6.18 A. A radiograph of the abdomen, with the baby supine, shows elevation of the diaphragms and air outlining the liver. **B.** With the baby erect, a massive pneumoperitoneum is seen.

Gastroesophageal Reflux

The differential diagnosis of vomiting in infancy includes gastroesophageal reflux. It can present as projectile vomiting, mimicking pyloric stenosis. Certain apneic episodes and "near-miss" sudden infant death syndrome (SIDS) have been postulated to result from laryngospasm following acid regurgitation. Chronic pulmonary infection may occur from repeated episodes of vomiting and aspiration. Inadequate nutrition and "failure to thrive" can be the consequence of repeated vomiting of feedings. Chronic reflux may result in esophagitis and esophageal stricture. Brain-damaged children have a high incidence of gastroesophageal reflux.

Confirming the diagnosis is often difficult. Barium swallow with fluoroscopy is not always confirmatory, even when performed by the most experienced radiologist. Esophagoscopy will show only the presence or absence of esophagitis or stricture. Radioactive scintiscan ("milk scan") may miss the reflux episodes. The most reliable diagnostic method is reported to be 24-hour pH monitoring with a fine probe in the esophagus. In case of potentially serious respiratory symptoms or malnutrition, therapy is mandatory even in the absence of confirmatory studies.

Initial conservative management consists of giving thickened feedings and maintaining upright position after feedings; some studies suggest that the prone position, with the baby's head elevated, is best for minimizing reflux. Metoclopramide (Reglan) has been administered to relax the pylorus and stimulate gastric emptying. Failure of medical therapy or persistence of serious symptoms, such as apnea, failure to thrive, or recurrent pulmonary infection, requires antireflux surgery. Intensive pulmonary therapy to clear secretions and infection may be necessary prior to any surgery.

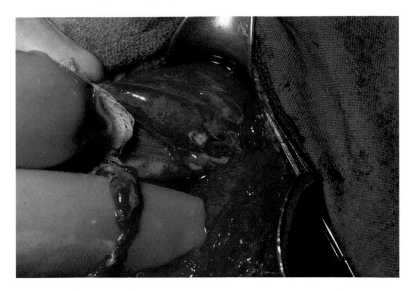

Figure 6.19 At abdominal exploration, air is decompressed from the abdomen and curds of formula are found in the peritoneal cavity. The ragged edges of the perforation in the greater curvature of the stomach are seen, as is the red rubber nasogastric catheter in the gastric lumen.

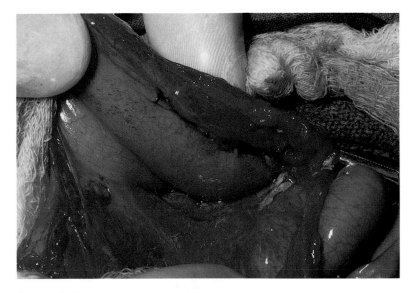

Figure 6.20 Suture closure of the gastric perforation and placement of a gastrostomy tube complete the emergency operation.

The author prefers the Nissen fundoplication as an antireflux procedure (Figs 6.21–6.24). A large-bore esophageal tube (#24 Fr in the infant and #28–32 Fr in the older child) is kept in place during the procedure to prevent too tight a plication ("wrap"), which could result in inability to expel gastric contents or air ("gas bloat"). Some surgeons advocate a Thal procedure, or "partial" plication, to avoid this problem. Brain-damaged children —especially those with muscle spasticity or seizures— commonly develop recurrent reflux at some time after surgery, despite the routine placement of a gastrostomy for decompression and for feeding.

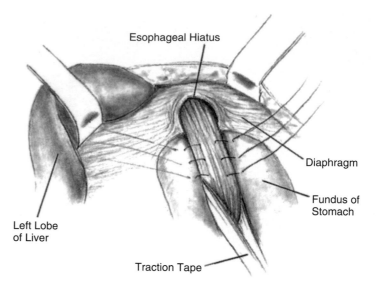

Figure 6.22 Sutures are placed from the seromuscular fundus anteriorly to the esophageal muscularis and then through the fundus posteriorly.

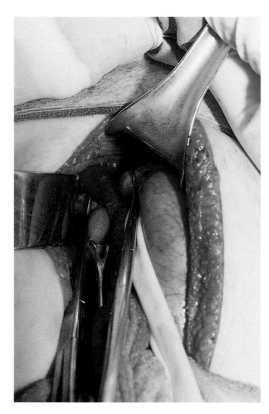

Figure 6.21 Technique for Nissen Fundoplication The left hepatic ligament is divided to allow exposure of the esophageal hiatus. A tape or rubber drain, for caudad traction, is placed around the gastroesophageal junction—care being taken to avoid vagus nerve damage—and the superior short gastric vessels to the spleen are divided. The esophageal hiatus is closed with sutures. As shown in this operative photograph, the fundus is grasped with Babcock clamps and is brought posteriorly and medially around the lower esophagus.

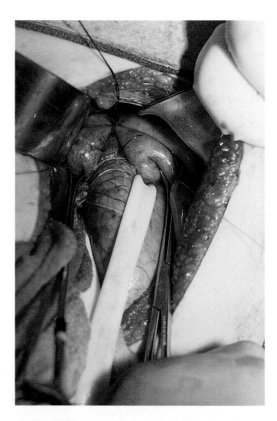

Figure 6.23 Placement of the sutures is seen at fundoplication for this 3½-year-old with multiple congenital anomalies. The superior suture has been tied.

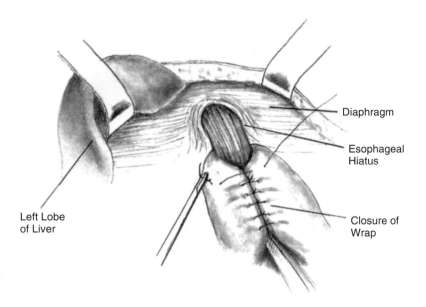

Figure 6.24 The sutures are tied to complete the fundoplication. Although multiple sutures are shown in this drawing, the author now rarely uses more than three.

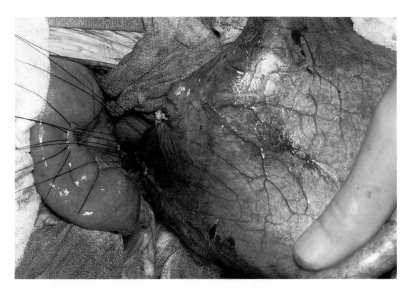

Figure 6.25 Surgery in this boy with Zollinger-Ellison syndrome consisted of total gastrectomy and esophagojejunostomy. The operative photograph shows the jejunum being sutured to the distal esophagus before complete division of the proximal stomach.

Peptic Ulceration

Acute gastric ulceration and bleeding may occur following stress in the neonate. Like spontaneous perforation, ulcerations are more common along the greater curvature. Such ulcers frequently respond to conservative management by gastric decompression, irrigation, and intravascular volume replacement. Persistent massive bleeding is rare; when it occurs, it requires laparotomy, gastrotomy, and direct suture ligation of the ulcers.

Other causes of acute ulceration in childhood include burns, shock, head or spinal cord injury, and caustic ingestion. Chronic gastric ulceration in the older child and teenager is less common than the same disease in adults; the symptoms, diagnostic findings, and response to therapy are similar.

Zollinger-Ellison syndrome, with measurable gastrin elevation and gastric hypersecretion, is associated with a secreting pancreatic tumor (gastrinoma), frequently with liver involvement (see Chapter 9). It is an unusual disease in the pediatric age group. In patients who do not respond to therapy with hydrogen ion–blocking agents (cimetidine), total gastrectomy is the therapy (Figs 6.25, 6.26); esophageal anastomosis to a jejunal pouch gives the best reported results.

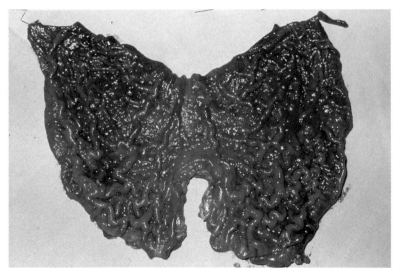

Figure 6.26 The gastrectomy specimen shows marked hyperemia and prominent folds of hypertrophied mucosa.

Intestinal Atresia, Stenosis, and Web

The most common form of congenital intestinal obstruction is atresia—a complete luminal discontinuity (Fig 6.27). Stenosis and perforate intraluminal web are forms of partial intestinal obstruction (Fig 6.28). Half of all atresias are ileal, and one fourth are duodenal, although any portion of the intestinal tract may be involved. Most duodenal obstructions are thought to result from a failure of complete canalization of the solid cord of embryonic cells that forms the intestine; atresia or stenosis of the second portion of the duodenum may be associated with annular pancreas. Distal to the ligament of Treitz, atresia is thought to be the result of a localized vascular compromise, as from a volvulus of the intestine.

Persistent vomiting is the primary symptom of all intestinal obstruction; the vomitus is bile-stained when the obstruction is distal to the ampulla of Vater. Abdominal distention is typical of obstructions beyond the mid-jejunum (Fig 6.29). A normal abdominal contour or a scaphoid abdomen is found in infants with ''high'' obstruction, in the duodenum or proximal jejunum (Fig 6.30).

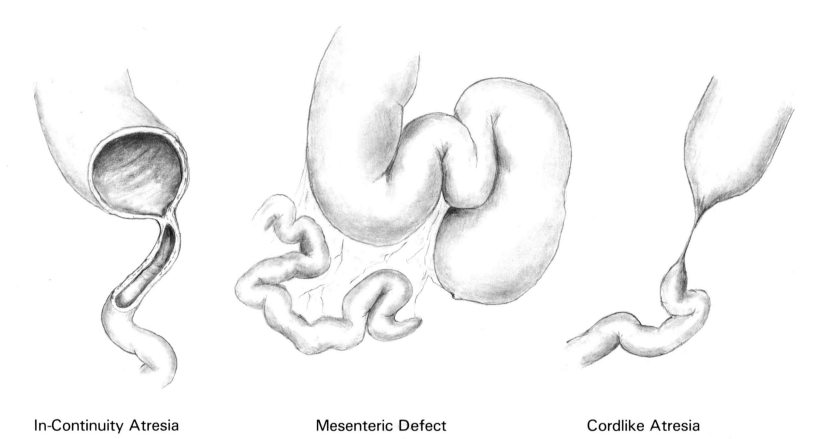

In-Continuity Atresia   Mesenteric Defect   Cordlike Atresia

Figure 6.27 Intestinal Atresia The types of intestinal atresia are illustrated: in-continuity, separated, and cordlike.

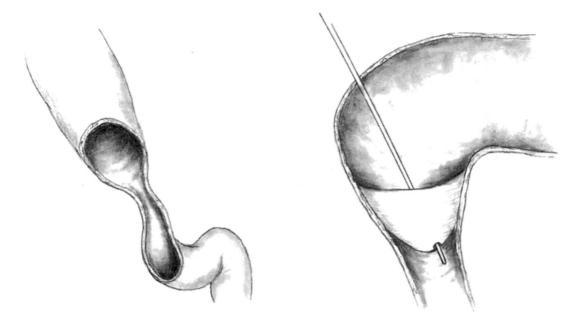

Figure 6.28 Intestinal Stenosis and Web Segmental narrowing or intraluminal membranous perforate webs may exist anywhere in the intestine as partial obstructions.

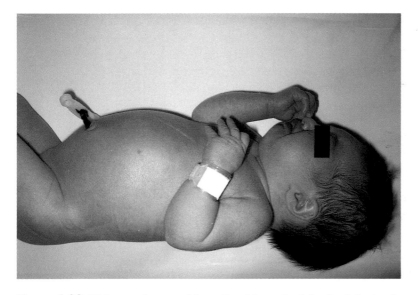

Figure 6.29 This newborn with a distal intestinal (colonic) atresia has a markedly distended abdomen.

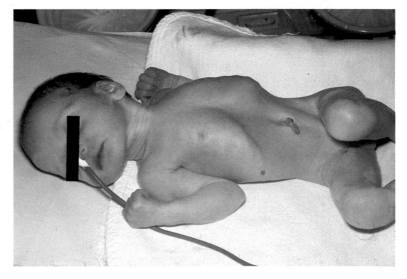

Figure 6.30 An unusually concave abdomen is seen in a 10-day-old girl with high (duodenal) atresia and bilious vomiting. The diagnosis was delayed because of absence of abdominal distention.

Radiographs of the abdomen will show distention of the bowel proximal to the obstruction. Air fills only the stomach and duodenum in duodenal atresia—the classic "double bubble" sign (Fig 6.31). In general, the greater the number of dilated bowel loops, the more distal is the obstruction (Figs 6.32, 6.33). Air, swallowed by the infant or injected through a nasogastric tube, is the safest initial "constrast material" to help in the radiographic diagnosis of neonatal intestinal obstruction. Instillation of barium or water-soluble contrast medium into the stomach is required only for the delineation of a partial upper gastrointestinal obstruction (see later). A contrast enema, indicated in lower obstructions, shows a narrow "unused" colon in most babies with complete congenital intestinal obstruction (Fig 6.34).

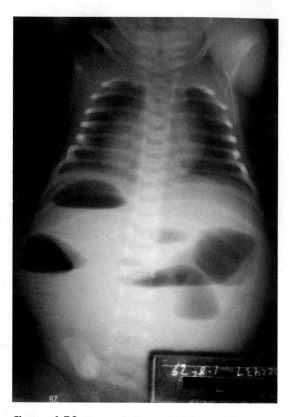

Figure 6.32 Several distended bowel loops, with no air distally, are seen in the abdominal radiograph of a newborn with jejunal atresia.

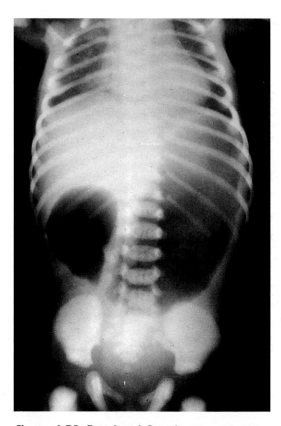

Figure 6.31 Duodenal Atresia The "double bubble" sign of air-distended stomach and duodenum is pathognomonic of duodenal atresia. There is no air visible distal to the duodenum.

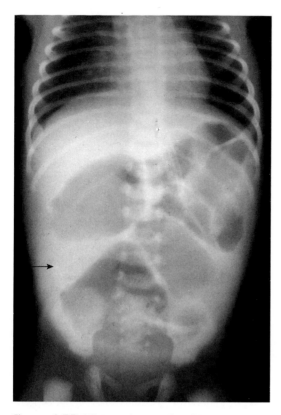

Figure 6.33 This radiograph of a 2-day-old girl shows multiple air-filled segments of intestine characteristic of distal atresia. In addition, a calcified circle of necrotic bowel *(arrow)* is seen at the site of the ileal atresia—the result of an intrauterine volvulus.

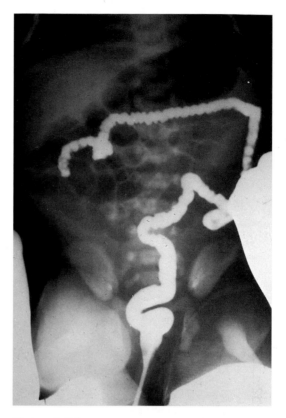

Figure 6.34 The narrow unused colon demonstrated on this contrast enema is associated with a meconium ileus, although it would have the same appearance with any complete congenital obstruction. There is no intrinsic abnormality of the colon, and it will distend to normal caliber once the obstruction is relieved.

Congenital Duodenal Obstruction

Vomiting occurs in the first few days of life in infants with duodenal atresia, and somewhat later in those with partially obstructing stenosis or web. A partial obstruction may not become evident in some infants until they begin taking solid foods. One third of babies with duodenal obstruction at birth have Down syndrome.

Radiographic studies confirm the diagnosis (Figs 6.31, 6.35). Following nasogastric decompression and fluid and electrolyte replacement through an adequate intravenous line, surgical correction is undertaken. The choice of pro-

cedure depends on the anatomy of the defect. Primary duodenoduodenostomy is possible for atresia of contiguous segments, especially when the dilated proximal duodenum overlaps the distal segment (Figs 6.36, 6.37). Duodenojejunostomy is preferable when the duodenal segments are separated, in the presence of annular pancreas (Figs 6.38–6.40), or for duodenal stenosis (Fig 6.41), which is rarely amenable to direct duodenoplasty. Gastrostomy is performed for decompression following repairs of all congenital duodenal obstructions, because they frequently take longer to "open up" than more distal anastomoses.

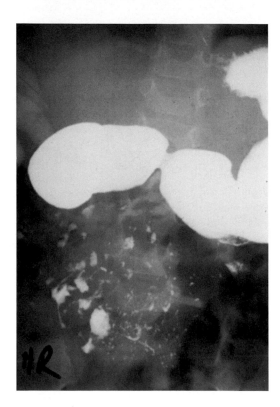

Figure 6.35 Duodenal Web Instillation of barium into the stomach and duodenum delineates the exact nature of this partial duodenal obstruction. The duodenum is dilated proximal to the obstruction, and only a few flecks of barium can be seen distal to the perforate web in an infant with Down syndrome.

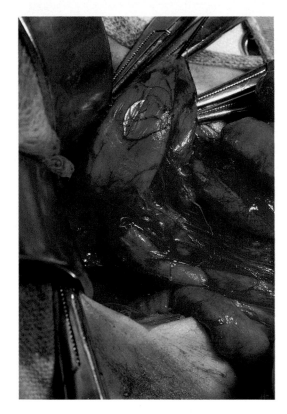

Figure 6.36 Duodenal Atresia At operation for duodenal atresia, the proximal duodenum is seen to be greatly dilated and to overlap the distal duodenum.

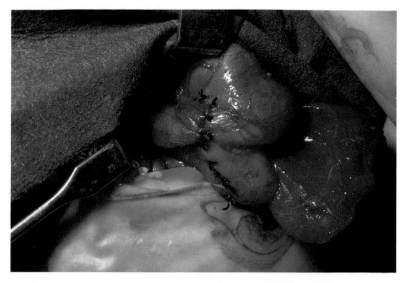

Figure 6.37 A linear duodenoduodenostomy has been created between the overlapping proximal duodenum and the narrow distal duodenum. The anastomotic length is almost 2 cm, permitting a nonobstructing two-layer closure.

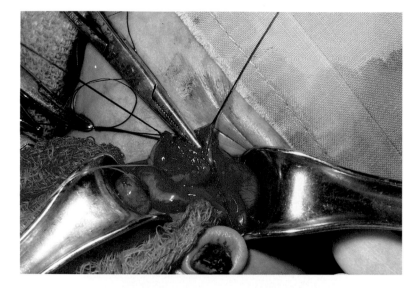

Figure 6.39 A duodenojejunostomy is performed between the dilated duodenum, just proximal to the site of atresia, and the side of a loop of jejunum, brought through the colonic mesentery in a retrocolic position. The hemostat tip is in the open duodenum.

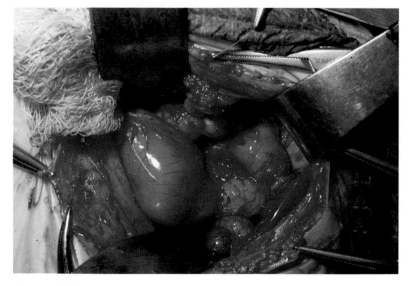

Figure 6.38 Light-colored pink pancreatic tissue surrounds the duodenum at the site of a congenital obstruction.

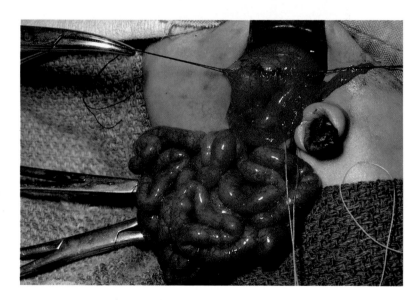

Figure 6.40 The anastomosis is completed with an inner layer of running 5-0 chromic gut and seromuscular interrupted 5-0 silk.

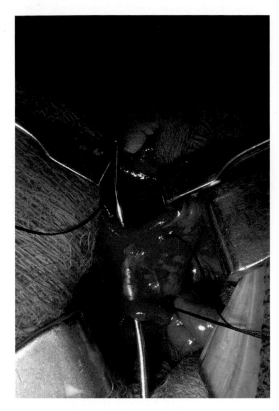

Figure 6.41 Duodenal Stenosis A probe is passed through the area of narrowing in a congenital duodenal stenosis.

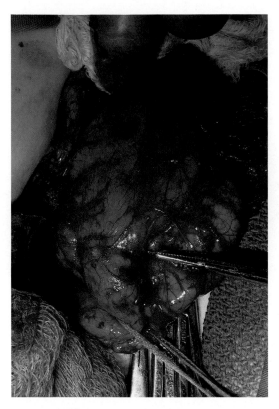

Figure 6.42 Duodenal Web The hemostat points to the junction between the dilated first portion of the duodenum and the narrower distal duodenum, corresponding with the radiograph in Figure 6.35.

Membranous webs may be excised primarily, once the ampulla of Vater has been shown not to enter the web (Figs 6.42–6.47). In the case of an elongated "windsock" web, pressure on the distal web by a catheter or probe passed into the lumen from above will cause indentation of the duodenal wall at the point of origin of the web; the duodenal incision for repair must be at this location (Fig 6.48).

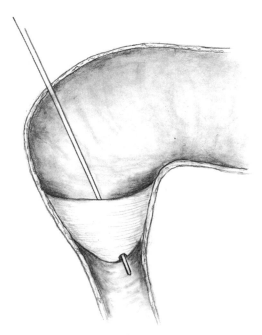

Figure 6.43 The anatomy of the membranous web and eccentric perforation is illustrated.

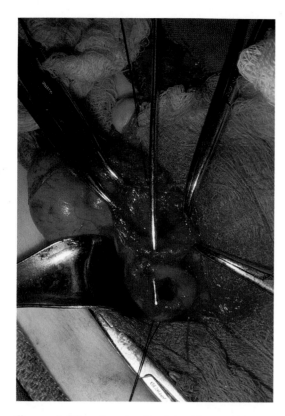

Figure 6.44 A longitudinal incision exposes the web. A probe passes through the small central perforation.

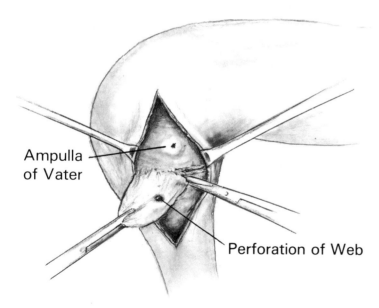

Ampulla of Vater

Perforation of Web

Figure 6.45 The web is carefully excised circumferentially, after identification of the ampulla of Vater.

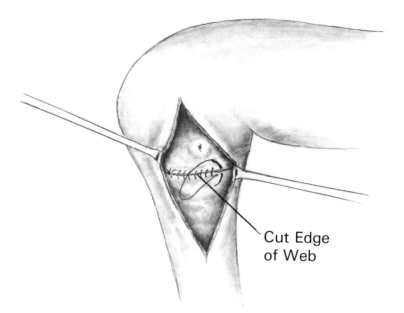

Cut Edge of Web

Figure 6.46 Fine suture—5-0 or 6-0 chromic gut—is used in a running stitch to approximate the cut edges of the mucosa and to achieve hemostasis.

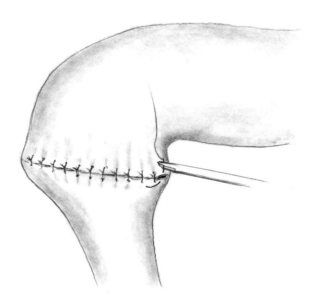

Figure 6.47 A transverse closure of the longitudinal incision (duodenoplasty) maximizes the luminal diameter.

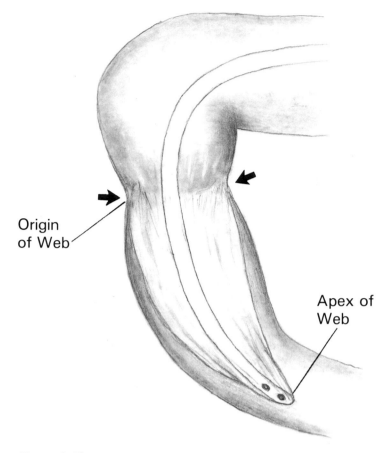

Origin
of Web

Apex of
Web

Figure 6.48 The "wind-sock" web extends distally from the point of mucosal origin. Pressure on the apex of the web causes the point of origin to indent, thus identifying the site for duodenotomy.

Pressure on the duodenum from extrinsic peritoneal bands—usually, but not always, associated with intestinal malrotation—may also result in partial obstruction (Fig 6.49). A typical "bird's beak" appearance is seen at the point of obstruction on contrast radiographs (Fig 6.50). Obstructing bands are divided at surgery (Fig 6.51). When malrotation is the diagnosis, correction is urgent because of the possibility of development of midgut volvulus (see Chapter 7).

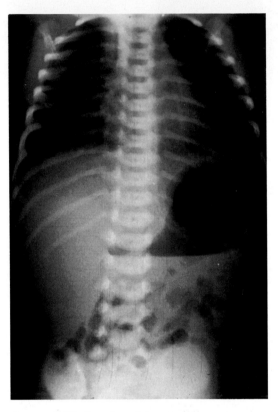

Figure 6.49 Duodenal Band A partial proximal intestinal obstruction is strongly suggested by this plain abdominal radiograph, showing a dilated stomach and very little air beyond the duodenum.

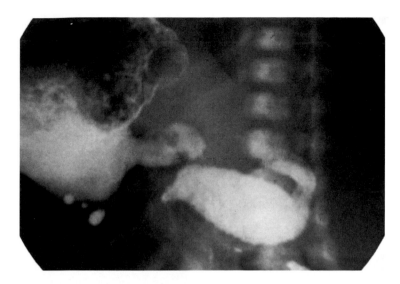

Figure 6.50 Contrast introduced into the stomach demonstrates the typical "bird's beak" appearance of an extrinsic band across the third portion of the duodenum.

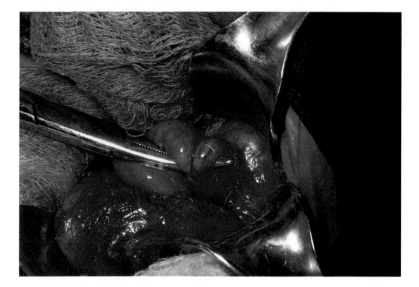

Figure 6.51 The duodenum is dilated proximal to the obstructing band, which produces a kink in the distal duodenum. There is no associated malrotation in this case.

Jejunoileal Atresia

Abdominal distention and bilious vomiting characterize jejunoileal atresia. The presence of distended, air-filled intestinal loops proximal to the atresia can be confirmed radiographically and at surgery (Figs 6.52, 6.53). Occasionally, abdominal radiographs of a neonate will show the intraperitoneal calcifications resulting from prenatal meconium peritonitis or devitalization of intestine by an intrauterine volvulus (Figs 6.33, 6.54–6.56).

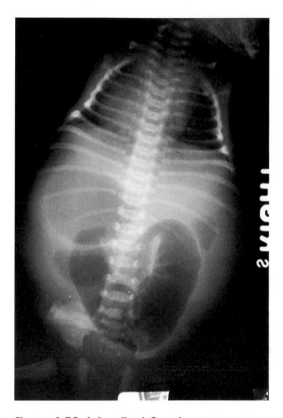

Figure 6.52 Jejunoileal Atresia The plain radiograph shows only a few loops of greatly dilated intestine in this neonate.

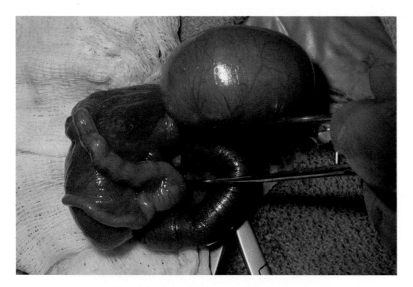

Figure 6.53 A midjejunal atresia, secondary to antenatal volvulus, is shown. The most dilated segment is proximal to the atresia.

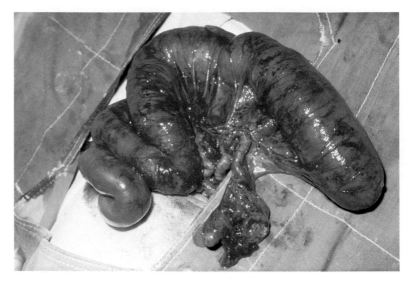

Figure 6.55 At surgery, the ileal atresia with mesenteric defect is found, along with the twisted, calcified intrauterine volvulus that must have caused the atresia.

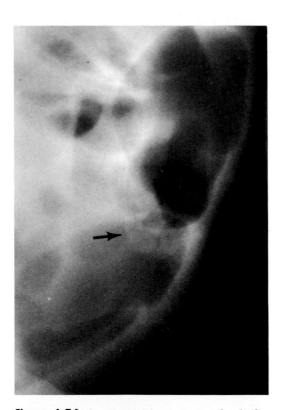

Figure 6.54 A concentric pattern of calcification at the site of an ileal atresia is seen on this lateral radiograph as well as in the anteroposterior view in Figure 6.33. Devitalized tissue and extravasated meconium in the fetal peritoneal cavity have become calcified (meconium peritonitis) and are radiopaque.

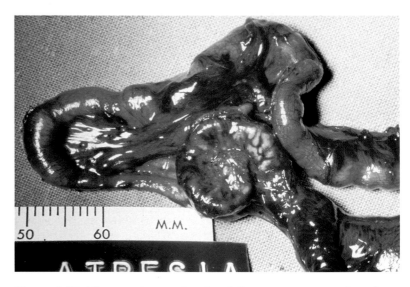

Figure 6.56 The specimen of twisted ileum was resected, and a primary anastomosis was performed.

Placement of a nasogastric tube and an adequate intravenous line is indicated in treating all cases of intestinal obstruction. The author gives prophylactic antibiotics in neonates. A transverse supraumbilical incision in the right side of the abdomen will give exposure to almost all intestinal obstructions beyond the ligament of Treitz; the incision can be extended across the midline for additional abdominal exposure. Isolated atresia is usually handled by primary end-to-end or end-to-oblique anastomosis. Most repairs can be performed with a two-layer closure. When there is a very narrow anastomosis, the surgeon may elect to turn in as little "cuff" as possible by using a single-layer closure with fine suture material. The techniques for anastomosis of infant intestine of greatly disparate diameters are illustrated and described (Figs 6.57–6.59).

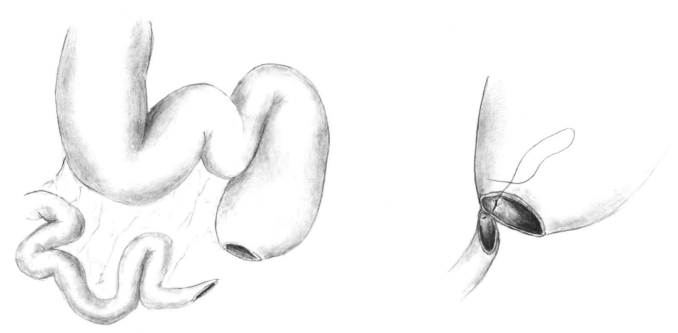

Figure 6.57 Anastomotic Techniques in the Infant The diagram illustrates the method of excising a central "button" from the end of the dilated proximal bowel for anastomosis to the obliquely divided, unused distal bowel. The obliquity is always toward the antimesenteric border, to ensure adequate blood supply.

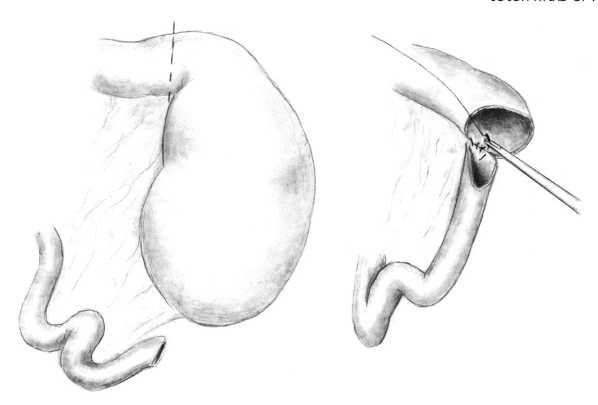

Figure 6.58 Some intestine proximal to an obstruction is so dilated that resection back to more normal-caliber bowel is desirable for anastomosis.

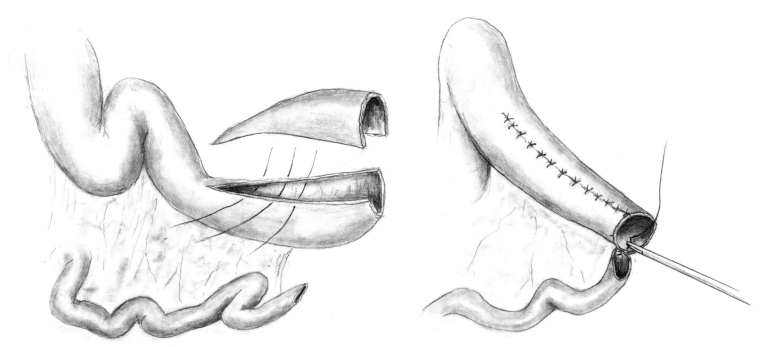

Figure 6.59 Tapering of the dilated, congenitally obstructed bowel will facilitate the anastomosis without sacrificing intestinal length.

Side-to-side anastomoses are avoided because they may lead to a "blind-loop" syndrome. Multiple atresias are more difficult to repair. Clinical judgment determines whether small segments of intestine are excised or are retained and connected with multiple anastomoses. The total length that must be preserved for future absorption is at least 20 cm of small intestine if there is an intact ileocecal valve.

The surgeon who is correcting one congenital intestinal obstruction must always be alert to additional, distal obstructions, especially as there is no change in bowel caliber to indicate their location (Fig 6.60). When the intestine is divided at the point of primary obstruction, normal saline is instilled and gently "milked" distally to ensure patency of the remainder of the bowel. Most distal intestinal anastomoses in infants can be protected with nasogastric tube decompression for the 3–5 days generally required for intestinal healing and return to function.

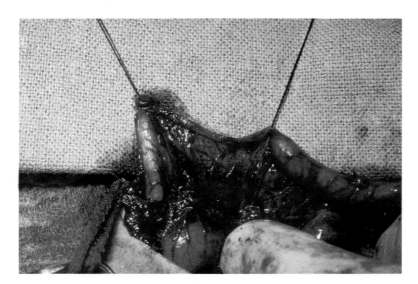

Figure 6.60 Colonic Atresia This cordlike atresia of the transverse colon was found on careful inspection during laparotomy for a duodenal atresia. The colon is of equally small caliber on both sides of the atresia.

Meconium Ileus

Meconium ileus is a congenital obstruction of the distal ileum by intraluminal, inspissated meconium in babies with cystic fibrosis. The meconium is abnormally thick because of the unusually viscid intestinal secretions and the lack of pancreatic digestive enzyme that are characteristic of cystic fibrosis. A family history of this recessive genetic disease will alert one to the diagnosis of meconium ileus in the newborn who presents with abdominal distention, bilious vomiting, and scant or absent stools.

The examiner may detect a "doughy" consistency to the palpably distended loops of small intestine in some infants with this condition. However, the diagnosis is best confirmed by supine and erect abdominal radiographs. The films with the baby in erect position are remarkably similar to those taken with the baby supine; there are no air-fluid levels seen on the erect films because the abnormally thick meconium cannot layer out in the short time the baby is held upright (Fig 6.61). In addition, a

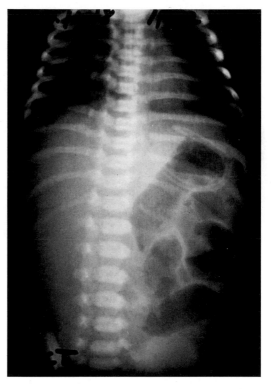

Figure 6.61 Meconium Ileus The erect abdominal radiograph in a 2-day-old with vomiting and abdominal distention shows dilated bowel loops without air-fluid levels and absence of air in the right side of the lower abdomen.

"ground-glass" appearance of air mixed with stool—or a complete absence of bowel gas—may be seen in the right lower quadrant on the abdominal films. A water-soluble contrast enema with diatrizoate sodium or diatrizoate meglumine (Hypaque or Gastrografin) will show a narrow unused colon (see Fig 6.34). In more than half the cases, the contrast enema may also be therapeutic, washing out the inspissated meconium from the terminal ileum and relieving the intestinal obstruction (Figs 6.62, 6.63). It is of utmost importance that the infant who is undergoing water-soluble contrast enema "washout" for meconium ileus have appropriate intravenous fluid running at 150%–200% of the maintenance rate both during and immediately after the procedure. Water-soluble contrast material has a high osmolality and draws considerable amounts of fluid into the intestinal lumen. The baby will go into severe hypovolemic shock if the fluid lost to the circulation is not promptly replaced.

When contrast "washout" is unsuccessful, or if another complication associated with meconium ileus—such as perforation, atresia, or volvulus—is suspected, surgical exploration is indicated. The typical operative findings (Figs 6.64–6.66) confirm the diagnosis of meconium ileus. If there are no associated complications, such as the volvulus or perforation pictured in Figures 6.67–6.69, there is no need for intestinal resection. The object of surgery is to relieve the obstruction by clearing the inspissated meconium from the distal ileal segment. Some surgeons perform a primary anastomosis after irrigating the distal bowel at the operating table. Others prefer to vent the ileum proximal to the obstruction; the Bishop-Koop end-to-side anastomosis, with exteriorization of the distal segment, is the preference of most pediatric surgeons (Fig 6.70). One may also use the Mikulicz double-barreled ileostomy or the Santulli side-to-end anastomosis.

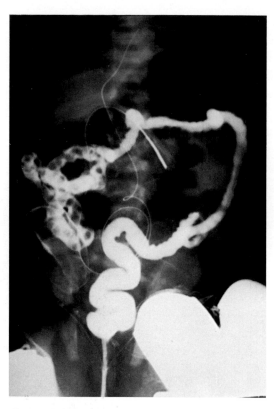

Figure 6.62 The water-soluble contrast enema is made to reflux into the terminal ileum to wash out the visible plugs of inspissated meconium.

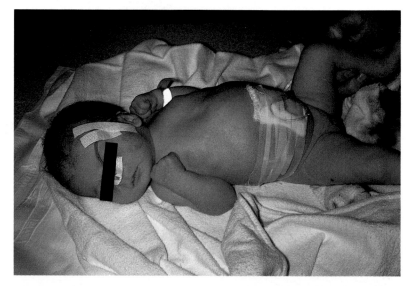

Figure 6.63 The "washout" of obstructing meconium is successful in this newborn girl, relieving her intestinal obstruction.

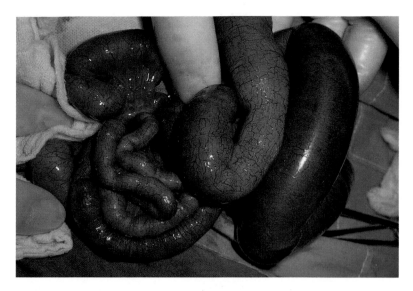

Figure 6.64 Typical of the operative findings in meconium ileus are the following: narrow distal ileum containing pellets of inspissated meconium; thick-walled muscular hypertrophy of the mid ileum; and thin-walled, dilated proximal intestine filled with air and liquid contents.

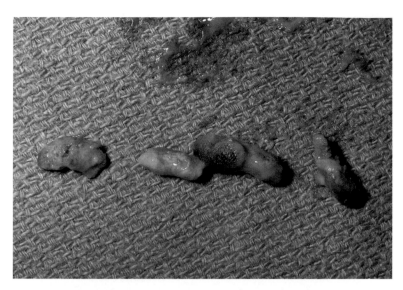

Figure 6.66 These pale pellets of obstructing, inspissated meconium have been milked out of the distal ileum; most of the water and bile has been absorbed from them.

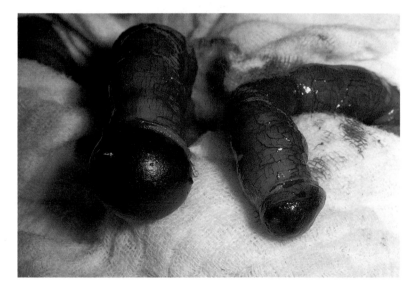

Figure 6.65 Division of the ileum, preparatory to a Bishop-Koop anastomosis, shows the abnormal, tarlike meconium.

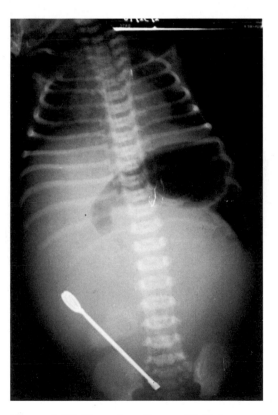

Figure 6.67 Meconium Ileus with Volvulus Intestinal obstruction and an abdominal mass were all that could be determined from this abdominal radiograph of a newborn.

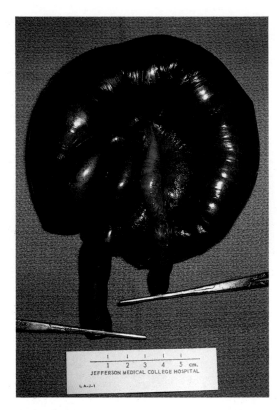

Figure 6.68 At surgery, there was evidence of meconium ileus and a necrotic volvulus of the heavy, meconium-filled ileum; the photograph is of the resected ileal volvulus.

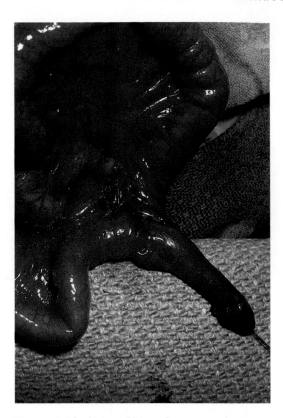

Figure 6.70 Bishop-Koop Anastomosis The divided ileum is anastomosed in an end-to-side Bishop-Koop anastomosis. The proximal end of the distal segment is brought out to the skin as a "vent."

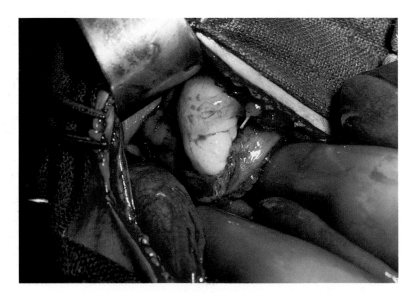

Figure 6.69 Meconium Ileus with Distal Perforation A large pellet of abnormal meconium is found to have perforated the sigmoid colon in this infant who underwent surgical exploration for meconium ileus.

If a catheter is left in the exteriorized segment, it is used to irrigate the distal ileum clear of meconium, with a solution of pancreatic enzyme or dilute mucolytic agent (Fig 6.71). Once the distal obstruction is cleared, the infant may be fed. Pancreatic enzyme is added to the feedings. The postoperative care of these infants must take into account the possible pulmonary problems to which they are subject. Humidified air, pulmonary physiotherapy, and prophylactic antibiotic therapy are used. A sweat test or antifibrinogen isoenzyme level will confirm the diagnosis of cystic fibrosis.

Mikulicz ileostomy segments are anastomosed by application of a crushing clamp. The Bishop-Koop and Santulli enterostomies stop draining as soon as bowel contents pass distally; they may be closed extraperitoneally, frequently under local anesthesia.

Meckel's Diverticulum

Meckel's diverticulum is an antimesenteric outpouching of the midileum that is a remnant of the embryologic vitelline (omphalomesenteric) duct. It is found in approximately 2% of the population and, in the adult, lies about 2 feet proximal to the ileocecal valve. It is a potential source of several problems in children: bleeding, two types of intestinal obstruction (intussusception and volvulus), and inflammation.

Totipotential embryonic tissue in the developing Meckel's diverticulum may form gastric mucosa or pancreatic tissue. The ectopic gastric mucosa secretes acid, responds to gastrin stimulation, and concentrates the radioactive compound sodium pertechnetate technetium 99m. Acid secretion from the diverticulum ulcerates the mucosa of the adjacent ileum, leading to significant, and even massive, painless lower gastrointestinal bleeding. It occurs most often in the child younger than 2 years, but may occur at any age. Persistent massive hemorrhage requires emergency abdominal surgery. Moderate bleeding allows time for diagnostic confirmation of the source. Technetium scan is the most reliable study, with approximately 70%–80% accuracy (Fig 6.72). A barium gastrointestinal series rarely demonstrates the lesion. Surgical excision of the diverticulum is the treatment (Figs 6.73–6.76). The laparoscopic excision of a Meckel's diverticulum is shown in Chapter 8.

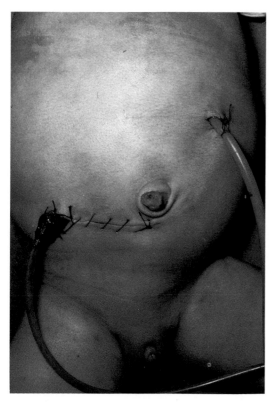

Figure 6.71 A tube for irrigation of residual meconium is left in the distal ileum and is sutured to the skin. A gastrostomy is performed for postoperative decompression, to avoid having a tube through the nasopharynx in a baby with the potential pulmonary problems of cystic fibrosis.

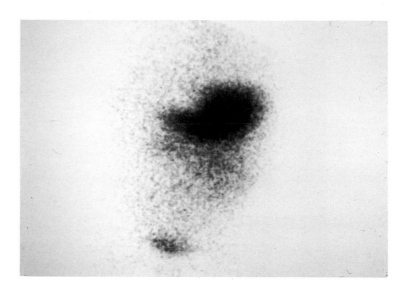

Figure 6.72 Meckel's Diverticulum Technetium radionuclide scan demonstrates concentration in the mucosa of the stomach and in the right lower abdomen—the location of a Meckel's diverticulum.

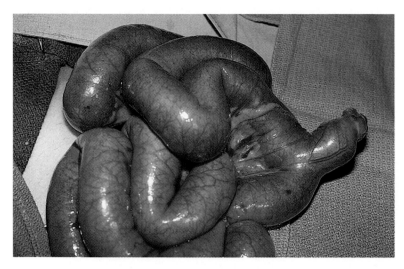

Figure 6.73 This Meckel's diverticulum is the source of massive, painless rectal bleeding in a 7-year-old. Blood can be seen within the distal ileum. A radionuclide scan failed to demonstrate the diverticulum in this patient.

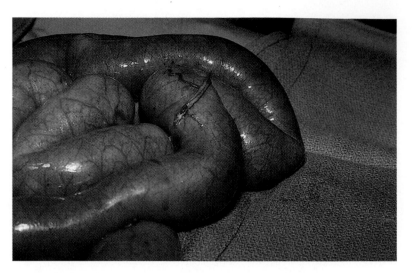

Figure 6.75 The stapled ileal closure is seen.

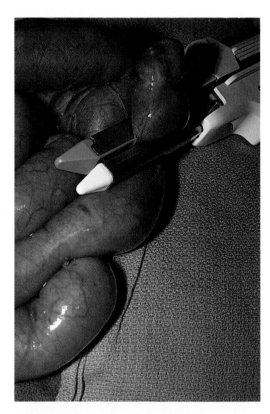

Figure 6.74 A GIA stapler is applied across the base of the diverticulum, oblique to the longitudinal axis of the intestine.

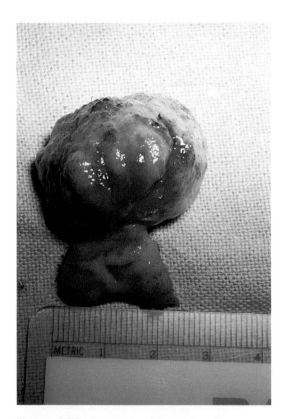

Figure 6.76 A resected Meckel's diverticulum is shown, with ectopic gastric mucosa.

Among the potential lead-points for intussusception is the Meckel's diverticulum, which invaginates at its ileal attachment and then is propelled distally by intestinal peristalsis. Patients have typical symptoms of intussusception, and the Meckel's diverticulum is resected at the time of operative reduction.

The Meckel's diverticulum may be adherent to the anterior abdominal wall at the umbilicus. This attachment is a possible focus for volvulus or internal hernia, similar to that formed by an intestinal adhesion, and is recognized only at surgery (Fig 6.77). The diverticulum may rarely become inflamed, producing a Meckel's diverticulitis that is clinically and pathologically very much like appendicitis; it may even rupture, with ensuing peritonitis (Figs 6.78, 6.79).

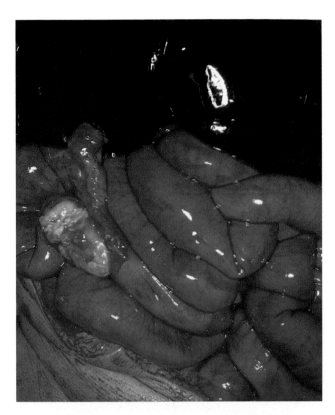

Figure 6.78 The perforation of an inflamed Meckel's diverticulum caused death from peritonitis in this infant.

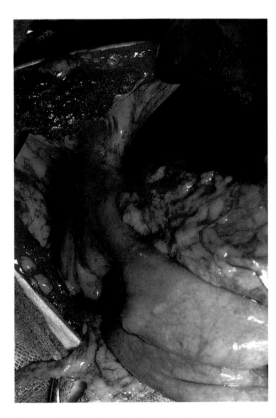

Figure 6.77 A Meckel's diverticulum is found adherent to the anterior abdominal wall at the umbilicus. Surgical exploration followed a bleeding episode.

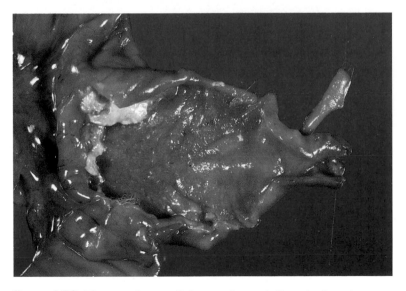

Figure 6.79 The specimen of the perforated diverticulum is shown.

There is no unanimity of opinion concerning the excision of a Meckel's diverticulum found incidentally during surgery for another problem (Fig 6.80). It has been the author's practice to remove the diverticulum, and there have been no known complications. Oblique excision at the base of the diverticulum, in a line at a 45° angle to the long axis of the ileum, is least likely to narrow the ileum. Resection of the ileum and attached diverticulum is necessary when there is extensive inflammation, questionable intestinal viability, or stenosis of the ileum at the origin of the diverticulum.

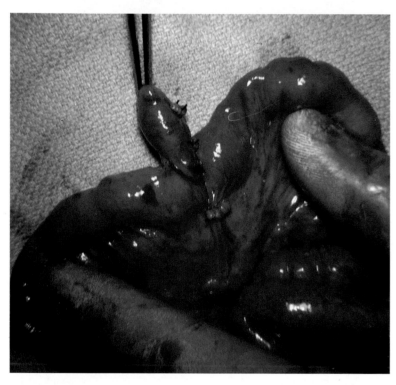

Figure 6.80 This Meckel's diverticulum was an incidental finding at surgery; it was excised.

Intussusception

Intussusception is an invagination, or "telescoping," of intestine into itself, usually in the direction of peristalsis. The invaginated component is called the *intussusceptum,* which is carried into the *intussuscipiens.* The cause can be demonstrated best in those cases with a lead-point, such as a polyp, tumor, or Meckel's diverticulum, attached to the intestinal wall. The lead-point is propelled distally and pulls the proximal intestine into the lumen of the distal bowel. Most often in children there is no demonstrable anatomic lead-point; this "idiopathic" intussusception is thought to result from hypertrophied submucosal lymphoid follicles—especially the Peyer's patches of the distal ileum—which act as a lead-point. Edematous mucosa, found in some malabsorption syndromes, may act as a lead-point in any portion of the intestine. Intussusception, especially of the small intestine, may also follow any major surgery in an infant. Transient intussusception has been observed to occur and to reduce spontaneously during abdominal surgery in some neonates.

Idiopathic ileocolic intussusception occurs typically in well-nourished children 6 to 24 months old, frequently following a viral infection. There is a seasonal prevalence, consistent with the peaks of upper respiratory infection. Classic symptoms include sudden onset of crampy abdominal pain, followed by reflex vomiting, and recurrent pain of regular periodicity with pain-free intervals of 15 to 30 minutes. Not all patients present in a typical manner. In an infant, the insidious onset of lethargy, with few other symptoms, should alert the physician to the possibility of intussusception.

The intussusception may be palpable as a sausage-shaped or oval nontender mass in the right upper abdomen. After several hours of symptoms, bloody mucus ("currant-jelly" stool) may be found on rectal examination (Fig 6.81). Rarely, the intussusceptum presents at the rectum as a palpable, or even visible, mass.

The diagnosis is confirmed radiographically. Some patients may be seen to have complete intestinal obstruction (Fig 6.82); the mass of telescoped intestine is visible on abdominal films in others (Fig 6.83). Ultrasonography has been used to demonstrate intussusception (Fig 6.84). In most children, the diagnosis is made—and there is an attempt at hydrostatic reduction—by barium enema (Figs 6.85, 6.86).

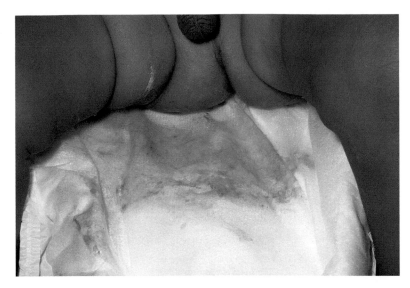

Figure 6.81 Intussusception A "currant-jelly" stool—blood mixed with mucus—was passed by this 6-month-old with intussusception.

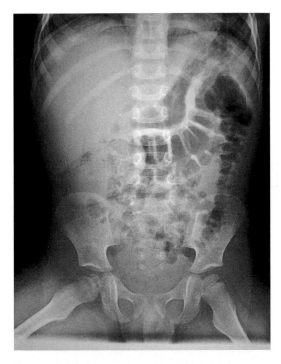

Figure 6.83 The right upper abdominal mass of an ileocolic intussusception can be seen inferior to the liver edge on the plain abdominal radiograph.

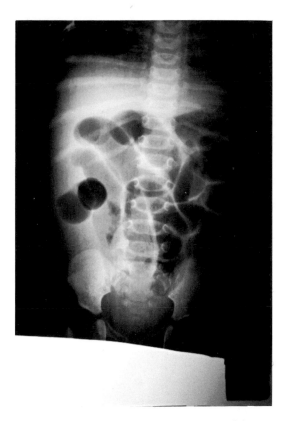

Figure 6.82 Multiple dilated intestinal loops represent a complete intestinal obstruction in a child with an irreducible intussusception.

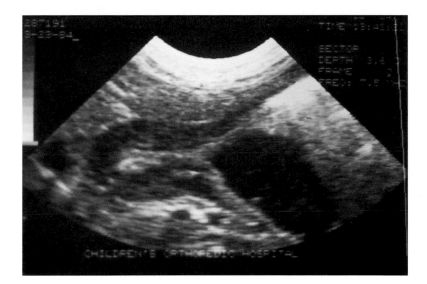

Figure 6.84 Ileum telescoping into colon is demonstrated here by abdominal ultrasonography.

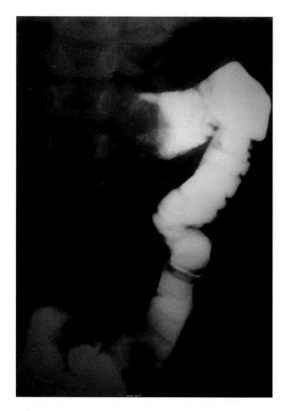

Figure 6.85 A barium enema outlines the mass of an intussusception in the left colon.

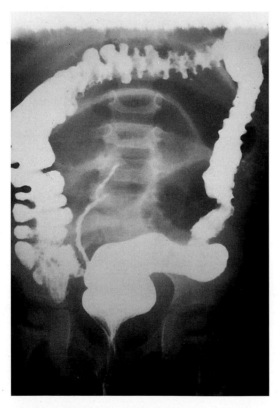

Figure 6.86 The pressure of barium has reduced the ileal mass to the cecum.

Barium Reduction

In the author's opinion, barium reduction should be attempted only under the following conditions: (1) duration of symptoms of less than 48 hours; (2) no clinical signs of peritoneal irritation; (3) no evidence in the child of a toxic condition, i.e., high fever or leukocytosis; (4) no evidence of complete intestinal obstruction; (5) regulation of the pressure of the column of barium mixture to no more than 36 inches above the level of the patient; (6) presence of a surgeon, in case the reduction attempt should fail or the colon be shown to have perforated; and (7) in-hospital observation for 24 hours after reduction to be sure that there is no residual ileoileal component or immediate recurrence of the ileocolic intussusception. Successful barium reduction is indicated by reflux of contrast material into the ileum after the intussusception has been completely reduced from the colon.

Surgical Reduction

Surgical exploration is indicated when an attempt at barium reduction is not safe or is not successful. The intussusceptum is gently "milked" from the distal bowel—as one expresses toothpaste from a tube (Figs 6.87–6.89).

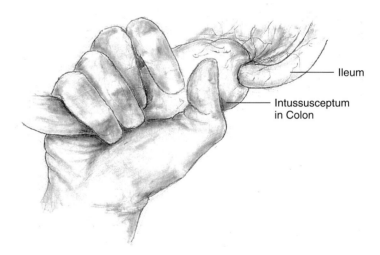

Figure 6.87 The gentle squeezing of intussuscepted ileum from the ascending colon is demonstrated in this illustration.

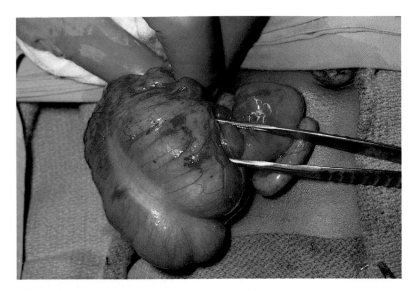

Figure 6.88 The actual surgical reduction, with the surgeon's hand expressing the intussusceptum from the ascending colon, is seen. The forceps follow the intussuscepted ileum into the cecum.

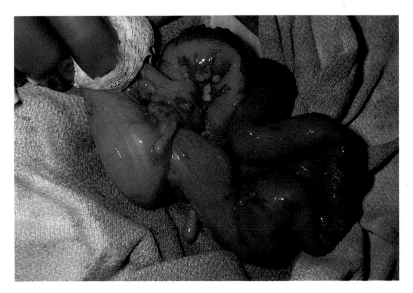

Figure 6.89 The intussusception is completely reduced. There is considerable edema of the ileal lead-point.

After reduction of the ileocolic component, any persistent ileoileal intussusception must be recognized and reduced (Fig 6.90). The vascular obstruction resulting from prolonged intussusception may lead to an irreducible or gangrenous intussusceptum, which must be resected (Fig 6.91). Other patients may develop necrosis and perforation of the intussuscipiens secondary to pressure from the intraluminal mass of intussusceptum (Fig 6.92); in these cases, an attempt at barium reduction can lead to barium peritonitis through areas of preexisting necrosis and perforation.

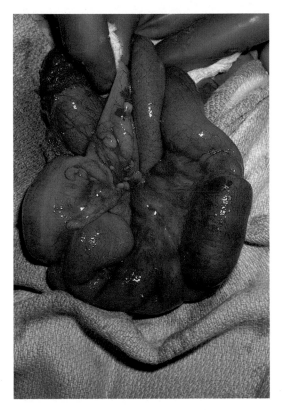

Figure 6.90 An ileoileal component remains after manual reduction of the ileocolic portion of this intussusception.

A child older than 3 years of age who develops an intussusception—or any child who has a recurrence of intussusception—must be suspected of having a specific anatomic lead-point. A Meckel's diverticulum or a polyp will produce recurrent episodes and should be excised (see Fig 7.55). In a child older than 5 years of age who develops an intussusception, surgical exploration is mandatory to rule out intestinal lymphoma as a lead-point—even if barium reduction has been successful. Benign lymphoid hyperplasia is also found as a cause at this age (Figs 6.93, 6.94).

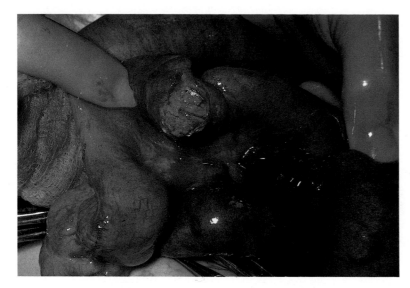

Figure 6.91 Gangrene of the wall of the ileal lead-point requires resection after reduction of the intussusception.

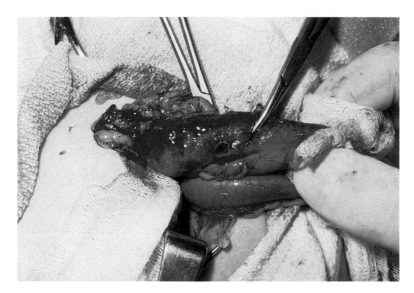

Figure 6.92 Punctate necrotic areas develop in the transverse colon at the site of the intussuscepted ileal mass. The ileal lead-point is also gangrenous in this patient.

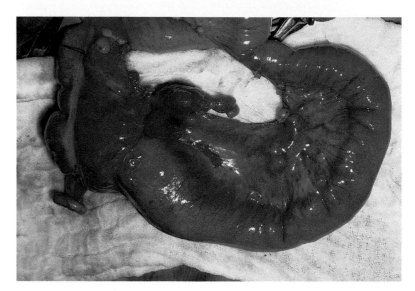

Figure 6.93 Thickening of the terminal ileum represents benign lymphoid hyperplasia in this 5-year-old whose intussusception was reduced with barium; laparotomy is to rule out lymphoma.

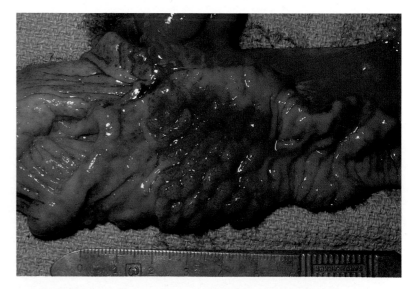

Figure 6.94 The submucosa is markedly hypertrophied and the mucosal folds prominent in the specimen resected from the patient in Figure 6.93.

In the case of spontaneous small bowel intussusception following major surgery in infants, the diagnosis may be suspected by clinical and radiologic evidence of intestinal obstruction. An upper gastrointestinal contrast study is often diagnostic (Fig 6.95), and surgical reduction is always indicated (Fig 6.96).

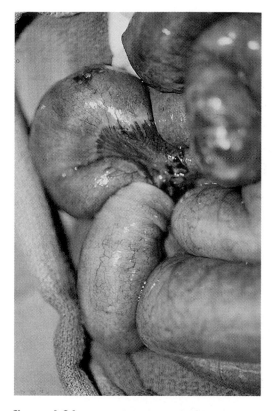

Figure 6.96 At exploration, the ileoileal intussusception was found and easily reduced.

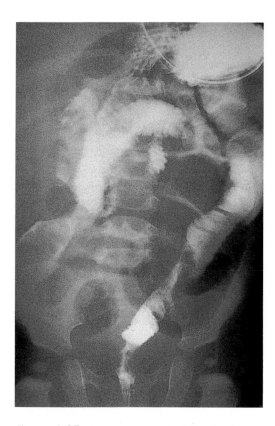

Figure 6.95 An upper gastrointestinal series with dilute barium demonstrates an ileoileal intussusception in this 1-year-old, with signs of partial intestinal obstruction following a pull-through for Hirschsprung's disease.

Intestinal Duplication

Duplications may occur on the mesenteric side at any point along the intestinal tract. They generally share part of the muscular wall of the adjacent intestine and have similar mucosa, although aberrant mucosa has been found in some duplications. Some exist as closed cysts; others communicate with the adjacent viscus in one or more places. Excision is advised, leaving the normal intestine intact when possible. Occasionally, anastomosis of a long duplication proximally and distally to the adjacent intestine allows egress of contents and prevents stasis and ulceration. In some, stripping the mucosa from the duplication is the best definitive treatment.

Gastric duplication is found in only a small percentage of cases. It presents most often as a palpable mass (Fig 6.97), as a source of upper gastrointestinal bleeding, or as a cause of partial obstruction at the pylorus. Excision is advised (Figs 6.98, 6.99).

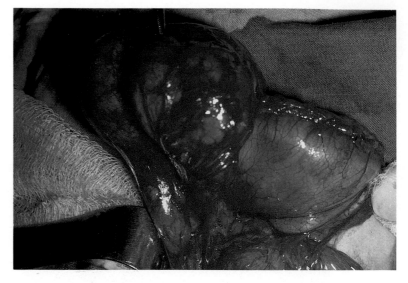

Figure 6.98 The stomach and mass are elevated, and the dissection of the mass is begun.

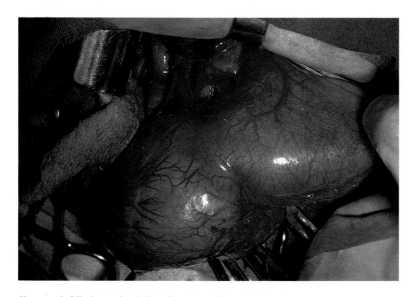

Figure 6.97 Intestinal Duplication This bilobed cystic mass was found attached to the greater curvature of the stomach, sharing part of its seromuscular wall.

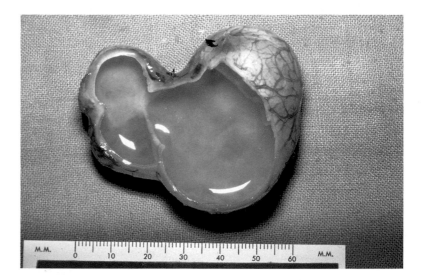

Figure 6.99 The excised, fluid-filled specimen is opened to show a duplicated body, antrum, and pylorus. Gastric mucosa lines the duplication.

Duplication of the terminal ileum may produce symptoms of partial obstruction or may be found as a mass on an abdominal radiograph (Fig 6.100). Resection of the duplication and adjacent ileum is the procedure of choice (Fig 6.101).

Microscopic examination demonstrates the relationship of the intestinal duplication to the normal bowel and the identical type of mucosa (Fig 6.102).

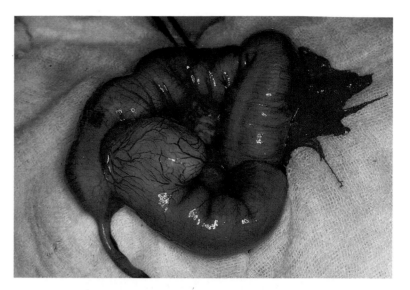

Figure 6.101 An ileocecal duplication, which communicated with the ileal lumen, was found and resected.

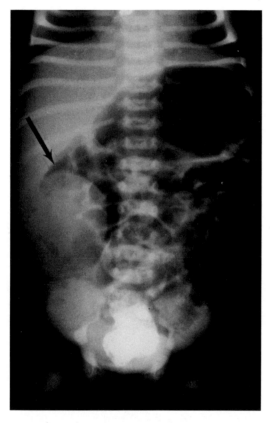

Figure 6.100 A radiograph of the abdomen clearly outlines a right-sided lower abdominal mass.

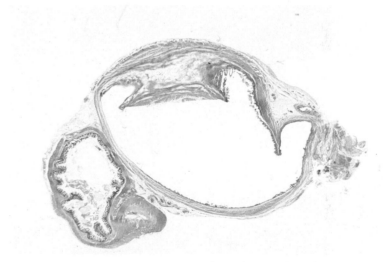

Figure 6.102 This microscopic cross-section of a colonic duplication shows identical mucosa in both lumina.

Foreign Bodies of the Gastrointestinal Tract

Children swallow many objects that do not belong in their intestinal tracts. Round or smooth objects, such as marbles, beads, or coins, will usually pass through the intestine without incident. Radiopaque foreign bodies may be followed through the intestine (Fig 6.103), some for up to 4–6 weeks, until they pass. Radiolucent ones are much more difficult to detect. Odd-shaped and sharp pointed objects are more dangerous, as they may stop at natural barriers—most often the pylorus and ileocecal

valve—or may perforate the intestine at any point (Fig 6.104). If such an object is known to have lodged in the esophagus or stomach, it should be removed endoscopically. When an irregular or pointed object has passed beyond the duodenum, the child must be observed closely and undergo abdominal exploration for any sign of perforation.

Small, flat hearing-aid batteries that are ingested are especially dangerous because of their corrosive alkaline contents. They must be removed, by endoscopy or surgery, if they do not pass promptly out of the gastrointestinal tract.

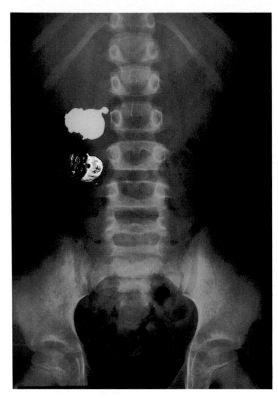

Figure 6.103 Gastrointestinal Foreign Bodies This composite photograph shows the outline of a radiopaque foreign body in its passage through the intestine, and the Santa Claus pin that eventually passed.

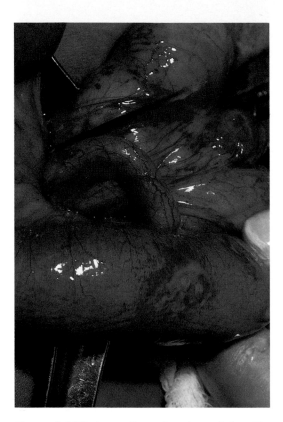

Figure 6.104 A small perforation of the distal ileum was discovered at laparotomy for possible appendicitis. The cause was a green broom-straw, swallowed several days before and found free in the abdomen next to the appendix.

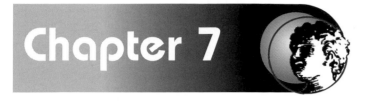

Chapter 7

Colon and Rectum

The colon and rectum are the sites of numerous congenital and acquired abnormalities. Correction often demands careful diagnostic evaluation and complex operative procedures.

Colonic Atresia

The colon is the least common site of intestinal atresia. The clinical picture is characterized by the development of massive abdominal distention in the neonate, as swallowed air fills the intestine proximal to the obstruction (Figs 7.1, 7.2). A contrast enema will demonstrate narrow unused colon distal to the obstruction (Fig 7.3).

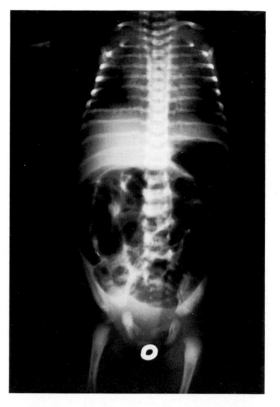

Figure 7.2 Multiple distended loops of bowel are seen on the plain abdominal radiograph.

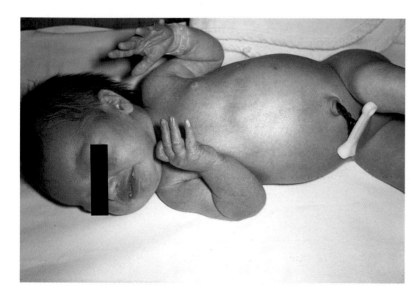

Figure 7.1 Colonic Atresia This infant girl with colonic atresia developed massive abdominal distention and vomiting during the first 36 hours of life.

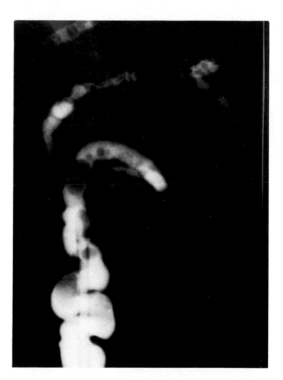

Figure 7.3 A contrast enema shows a distal unused colon with a few small flecks of meconium.

At exploration, the most dilated segment is generally found just proximal to the atresia (Fig 7.4). There may be multiple atretic segments, with no change in bowel caliber to indicate their location (see Fig 6.60). There is great disparity in diameter between the dilated proximal and unused distal colon. If an anastomosis cannot be created at the primary atresia site, the terminal ileum can be anastomosed to the distal colon, in an end-to-oblique fashion.

Colonic Stenosis

Colonic stenosis may be congenital or may follow neonatal necrotizing enterocolitis. It presents as a partial obstruction when the infant's stool becomes more firm; rarely it may lead to spontaneous colonic perforation (Figs 7.5–7.7).

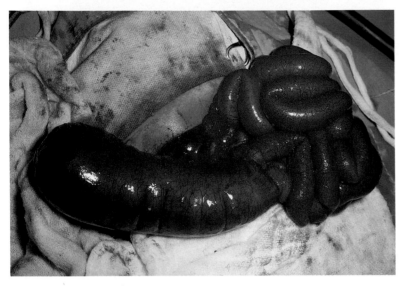

Figure 7.4 The huge, dilated right colon ends at the hepatic flexure. The narrow-diameter transverse colon can be seen in the midline, next to the liver. The atretic right colon is resected, and an anastomosis of terminal ileum to transverse colon is performed.

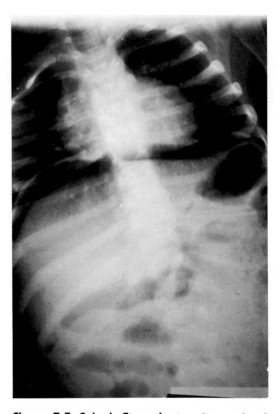

Figure 7.5 Colonic Stenosis A radiograph of this 14-month-old boy with fever and abdominal distention shows a pneumoperitoneum.

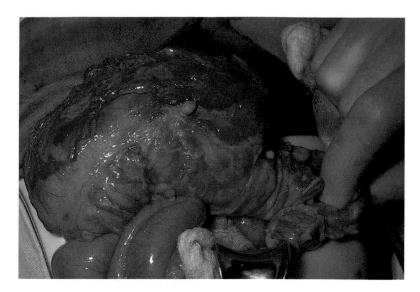

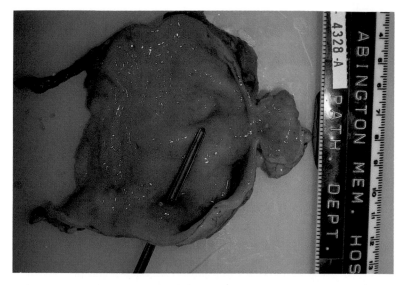

Figure 7.6 Stool is seen oozing from a small perforation in the dilated transverse colon, 3 cm proximal to a very narrow stenosis.

Figure 7.7 The resected specimen is opened to show the tight stenosis. A probe enters the site of spontaneous perforation.

Malrotation

The clinical presentation of malrotation (incomplete intestinal rotation) in the infant is that of a high partial obstruction, either duodenal (from extrinsic bands) or jejunal (secondary to a volvulus). There is bilious vomiting, without abdominal distention. Radiographs confirm the diagnosis (Figs 7.8–7.10). The older child most often presents with recurrent episodes of abdominal pain, chronic vomiting, and poor weight gain.

Malrotation classically involves incomplete embryologic rotation of both the colon and the duodenum and lack of normal fixation of the small bowel mesentery.

The cecum lies in the upper abdomen. The third portion of the duodenum lies completely to the right of the midline of the abdomen, and there is no ligament of Treitz. In that position, the duodenum is sometimes partially obstructed by peritoneal bands crossing it from the lateral abdominal wall to the malpositioned cecum in the epigastrium. The lack of fixation of the bowel mesentery allows the superior mesenteric vessels to become the axis for a midgut volvulus—a potentially fatal complication if the vascular supply to the entire small bowel is occluded (Fig 7.11).

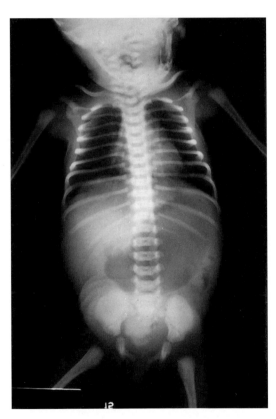

Figure 7.8 Malrotation The abdominal radiograph of a vomiting 3-day-old girl shows an air-distended stomach and very little small-intestinal air, characteristic of a high partial obstruction.

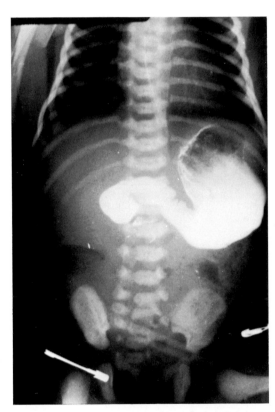

Figure 7.9 An upper gastrointestinal barium study demonstrates partial obstruction of the duodenum; the ''bird's-beak'' appearance is caused by an extrinsic peritoneal band, commonly associated with malrotation.

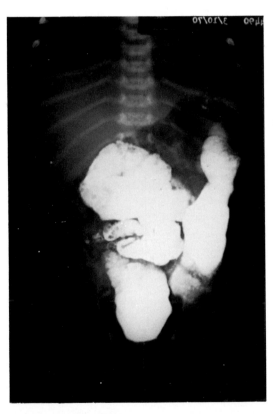

Figure 7.10 A barium enema shows the cecum to be in the right upper abdomen, another finding in malrotation. However, without other evidence of malrotation, this picture could represent a normal mobile cecum, frequently seen in infants.

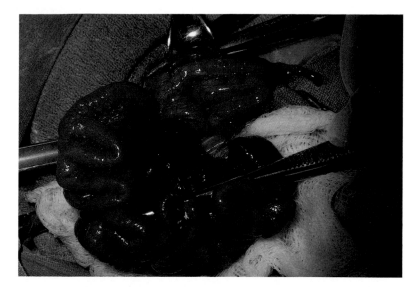

Figure 7.11 The entire small intestine is dusky because of a partial volvulus at the root of the mesentery in this infant with malrotation.

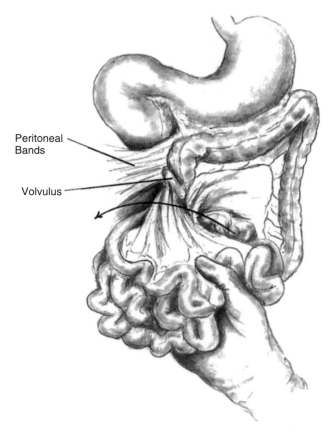

Peritoneal Bands

Volvulus

Figure 7.12 The intestinal volvulus is reduced in a counterclockwise direction.

Ladd Procedure

At surgical exploration, any volvulus is reduced by the manual untwisting of the small bowel in a counterclockwise direction (Fig 7.12). The position of the cecum and duodenum and the absence of a ligament of Treitz are determined (Fig 7.13). The peritoneal bands across the duodenum are lysed, freeing the duodenum from extrinsic pressure and allowing the cecum to be placed in the left lower quadrant of the abdomen (Figs 7.14–7.16); this maneuver also widens the base of the mesentery to prevent future volvulus. Elective appendectomy (see Figs 7.64–7.66) saves the patient from the possibility of a future left-sided appendicitis.

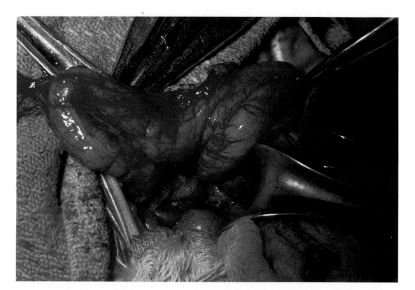

Figure 7.13 With the small bowel untwisted and returned to the abdomen, the cecum can be seen in the right upper abdomen.

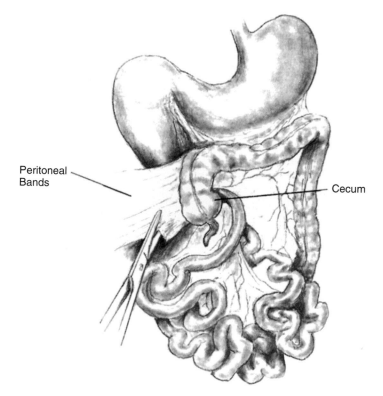

Peritoneal
Bands

Cecum

Figure 7.14 The peritoneal bands to the cecum are lysed, freeing the duodenum if it is obstructed and allowing the cecum to be placed in the left side of the abdomen.

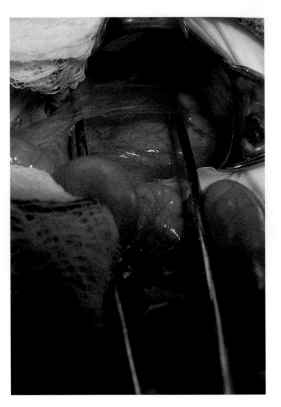

Figure 7.15 The peritoneal bands are exposed prior to lysis.

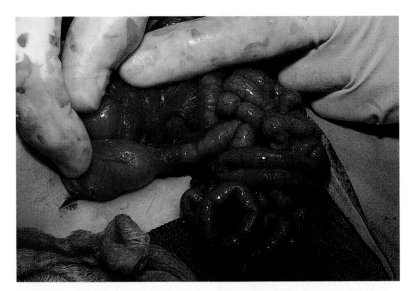

Figure 7.16 Following lysis, the dilatation of the duodenum proximal to the obstructing extrinsic bands can be seen in this infant.

Hirschsprung's Disease

Hirschsprung's disease is due to the congenital absence of ganglion cells in the muscular wall of the intestine, in both the deep myenteric plexus and the superficial Meissner's plexus. It is thought to be the result of an arrest in caudal migration of ganglion cells along the intestine during embryologic development. Occurring in approximately 1 in 5000 births, it has a male predominence of 3–4:1. The lack of ganglion cells results in absence of normal coordinated peristalsis and a functional mechanical obstruction at the transition zone between normal and aganglionic segments (Fig 7.17). Proximal to this obstruction, the bowel is dilated, giving rise to the term *megacolon*. The aganglionic bowel, usually of normal caliber, includes all of the intestine distal to the zone of transition (Fig 7.18). This transition zone is most often found in the sigmoid colon (see Figs 7.19, 7.20). In a few patients, only the rectum is involved—short-segment Hirschsprung's disease (see Fig 7.21). Rarely, the entire colon is affected (total colonic aganglionosis). Still rarer is involvement of the entire intestine, a condition usually incompatible with life.

Low intestinal obstruction in a neonate with a patent anus and rectum is assumed to result from Hirshsprung's disease until proved otherwise. Delayed or infrequent passage of meconium should also alert the pediatrician or neonatologist to this possibility. Chronic constipation in the infant or toddler must be investigated for the same diagnosis; the child's abdomen is usually moderately distended, and he or she may have poor appetite and weight gain. An infant with such a history may present with fever and explosive diarrhea, the sign of enterocolitis that is a complication of Hirschsprung's disease. Prompt diagnosis and treatment may prevent the child with enterocolitis from developing a potentially fatal septicemia or intestinal perforation.

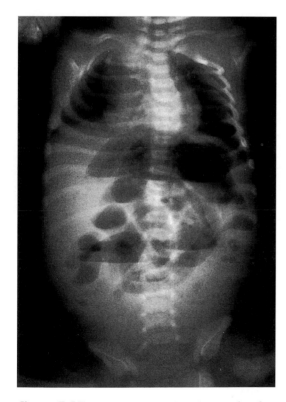

Figure 7.17 The abdominal radiograph of this newborn infant shows multiple loops of distended bowel and the granular appearance of meconium in the distal colon.

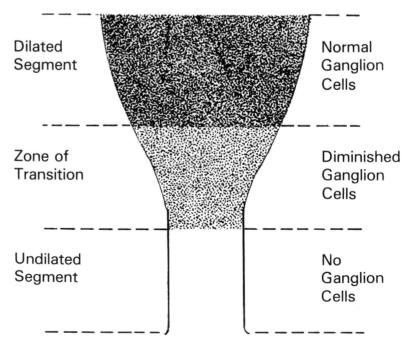

Figure 7.18 The proximal dilated intestine has a normal complement of ganglion cells. Distal to the transition zone the entire intestine lacks ganglion cells, leading to a functional obstruction.

Diagnosis

A contrast radiograph of the rectum and colon may be diagnostic (Figs 7.19–7.21). In equivocal cases, or if short-segment disease is suspected, a rectal biopsy is required. The biopsy must be taken 2–3 cm above the anal dentate line, because the number of ganglion cells normally decreases in the most distal rectum. The most reliable is a full-thickness biopsy that includes the myenteric plexus of the muscularis layer. Diagnosis from a suction biopsy is not always reliable, because it requires a deep enough specimen to include the muscularis mucosae and an experienced pathologist to read the slide. The suction biopsy is most useful if it definitely shows normal ganglion cells, thereby excluding the diagnosis of Hirschsprung's disease. Anal tonometry, which demonstrates the characteristic lack of normal relaxation of the internal anal sphincter in Hirschsprung's disease, has been used by some to clarify the diagnosis. The known presence of increased amounts of acetyl cholinesterase in the lamina propria and muscularis mucosae of the aganglionic rectum is the basis for a histochemical test on biopsy specimens that is used by some to help confirm the diagnosis.

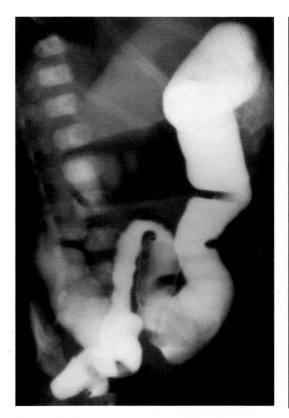

Figure 7.19 A sigmoid transition zone is clearly demonstrated on contrast enema in this 3-day-old infant with abdominal distention.

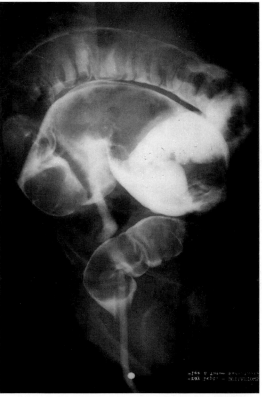

Figure 7.20 The colon proximal to this sigmoid transition zone has become massively dilated by the age of 4 months.

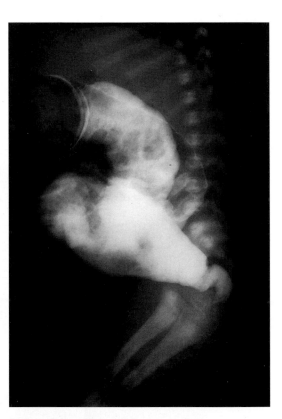

Figure 7.21 Hirschsprung's disease involves only the rectum of this 1-month-old boy, as seen in the lateral view of a barium enema. The dilated sigmoid colon narrows at the rectosigmoid transition zone.

Surgical Procedures

When imaging or other diagnostic studies are strongly suggestive of Hirschsprung's disease, a laparotomy is performed to establish the diagnosis, to identify the point of transition between normal and aganglionic bowel, and to exteriorize the intestine for decompression—at the most distal area of normal ganglion cells. At laparotomy, the transition zone may be apparent (Figs 7.22, 7.23, 7.27). Seromuscular biopsies are taken for frozen section, first in the distal segment to confirm the diagnosis by demonstrating the lack of ganglion cells, then at the proposed colostomy site to be sure that it contains normal ganglion cells (Figs 7.24–7.27). If a biopsy is taken at the transition zone, a diminished number of ganglion cells will be seen. A divided colostomy—or ileostomy in the case of total colonic aganglionosis—is then performed (Fig 7.28).

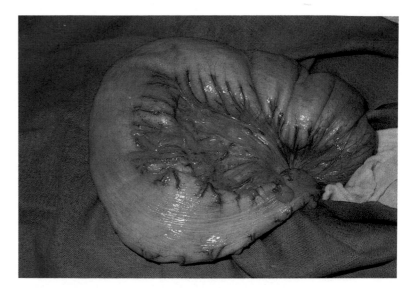

Figure 7.23 There is thick muscular hypertrophy in the colon proximal to the zone of transition at the time of diagnosis in this 2-year-old.

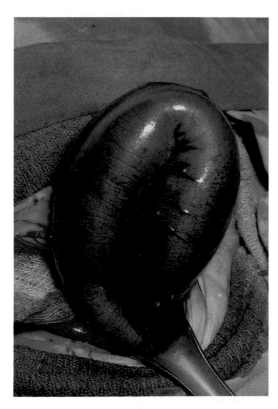

Figure 7.22 The transition zone in the colon is seen at surgery in this 1-day-old boy. The proximal colon is dilated but has not yet developed muscular hypertrophy.

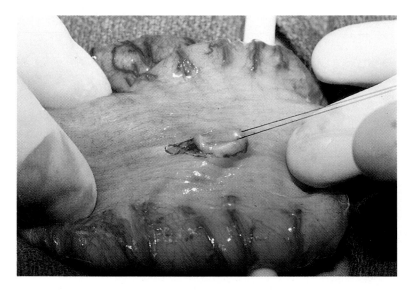

Figure 7.24 The author's technique of seromuscular biopsy is demonstrated. A fine suture (5-0 silk) is placed in the seromuscular layer of the colon. With traction on the suture, an elliptical incision is made in the seromuscular bowel at that site.

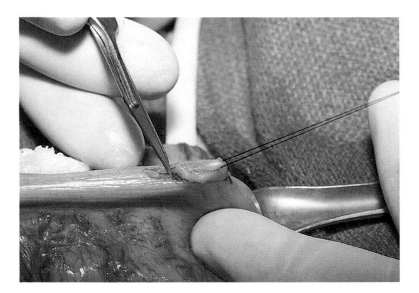

Figure 7.25 While traction is maintained on the fine suture, the blunt edge of a scalpel blade is used to tease the seromuscular specimen from the underlying muscularis mucosae and mucosa, which are not entered.

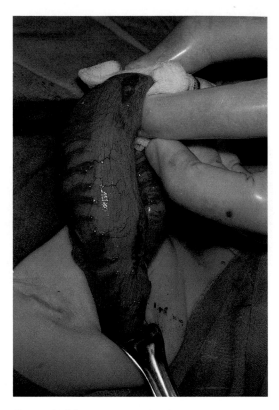

Figure 7.26 Seromuscular biopsy specimens for frozen section are taken from the distal aganglionic bowel, the proposed colostomy site, and the apparent transition zone. If there are no ganglion cells at the proposed colostomy site, more proximal biopsies are performed until ganglion cells are found, and the ostomy is created there. The biopsy sites are closed with fine seromuscular interrupted sutures.

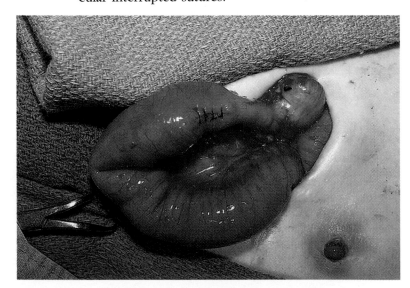

Figure 7.27 A transition zone in the terminal ileum is seen in this infant with total colonic aganglionosis. There are no ganglion cells in the wall of the excised appendix, and normal cells are found at the ileostomy biopsy site, proximal to the apparent transition zone.

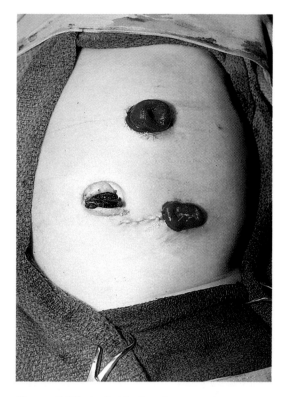

Figure 7.28 A divided colostomy is performed, with the proximal functioning segment brought out and matured through a separate incision in the upper abdomen for ease in applying a colostomy bag. The distal mucus fistula is matured at the corner of the low abdominal incision.

Pull-through Procedure for Hirschsprung's Disease

At a subsequent definitive procedure, the ostomy of ganglionated intestine is taken down and brought to the anus, and excess aganglionic bowel is excised. Most surgeons perform the definitive surgery when the child is 9–15 months old and use a variation of one of three standard abdominoperineal pull-through operations: (1) the Swenson low circumferential rectal dissection with an eversion of the full thickness of rectum—through which is pulled the ganglionated bowel for direct anastomosis to the distal rectum; (2) the Duhamel posterior pull-through with closure of the proximal rectum and side-to-side anastomosis of the normal bowel to the full length of posterior rectum; or (3) the Soave endorectal pull-through, which is the procedure preferred by this author (Figs 7.29–7.40).

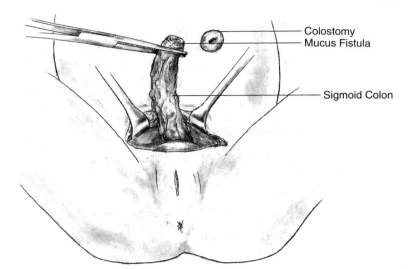

Figure 7.29 The transverse abdominal incision is re-entered and extended across the midline to the right. The mucus fistula is taken down and the distal sigmoid dissected free.

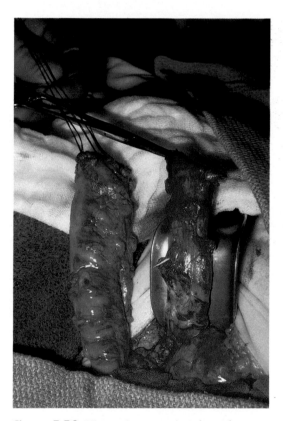

Figure 7.30 The colostomy is taken down, and the proximal end is sutured closed; the suture ends are left long. The closed colostomy and proximal ganglionated colon are seen on the left of this photograph; the mucus fistula and distal aganglionic sigmoid are on the right.

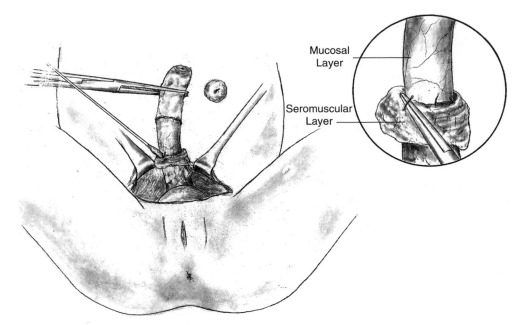

Mucosal
Layer

Seromuscular
Layer

Figure 7.31 Dissection of the mucosa from the rectal seromuscular cuff is illustrated. Injection of saline between the muscularis and the muscularis mucosae separates those layers prior to a circumferential seromuscular incision to begin the dissection. A cotton-tipped swab or small "peanut" aids in the separation of the layers.

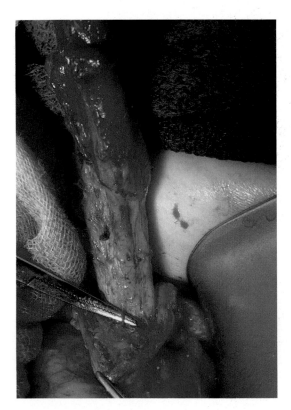

Figure 7.32 The mucosa of the distal colon and rectum is dissected from its seromuscular cuff in a 14-month-old boy. Small bridging vessels, as shown here and in the preceding drawing, are electrocoagulated.

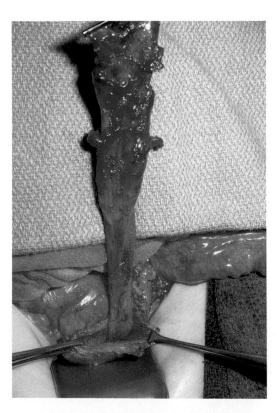

Figure 7.33 The circumferential mucosal dissection is carried distally to the level of the sphincter. Clamps hold the seromuscular cuff.

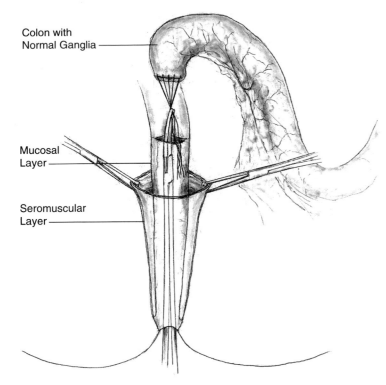

Colon with Normal Ganglia

Mucosal Layer

Seromuscular Layer

Figure 7.34 A long narrow hemostat is passed from the rectum into the mucosal sleeve. An incision in the mucosal sleeve allows the hemostat to grasp the sutures of the closed ganglionic bowel.

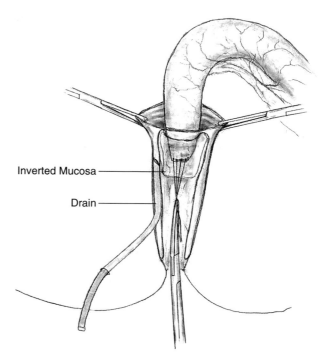

Inverted Mucosa

Drain

Figure 7.36 As the ganglionic colon is pulled through the seromuscular cuff, the mucosal sleeve—which remains after the more proximal aganglionic colon has been excised—is everted out the rectum.

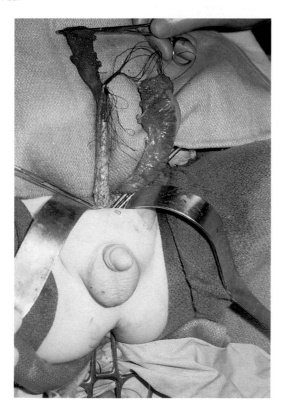

Figure 7.35 The procedure illustrated in Figure 7.34 is being performed. The ganglionic colon is on the right in the photograph. The sutures and colon will be pulled into the seromuscular cuff.

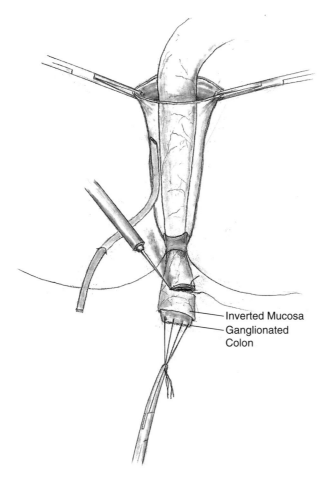

Inverted Mucosa
Ganglionated
Colon

Figure 7.37 The proximal colon is pulled through the seromuscular cuff, and the rectal mucosa is everted. The mucosal sleeve and pulled-through colon are divided with electrocautery approximately 1.5 cm from the anus. The first absorbable sutures of the anastomosis are placed before the division of the bowel is completed. A small rubber drain is placed in the space between the pulled-through colon and the cuff to prevent fluid accumulation and formation of a cuff abscess.

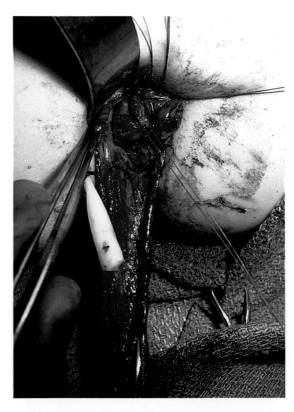

Figure 7.38 Several interrupted sutures are placed through the mucosal sleeve and the full thickness of ganglionic colon. The colon and the mucosal sleeve are not completely divided circumferentially.

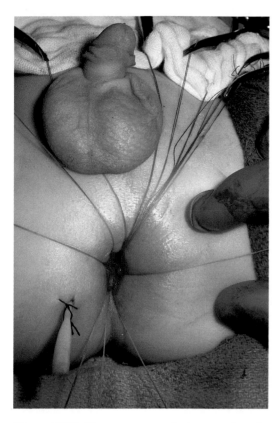

Figure 7.39 The anastomosis is completed with a single layer of sutures, after the excess colon and mucosal sleeve are excised. The anastomosis retracts, leaving a normal-appearing anus. The drain is left in place 3–5 days.

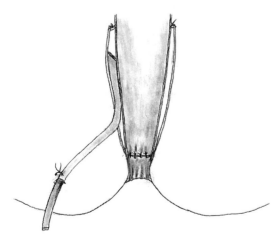

Figure 7.40 The completed anastomosis of ganglionated colon to distal rectal mucosa is shown.

Procedure for Total Colonic Agangliosis

Total colonic aganglionosis requires an ileal pull-through. Some surgeons perform a direct anastomosis of ileum to distal rectum, using one of the above-named procedures. Many pediatric surgeons prefer the Martin modification of the Duhamel procedure, a posterior pull-through with a long side-to-side ileocolic and ileorectal anastomosis; this procedure has proved most effective in relieving the obstruction, providing a reservoir for fecal storage, and maximizing intestinal fluid absorption. Because most of the significant maneuvers are intraabdominal or intrarectal and cannot be photographed adequately, the steps of the entire procedure are illustrated graphically (Figs 7.41–7.50).

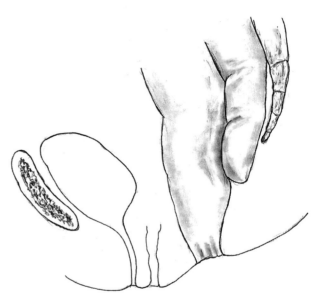

Figure 7.41 The patient is prepped and draped for an abdominoperineal procedure. The abdomen is opened, and the posterior peritoneal reflexion is incised. The surgeon's finger dissects a plane posterior to the entire length of the rectum, to the level of the internal sphincter.

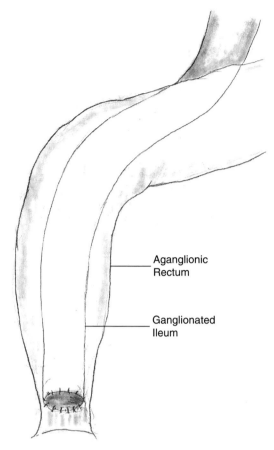

Aganglionic
Rectum

Ganglionated
Ileum

Figure 7.42 The ileostomy has been taken down, and the ileum is mobilized on its blood supply. An incision is then made from below in the posterior rectum, just proximal to the sphincter. The distal ileum is brought down through the posterior rectal plane, and a direct anastomosis of ileum to posterior rectum is performed. The anastomosis is shown from the anterior view.

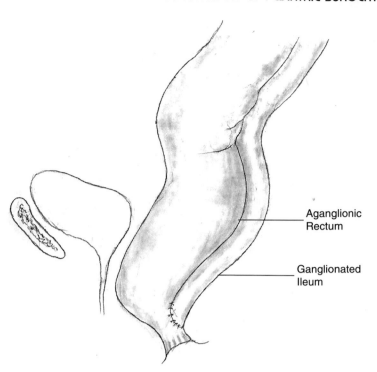

Aganglionic
Rectum

Ganglionated
Ileum

Figure 7.43 The position of the ganglionated ileal pull-through bowel and the distal ileorectal anastomosis are illustrated in lateral view.

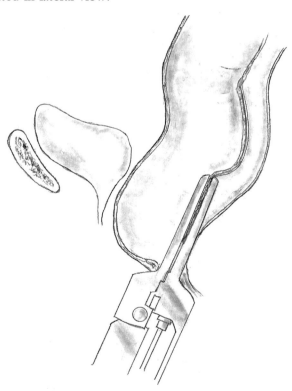

Figure 7.44 The blades of a GIA stapler are inserted carefully through the anus into the ileorectal anastomosis. One blade lies in the rectum, the other in the distal ileum. The stapler is fired, dividing the common wall and creating a long side-to-side anastomosis.

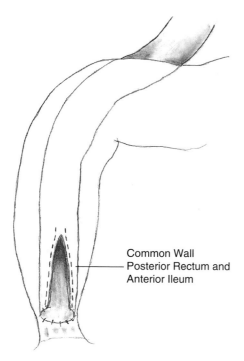

Common Wall
Posterior Rectum and
Anterior Ileum

Figure 7.45 The ileorectal anastomosis, with a row of fine staples on either side of the incision, is seen from the anterior view.

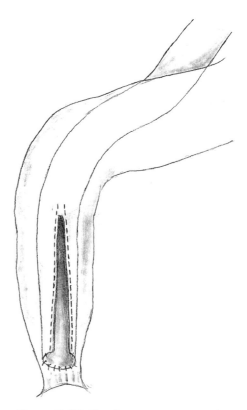

Figure 7.47 The longer anastomosis of ileum to sigmoid and rectum is shown from the anterior aspect in this drawing.

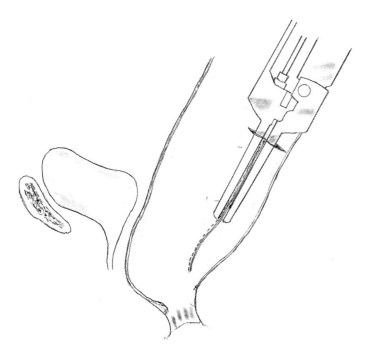

Figure 7.46 An incision is made in the posterior (aganglionic) sigmoid colon and the anterior ileum. The blades of the anastomotic stapler are inserted on either side of the common bowel wall, and the stapler is fired, extending the anastomosis.

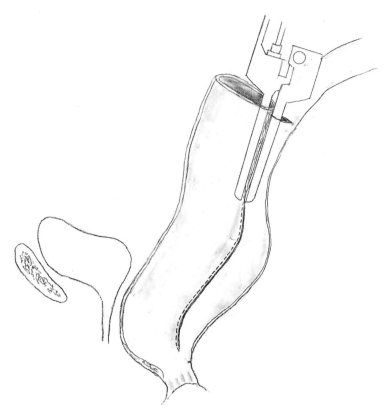

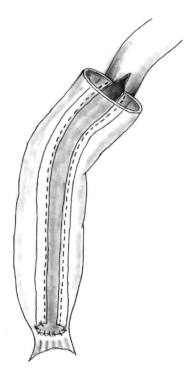

Figure 7.48 The blades of the stapler are placed through the open end of the divided colon, usually at the level of the mid or proximal sigmoid, and an incision in the anterior ileum. The common wall is again divided between rows of staples. It is important to be sure there are no undivided "bridges" between each stapled anastomosis.

Some pediatric surgeons advocate a definitive, one-stage procedure in newborns with Hirschsprung's disease, with no preliminary diverting colostomy. For surgeons who perform an endorectal pull-through, the mucosal dissection is reported to be easier in infants than in older children. This operation is a reasonable alternative to the two-stage procedure, if the proximal ganglionated bowel is not so dilated as to preclude being pulled through the rectum. The new technique of primary pull-through with preliminary laparoscopic dissection of the colon is illustrated in Chapter 8.

Figure 7.49 The completed long anastomosis is depicted in this drawing.

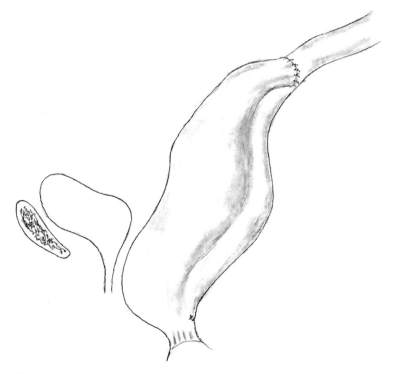

Figure 7.50 The proximal colon is anastomosed with sutures to the ileal incision, completing the long side-to-side anastomosis.

Meconium Plug Syndrome

An inspissated plug of meconium in the rectum of a newborn infant may produce intestinal obstruction similar to that of Hirschsprung's disease (Fig 7.51). This obstruction is relieved with a simple saline, or soluble contrast, enema (Fig 7.52).

A small percentage of infants with meconium plug syndrome have Hirschsprung's disease and should be observed for signs of bowel difficulties if a contrast enema fails to confirm that diagnosis in infancy. Routine rectal biopsy of all infants with meconium plug syndrome is *not* recommended.

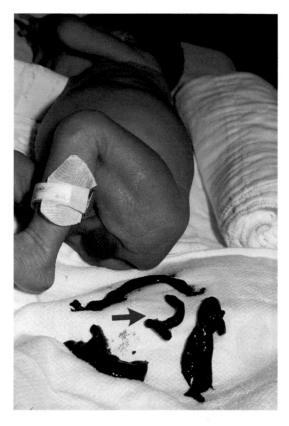

Figure 7.52 A large plug of inspissated meconium *(arrow)*, followed by copious normal meconium, is washed out by a diatrizoate (Hypaque) enema. The infant has no other intestinal problems.

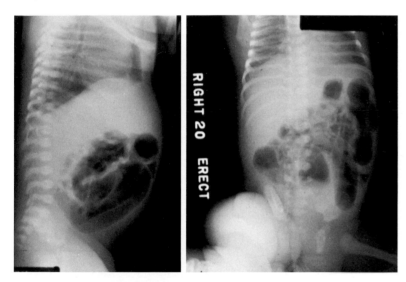

Figure 7.51 The anteroposterior and lateral radiographs of this neonate's abdomen show multiple air-filled loops, indicative of a low intestinal obstruction.

Intestinal Polyps

Bleeding and intussusception are the two primary presentations of intestinal polyps in childhood. Single pedunculated polyps are usually termed *juvenile, retention,* or *inflammatory* polyps; the etiology is unknown. They are not premalignant. Blood streaking on the stool is usually the first sign. If sigmoidoscopy fails to show the polyp, then a contrast enema may do so (Fig 7.53).

Colonic polyps on a stalk may slough spontaneously, with or without significant bleeding from the base. Others may be removed through a colonoscope, or surgically when identified as the lead-point of an intussusception. Some present at the anus for simple excision (Fig 7.54). Sessile polyps (Figs 7.55, 7.56) are less common in children and require surgical excision (Fig 7.57). Multiple polyposis associated with melanotic spots of the lips and oral mucous membranes constitutes the Peutz-Jeghers syndrome. Only familial adenomatous polyposis has a known premalignant potential, for which total colectomy or subtotal colectomy, with ileal endorectal pull-through similar to that for Hirschsprung's disease, is recommended (Figs 7.58, 7.59).

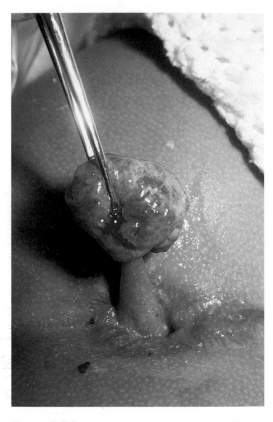

Figure 7.54 This rectal polyp on a stalk is typical of the retention polyp seen in children. It is easier to remove than most.

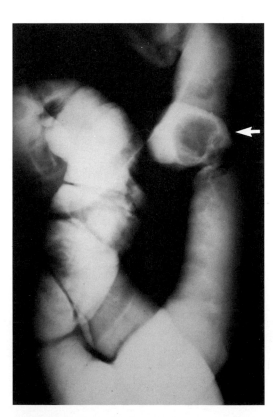

Figure 7.53 A polyp *(arrow)* just distal to the splenic flexure is seen on barium enema.

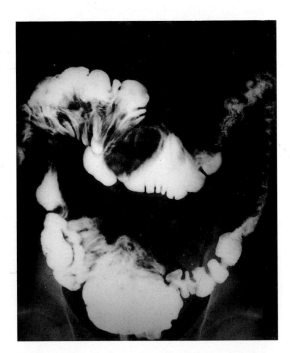

Figure 7.55 This student was given psychotherapy for "school problems" because of recurrent attacks of crampy abdominal pain. The barium enema study demonstrates an ileocolic intussusception.

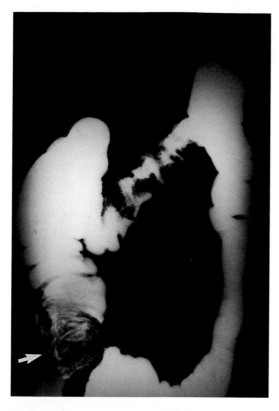

Figure 7.56 A filling defect is seen in the cecum, following reduction of the intussusception.

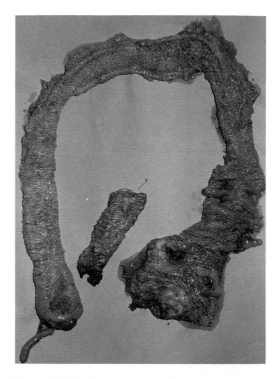

Figure 7.58 The operative specimen of a subtotal colectomy for familial polyposis is seen. The entire colon is involved.

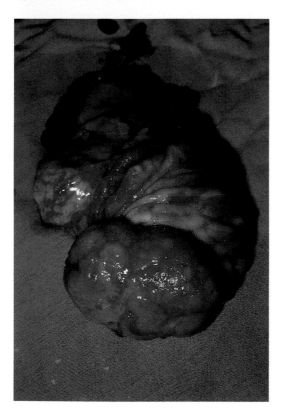

Figure 7.57 The resected cecal mass, a benign sessile polyp, is shown at surgery.

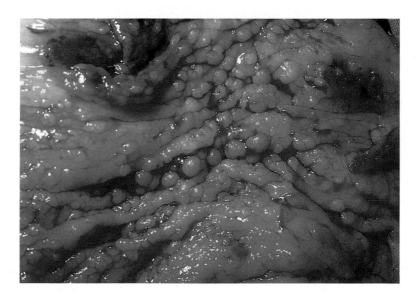

Figure 7.59 There are many adenomatous polyps of varying size seen in this close-up of a portion of the left colon.

Appendicitis

Acute appendicitis is one of the most common problems that bring children to surgery. It may also be one of the most difficult clinical diagnoses in the pediatric age group. The typical history and the classic findings on examination are not found in all children. Other clues to diagnosis may be needed, such as the child's stooped walk, reluctance to hop on one foot, or involuntary flexion of the thigh onto the abdomen.

Point tenderness, involuntary muscular guarding, and rebound tenderness referred to the right side of the lower abdomen are the principal findings—when they can be elicited. The child younger than 6 years of age, if frightened or unable to cooperate, will be easier to examine following mild sedation. Localized tenderness on rectal examination is highly significant, but the unhappy response of many children to this examination makes interpretation difficult.

There is often low-grade fever. Moderate leukocytosis with a predominance of polymorphonuclear leukocytes, and an increased percentage of band forms, is common but is not invariable. Radiographs are helpful only when they demonstrate a fecalith (Fig 7.60) or an appendiceal abscess (Fig 7.61)—certain indications for surgery.

If preoperative findings indicate the possibility of a gangrenous or perforated appendicitis, administration of intravenous antibiotics is begun, to cover gram-negative and anaerobic organisms. The author prefers aminoglycoside and clindamycin, or cefoxitin alone (intravenous aminoglycoside 7.5 mg/kg/d and clindamycin 40 mg/kg/d, or cefoxitin 100–150 mg/kg/d). Correction of dehydration and electrolyte abnormalities must be carried out and high fever should be brought down prior to the induction of anesthesia.

The preferred approach is a transverse (Rockey-Davis) abdominal incision, which can be extended to, or across, the midline if further intraperitoneal exposure is required. Removal of the appendix can almost always be accomplished, even in the presence of an appendiceal abscess. Cultures of gross pus or cloudy peritoneal fluid are obtained; none are needed for uncomplicated appendicitis.

Using an appropriate antibiotic regimen for gangrenous (Fig 7.62) or perforated (Fig 7.63) appendicitis, the author closes all incisions primarily, with complication rates only slightly higher than for uncomplicated appendicitis.

Intraperitoneal drains are placed only for localized intra-abdominal abscesses. If aminoglycoside is prescribed, serum peak and trough levels of the antibiotic, as well as blood urea nitrogen and serum creatinine levels, should be determined at regular intervals, both to ensure adequate therapeutic antibiotic levels and to avoid renal toxicity from excessive drug levels.

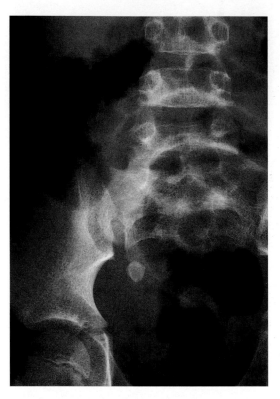

Figure 7.60 Appendicitis The fecalith seen in the right lower abdomen of this boy with abdominal pain is sufficient evidence to prompt appendectomy.

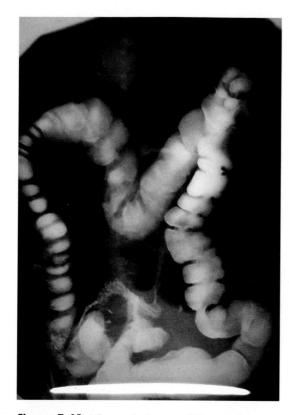

Figure 7.61 The radiolucent filling defect next to the barium-filled cecum is an appendiceal abscess. Signs of intestinal obstruction were the reason for performance of the barium enema.

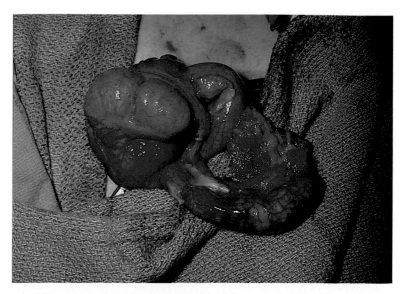

Figure 7.62 Areas of dark discoloration in this inflamed appendix indicate a gangrenous appendicitis.

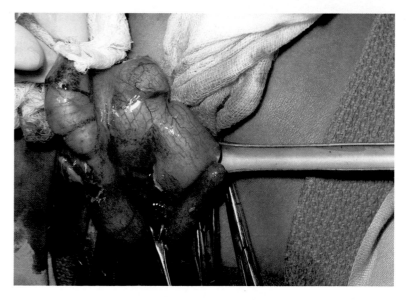

Figure 7.63 There is a frank perforation in the wall of this appendix, near its base. The fecalith seen in Figure 7.60 lies free in the abdomen.

Because appendicitis occurs frequently, many surgeons perform an incidental appendectomy at surgery for other, noninflammatory problems. The author uses the technique of inversion appendectomy (Figs 7.64–7.66) to avoid contamination of an otherwise ''clean'' operative field.

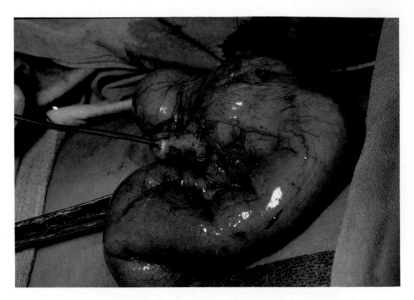

Figure 7.65 All but 1.5 cm of the appendix is inverted into the cecum. A heavy (0 to 2-0) ligature of plain catgut is then tied tightly at the base of the appendix to occlude its circulation.

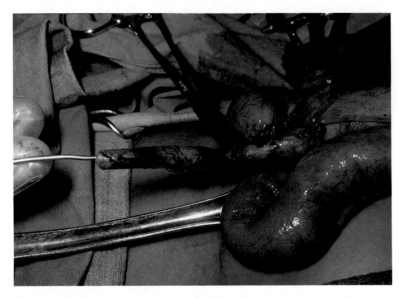

Figure 7.64 Inversion of the Appendix The mesentery is dissected and vessels are divided close to the appendix. The tip is squeezed for several minutes to facilitate inversion with a blunt-tipped probe.

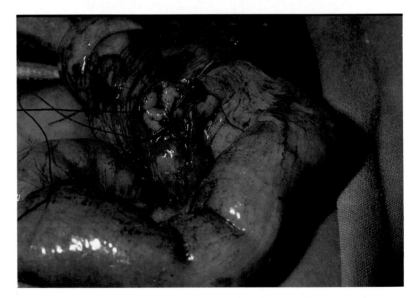

Figure 7.66 The appendix is completely inverted, and a nonabsorbable pursestring suture is tied to complete the procedure. The appendix sloughs and appears in the stool in 5–7 days.

Inflammatory Bowel Disease

Surgery is indicated for the complications of inflammatory bowel disease (ulcerative colitis, Crohn's disease). Colectomy and ileostomy are indicated for ulcerative colitis that progresses to uncontrolled bleeding, toxic dilatation of the colon, perforation, systemic sepsis, or growth retardation (Figs 7.67–7.69). Prolonged, active ulcerative colitis may lead to colonic malignancy in adult life. If the rectum can be preserved and the rectal mucosal disease can be healed, an endorectal ileal pull-through with proximal pouch reservoir will provide appliance-free continence.

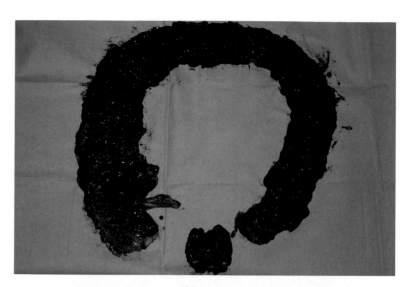

Figure 7.68 The opened specimen of her colon shows hemorrhagic mucosal ulceration throughout.

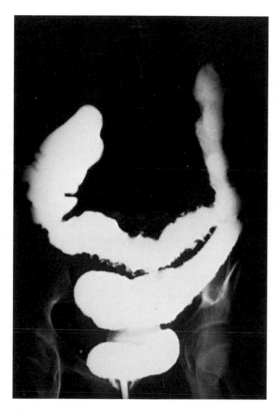

Figure 7.67 Ulcerative Colitis The barium enema findings of mucosal involvement of almost the entire colon are consistent with the explosive bloody diarrhea and rapid clinical deterioration of this 13-year-old girl with ulcerative colitis.

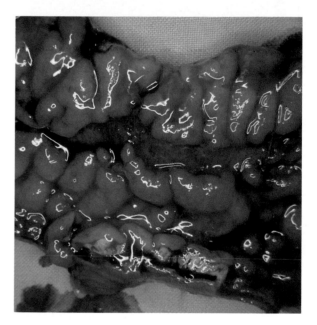

Figure 7.69 This close-up of the urgently removed colon of another patient shows the deep ulcerations and pseudopolyp formation characteristic of the disease.

Crohn's disease of the small or large intestine may result in obstructive stricture, enteroenteral and enterocutaneous fistulas, abscess formation, and failure to grow or mature. Resective surgery of the most seriously involved intestine does not ''cure'' the disease, but it may give a chance for successful suppression of residual disease by medical therapy (Figs 7.70–7.74).

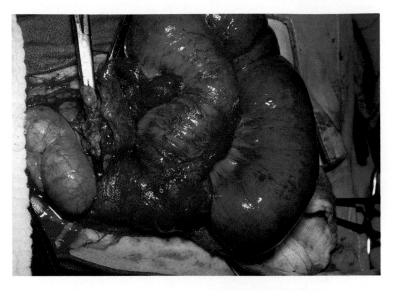

Figure 7.71 At surgery, there is inflammation of the terminal ileum, thickening and adherence of the mesentery, and an abscess adherent to the bladder.

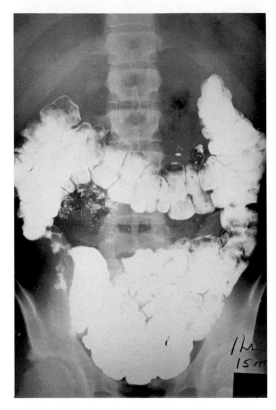

Figure 7.70 Crohn's Disease Severe localized stenosis and partial obstruction of the terminal ileum accompany symptoms of recurrent pain, fever, and weight loss and warrant ileal resection in this boy of 14.

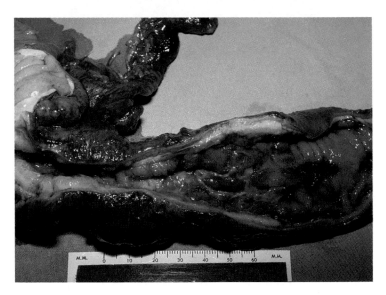

Figure 7.72 The resection specimen has thick fibrotic walls and severe narrowing.

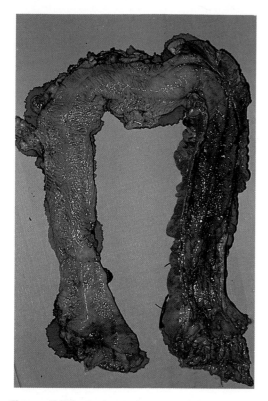

Figure 7.73 Crohn's disease of the colon, formerly termed "granulomatous colitis," is also amenable to resection in some cases.

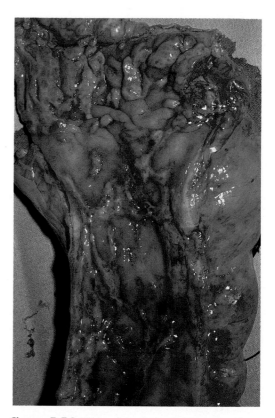

Figure 7.74 This close-up of the operative specimen shows longitudinal ulceration and submucosal granuloma formation and fibrosis.

Necrotizing Enterocolitis

Developing in stressed premature—and some full-term—neonates, necrotizing enterocolitis has no clear etiology. It produces mucosal inflammation and necrosis of the small and large intestine. The presenting signs are those of abdominal distention and mucoid diarrhea, frequently with blood. Some cases resolve on gastric decompression and parenteral antibiotics. Progression may lead to focal or extensive intestinal infarction and perforation, the complications that require urgent surgical intervention. Intestinal stricture is a late complication of healed enterocolitis, and resection may be indicated. Transluminal balloon-catheter dilatation, through an established enterostomy, is a technique that has been used successfully for some structures.

The premature newborn who develops bloody mucoid stools and a distended abdomen is likely to have necrotizing enterocolitis. Initial therapy consists of nasogastric decompression, fluid resuscitation and maintenance, and intravenous antibiotics. The development of abdominal-wall erythematous or bluish discoloration (Fig 7.75), abdominal tenderness, metabolic acidosis, and progressive thrombocytopenia are signs of intestinal compromise. The presence of subserosal gas (pneumatosis intestinalis) on abdominal radiographs confirms the diagnosis (Fig 7.76). Subsequent films may show (1) portal venous gas (Fig 7.77), not necessarily an ominous sign; (2) a fixed, dilated loop of intestine indicative of gangrene; or (3) pneumoperitoneum secondary to intestinal perforation. Resection of frankly gangrenous bowel and exteriorization of the viable proximal and distal ends are the objects of surgery (Fig 7.78). Extensive involvement, especially of small intestine, may require excision of only the clearly devitalized bowel and a "second-look" operation within 24 hours, at which time the demarcation between viable and necrotic intestine will be clearer. Despite adequate surgical therapy, many infants with this serious problem do not survive.

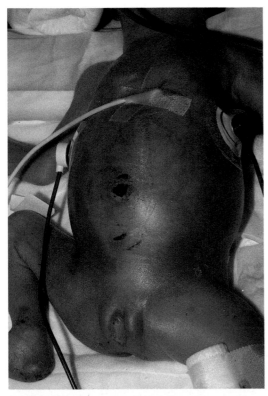

Figure 7.75 Necrotizing Enterocolitis The distention and bluish discoloration of the abdomen in this premature neonate are signs of possible intestinal gangrene.

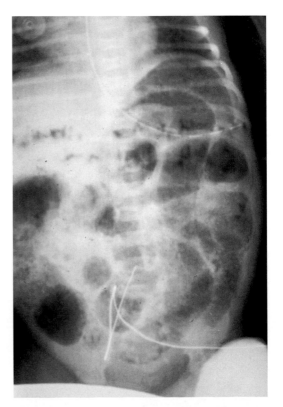

Figure 7.76 Subserosal gas (pneumatosis intestinalis) on the abdominal radiograph is characteristic of necrotizing enterocolitis.

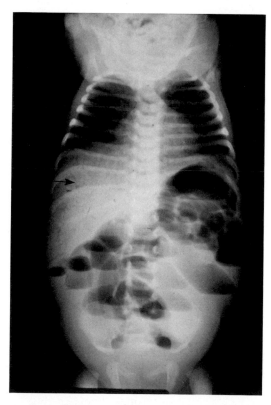

Figure 7.77 Gas in the portal venous system can be seen in the liver of this infant.

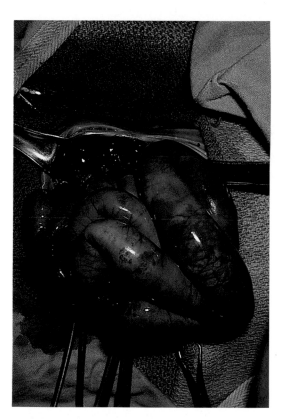

Figure 7.78 Gangrenous intestine is found at exploration of the abdomen of the infant in Figure 7.75. It is resected, with a successful outcome in this case.

Imperforate Anus and Rectal Fistula

Imperforate anus is a visual diagnosis: there is no anal opening in the normal position, and there may be an abnormal opening elsewhere—perineum, scrotum, vaginal fourchette, vaginal canal, urethra, or bladder (Figs 7.79–7.82). Ascertaining the level at which the bowel ends—a "high" or a "low" imperforate anus—determines the need for an immediate colostomy or the possibility of perineal repair. So that swallowed air can get to the rectum for diagnostic radiographs (Figs 7.83, 7.84), nasogastric decompression is delayed until 8 hours after birth. Some pediatric surgeons perform a colostomy on all infants who do not have a situation clearly amenable to perineal repair, such as a low fistula or membranous "covered anus."

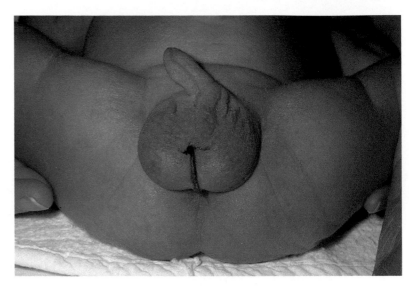

Figure 7.80 A meconium-filled rectal fistula tracts anteriorly along the medial raphe of the scrotum.

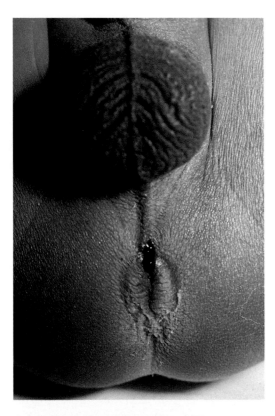

Figure 7.79 Imperforate Anus This male infant has an imperforate anus with a tiny perineal fistula in which meconium can be seen. Only skin covers the very low rectal pouch, in what some call a "covered anus."

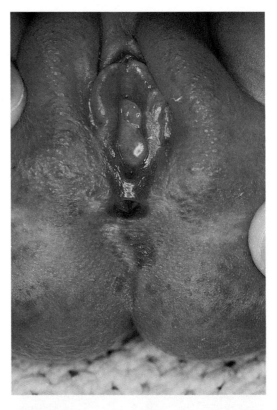

Figure 7.81 A perineal fistula, just posterior to the vagina, is present. A low imperforate anus with external rectal fistula—to the perineal skin or the vaginal fourchette—is the most common situation in girls.

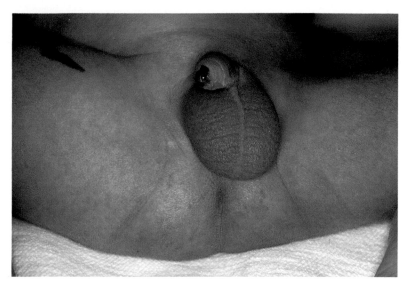

Figure 7.82 Meconium and a bubble of air are seen at the urethral meatus of this infant boy. Most boys have a high imperforate anus, with or without a patent fistula to the urethra or bladder.

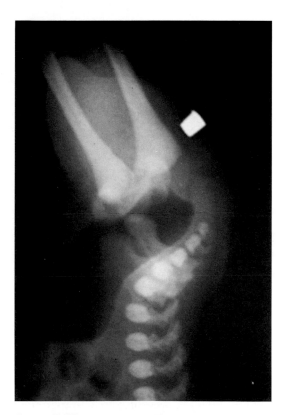

Figure 7.83 This lateral film of the inverted baby at 6 hours of age shows a distance of more than 2 cm from the bowel to the anal marker. The air has not yet displaced all the distal meconium.

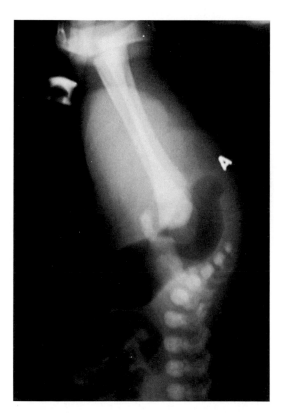

Figure 7.84 A radiograph of the same infant at 24 hours of age shows the bowel within 1 cm of the anus—a situation amenable to perineal anoplasty, with an expected good result.

Other congenital anomalies commonly associated with
imperforate anus include those of the urinary and gastrointestinal tracts. At birth, the simple passage of a catheter
into the newborn's stomach ensures the absence of
esophageal atresia; no newborn should be turned head-
down for radiographic studies until this maneuver has
been performed (see Fig 4.66). Aspiration of a large
volume (more than 35 ml) of gastric contents should
raise suspicion of more proximal intestinal obstruction.
Abdominal sonography for screening may be followed by
intravenous pyelography and cystourethrography, as indicated, for urinary tract evaluation.

A perineal or fourchette fistula generally indicates a
low imperforate anus, amenable to perineal repair (Figs
7.85–7.89). For a high imperforate anus—or a complicated anomaly, such as a cloaca or exstrophy of the
bladder—an initial divided colostomy decompresses the
intestine (Fig 7.90). The timing of definitive repair, at 6
months to 1 year of age, is determined by the specific
anomaly and the size and health of the baby.

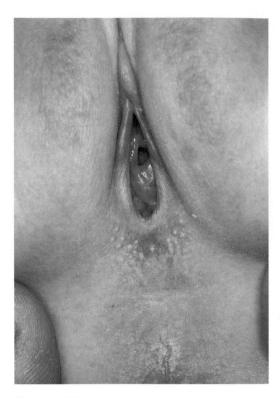

Figure 7.86 This female infant has a rectal
fistula into the vaginal fourchette, posterior
to the hymenal ring.

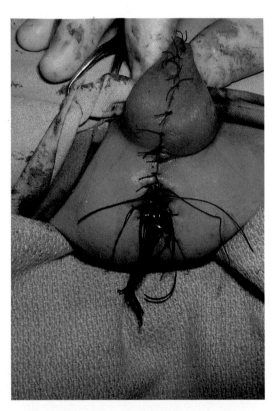

Figure 7.85 The scrotal fistula (see Fig
7.80) is excised, and the bowel is dissected
free and sutured to the skin. Great care is
taken to identify the subcutaneous (external) sphincter and to bring the bowel
through the center of it, without damage
to the muscle. The definitive perineal operation is performed early, in this case when
the infant is 1 day of age.

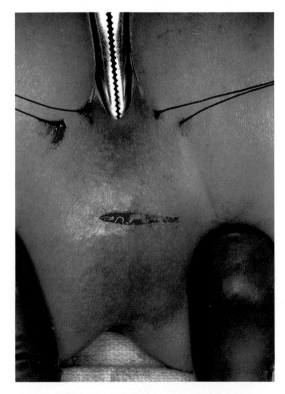

Figure 7.87 A hemostat inserted into the
fourchette fistula demonstrates the bowel
just beneath the skin. An incision is made
at the anal dimple, at the site of the external sphincter.

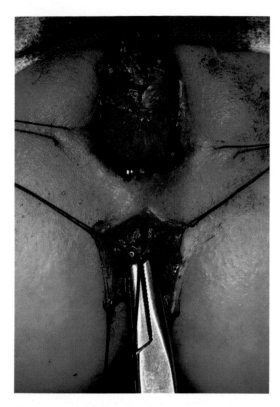

Figure 7.88 The fistula is dissected free; it sometimes requires great care to separate the fistula from the vaginal wall. A hemostat is passed in the subcutaneous tissue anteriorly, through the center of the sphincter muscle, to grasp the multiple traction sutures placed around the fistula opening.

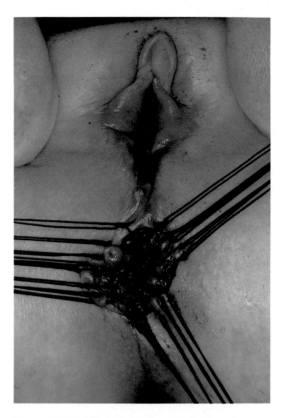

Figure 7.89 The fistula is withdrawn into the anal incision, is trimmed or opened as needed, and is sutured to the skin circumferentially to form a new anus.

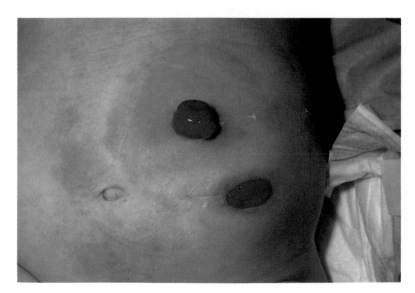

Figure 7.90 A diverting colostomy is created in the infant with a high imperforate anus or a complex anomaly. This girl has a persistent cloaca, with only one visible opening for urethra, vagina, and rectal fistula.

Repair of High Imperforate Anus

The object of repair is to bring the bowel through whatever control muscles are present and to have it exit on the perineal skin with a normal appearance. The association of a myelomeningocele or the absence of a well-defined natal cleft—termed a "rocker-bottom"—makes it unlikely that functional control muscle is present; these patients require more extensive neuromuscular evaluation to determine whether they are candidates for anoplasty.

The Peña-DeVries posterior sagittal rectoanoplasty has become the preferred procedure for repair of high imperforate anus. It gives exposure of the entire control muscle mechanism and allows careful closure of an associated anterior fistula or mobilization and repair of the components of a cloacal anomaly (Figs 7.91–7.107).

Text continued on page 205

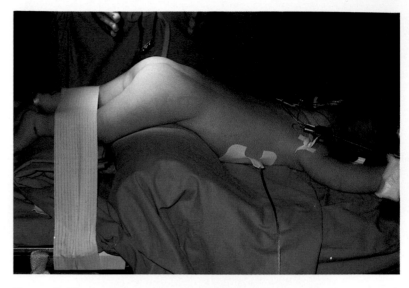

Figure 7.92 For the posterior sagittal repair, the patient is placed prone with the pelvis over a well-padded, elevated kidney rest.

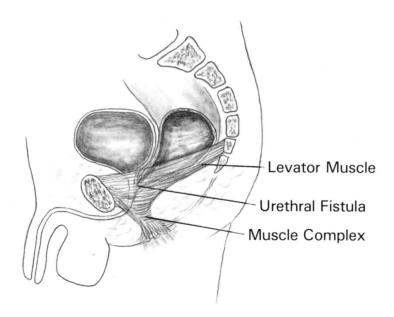

Figure 7.91 This drawing of a sagittal pelvic cross-section illustrates a high imperforate anus with a narrow fistula into the urethra, the transverse levator muscle, and the funnel of muscle—the "muscle complex"—that extends from the levator to the subcutaneous (external) sphincter at the anal dimple.

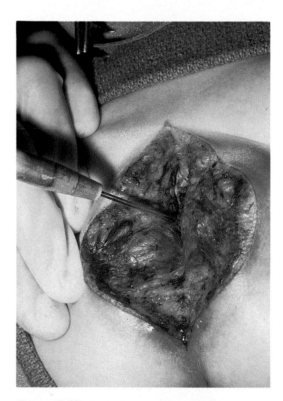

Figure 7.93 The dissection is carried out with a needle-tipped electrocautery; the skin is incised, and the muscle is split exactly in the midline, from the level of the fifth sacral vertebra to a point 2–3 cm anterior to the anal dimple. Before the incision is made, and during the entire dissection, the location and function of the muscles are confirmed with a bipolar nerve stimulator, as seen here; stimulation through the skin requires close to 200 mA, and direct muscle contact only 60–75 mA.

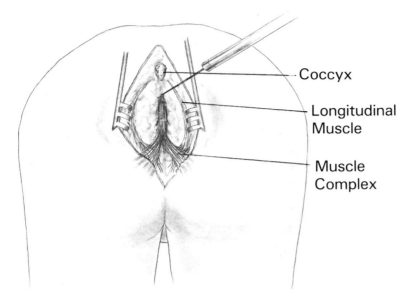

Coccyx

Longitudinal
Muscle

Muscle
Complex

Figure 7.94 The longitudinal subcutaneous muscle, and the vertical muscle complex that interdigitates with it, are split in the midline to the level of the levator.

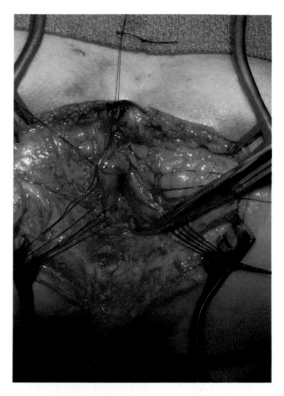

Figure 7.96 The bowel is found deep to the levator. It is opened vertically, and fine silk traction sutures are placed around the entire open margin. The tip of the hemostat points to the opening of the rectourethral fistula.

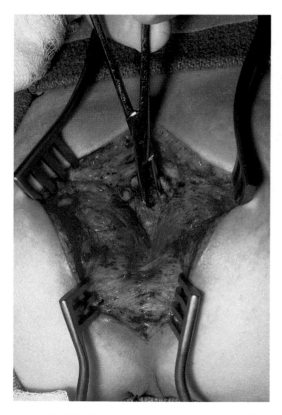

Figure 7.95 The cartilaginous coccyx is divided in the midline, and a right-angle hemostat is placed deep to the posterior portion of the levator to expose it. The levator is divided in the midline.

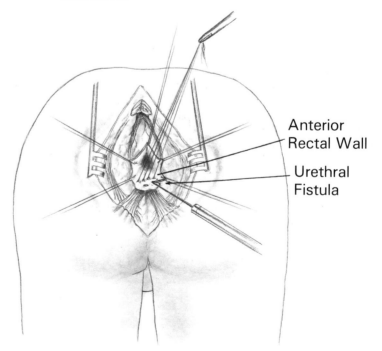

Anterior
Rectal Wall

Urethral
Fistula

Figure 7.97 A row of fine sutures is placed in the mucosa of the anterior bowel wall, just proximal to the urethral fistula. With traction on the sutures, the mucosa and the bowel wall are freed from the urethra and prostate by meticulous cautery dissection. Interrupted sutures then close the fistula.

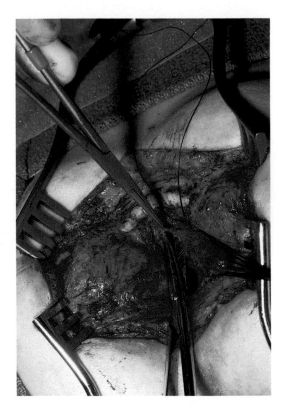

Figure 7.98 The lateral bowel wall is dissected free. Numerous vascular bands to the intestinal wall are identified, electrocoagulated, and divided, as shown here. The bowel is mobilized in this manner to the level of the peritoneal reflection, giving maximal length for the reconstruction.

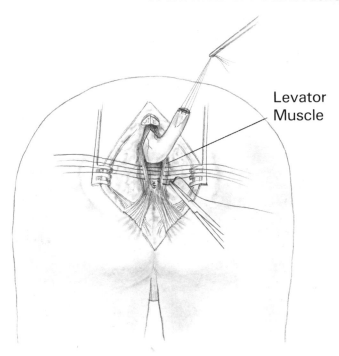

Figure 7.100 The edges of the levator are then approximated. The tapered bowel is then placed deep to the levator, and the sutures are tied. The anteriormost suture is left long as a marker.

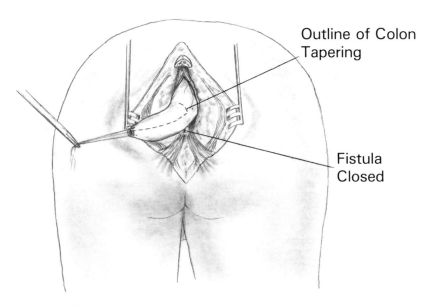

Figure 7.99 In most cases, the rectal segment must be tapered so it may lie completely within the muscle complex. The dotted line shows the portion to be removed for tapering.

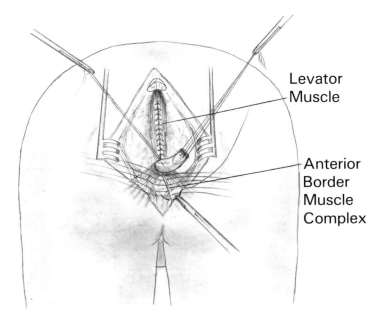

Figure 7.101 Sutures are passed carefully through the anterior edges of the two sides of the vertical muscle complex. When all are placed and proper alignment is ensured, they are tied.

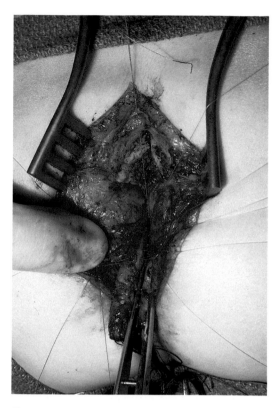

Figure 7.102 The tapered rectum is then placed within the muscle complex. Individual sutures are passed through the posterior edge of the muscle complex on one side, a seromuscular bite of rectal wall, and the opposing posterior edge of the muscle complex. Forceps between the rectum and the right wall of the muscle complex show the sutures in place.

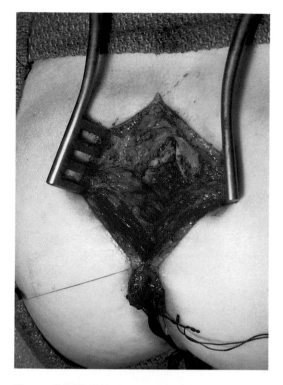

Figure 7.103 All the posterior sutures are tied. The rectum now comes to the skin entirely within the vertical muscle complex, giving the best chance for future control.

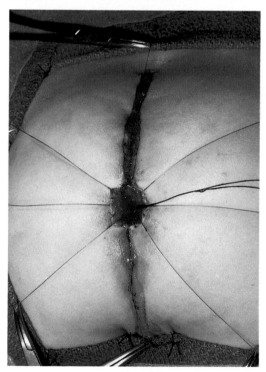

Figure 7.104 The procedure is completed with trimming of any excess rectum, circumferential suturing of full-thickness bowel to the skin (anoplasty), approximation of the subcutaneous longitudinal muscle, and subcuticular closure of the incision.

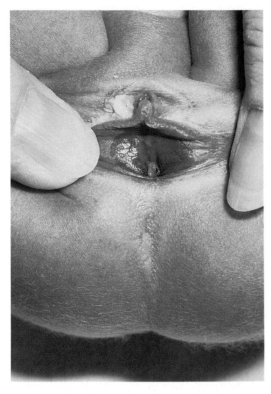

Figure 7.105 Cloaca This infant girl with an imperforate anus has only one opening for the urethra, vagina, and rectovaginal fistula.

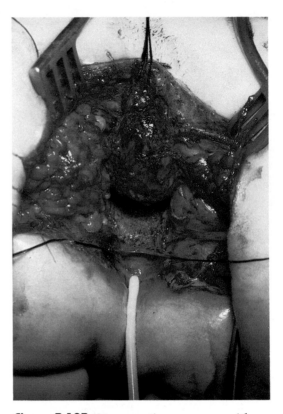

Figure 7.107 At corrective surgery, with the posterior sagittal Peña-DeVries approach, the rectum is mobilized in the posterior part of the dissection, the vaginal opening is seen, and there is a catheter in the urethral orifice. In this case, the urethral meatus is close enough to the perineum that it is not repaired.

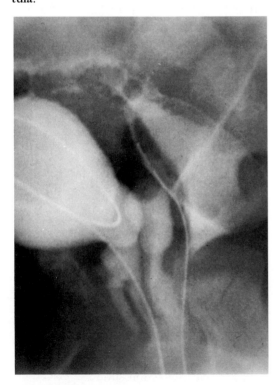

Figure 7.106 A contrast radiograph of the cloaca shows the rectum and rectovaginal fistula posteriorly (to the right as shown here), the vagina centrally, and the bladder and duplicate urethras anteriorly. Only one urethra opens into the perineum.

Anal Stenosis

The properly placed anus that is congenitally stenotic may require repeated gentle dilatation to allow normal passage of stools. Surgical anoplasty is rarely indicated.

Anal Fissure

The most common cause of blood in the stool in infancy is anal fissure, a split in the anal mucosa from stretching—usually after a hard or bulky stool. When the stool is kept soft and easy to pass, warm sitz baths and topical anesthetics aid in spontaneous healing. Simple excision is reserved for chronic fissures that do not heal (Fig 7.108).

Anal Fistula

The appearance of a small abscess next to the infant anus is the first sign of an anocutaneous fistula. Originating in an anal crypt, the inflammatory process tracts to the skin. The abscess may require surgical drainage, or it may drain spontaneously after warm compresses or baths. When a chronic fistula tract has become established, purulent drainage recurs. Antibiotics are of little help. Excision, or surgical unroofing and curetting, of the tract is curative (Figs 7.109, 7.110). Development of an anal fistula in an older child should raise the possibility of Crohn's disease of the rectum.

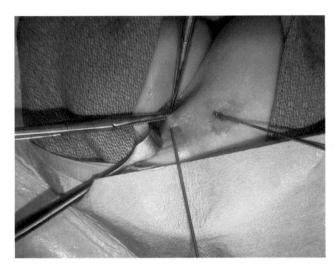

Figure 7.109 A probe is placed in each of two anal fistulas in this infant.

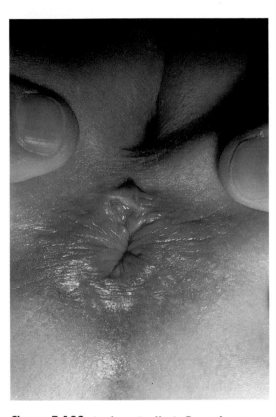

Figure 7.108 A chronically inflamed anterior anal fissure in this girl requires surgical excision.

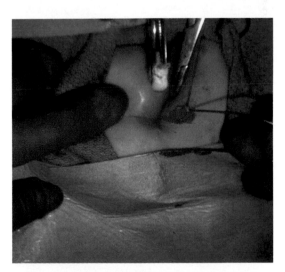

Figure 7.110 A traction suture is placed in the cutaneous end of the fistula tract, and the tract is dissected free along the length of the probe. The anorectal mucosa is closed with an absorbable suture; the lateral part of the skin incision is left open, for drainage, and heals rapidly.

Chapter 8

Laparoscopic and Thoracoscopic Procedures in Pediatric Surgery

Thom E Lobe, M.D.

In the late 1980s, a virtual revolution occurred in general surgery after which the number and variety of endoscopic, minimally invasive procedures performed increased dramatically. Although pediatric surgeons were slower to adopt some of these procedures into their practices, sufficient time has now passed to allow us to determine which of these endoscopic procedures are suitable for surgery on infants and children.

Laparoscopy

Inguinal Exploration

Infants and children with unilateral symptomatic inguinal hernias can now undergo safe and accurate exploration of the contralateral groin using laparoscopic techniques. The patients are usually anesthetized under general anesthesia using endotracheal intubation. The stomach is emptied with a suction catheter, and the bladder is emptied by a Credé maneuver. The symptomatic side is explored in the normal open fashion, and the hernia sac is dissected free from the cord structures and divided. A 4-mm laparoscopic cannula is passed into the peritoneal cavity via the hernia sac and is secured in position with a 2-0 silk suture to prevent it from slipping. The abdomen is then insufflated with carbon dioxide (CO_2) to a pressure of 8–10 torr, a 70° telescope (that usually used for bronchoscopy) is passed into the peritoneal cavity via the cannula, and the peritoneal aspect of the contralateral internal inguinal ring is inspected. In the normal male patient, the vas deferens and spermatic vessels can be seen passing through the internal ring, where it can be determined either that there is no hernia defect (Fig 8.1) or that there is an obvious hernia (Fig 8.2).

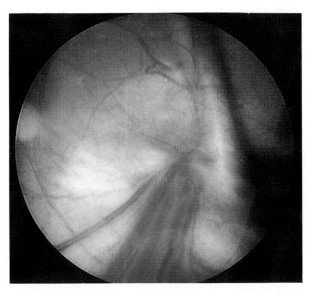

Figure 8.1 Normal Internal Ring A normal left internal inguinal ring is inspected laparoscopically from a right-sided hernia sac.

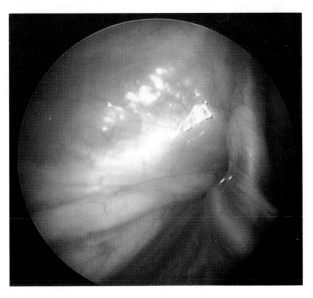

Figure 8.2 Hernia Defect An asymptomatic defect in the left internal inguinal ring is visualized laparoscopically from the right.

When no hernia is found, the CO_2 is evacuated and the ipsilateral hernia repair is completed. When a contralateral hernia is discovered, it is repaired in the normal (open) fashion after completing the repair of the symptomatic side.

Undescended Testes

Many surgeons believe the best way to assess a nonpalpable testis is to perform a laparoscopic exploration. For these cases, the patient is anesthetized using general anesthesia with endotracheal intubation. The stomach and bladder are emptied as described previously, and the abdomen is insufflated with CO_2 to a pressure of 10–12 torr using either a Veress needle inserted through a small umbilical stab wound or a 4- or 5-mm cannula inserted under direct vision via an enlarged umbilical stab wound. In either case, a cannula is inserted into the abdomen at the umbilicus. Some patients have a small umbilical hernia defect through which the cannula can be passed, which avoids the use of the blind, Veress needle technique. The patient is placed in Trendelenburg position and a 0° telescope is inserted to inspect the abdomen for the presence of an intraabdominal testis (Fig 8.3). One can generally see whether the vas deferens and/or the spermatic vessels end blindly or whether there is a testicle hiding just inside the internal inguinal ring (Fig 8.4).

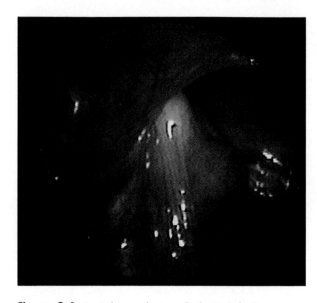

Figure 8.4 A right undescended testicle is seen high in the inguinal canal, at the internal ring, in another child.

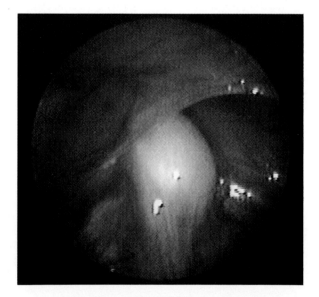

Figure 8.3 Undescended Testis A right undescended testicle is noted to be predominantly within the abdomen at the internal inguinal ring.

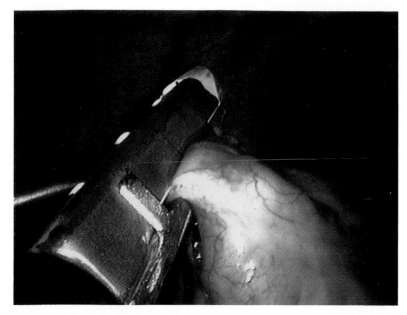

Figure 8.10 The endoscopic stapler transects the appendix at its junction with the cecum.

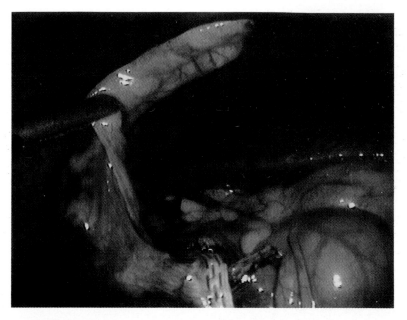

Figure 8.12 The freed appendix is held by an endoscopic grasper and will be removed through the 12-mm, left lower quadrant cannula.

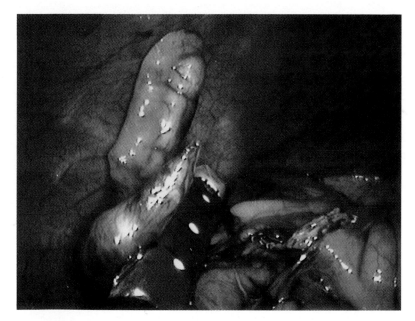

Figure 8.11 The mesoappendix is transected with the endoscopic stapler after the appendix has been divided.

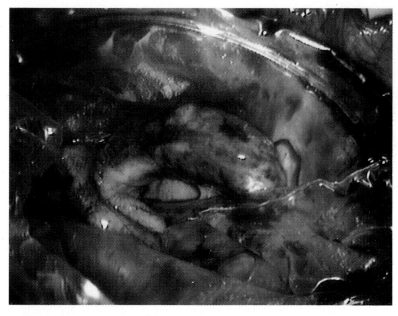

Figure 8.13 In this case, the freed appendix is placed in the opening of an endoscopic pouch before removal through the left lower quadrant trocar site.

Meckel's Diverticulum

A Meckel's diverticulum may be found as an incidental finding at laparoscopy (Fig 8.14) or as the source of inflammation or acute bleeding (see Chapter 6). Laparoscopic resection at the base of the diverticulum with an endoscopic stapler can be achieved in most cases (Fig 8.15).

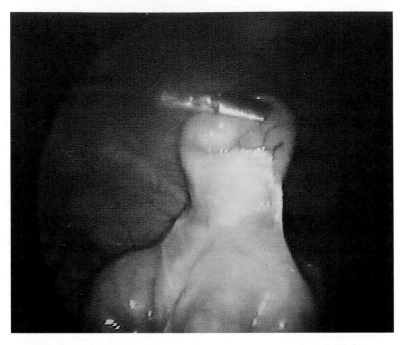

Figure 8.14 Meckel's Diverticulum This Meckel's diverticulum was an incidental finding at laparoscopy. (Courtesy of Steven Stylianos, M.D.)

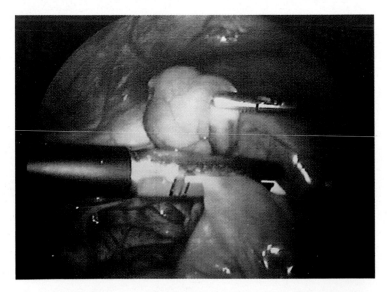

Figure 8.15 With the diverticulum held by a grasper placed through a left lower abdominal port, the endoscopic stapler is applied across the base for resection. (Courtesy of Steven Stylianos, M.D.)

Cholecystectomy

Now a standard of care in adult general surgery, laparoscopic cholecystectomy is being performed by increasing numbers of pediatric surgeons.

The child is anesthetized under general anesthesia, the stomach is emptied with a tube, and the bladder is emptied either by a Credé maneuver or by catheterization with a Foley catheter. Access is usually gained via an umbilical stab wound with direct placement of a 10-mm umbilical cannula for insertion of the telescope. Three additional cannulae are inserted: a 10-mm cannula is inserted either in the midline below the xyphoid (in large patients) or to the left of the midline below the costal margin (in smaller patients), one 5-mm cannula is inserted in the right midclavicular line below the costal margin, and one cannula is inserted in the right anterior axillary line above the iliac crest (Fig 8.16).

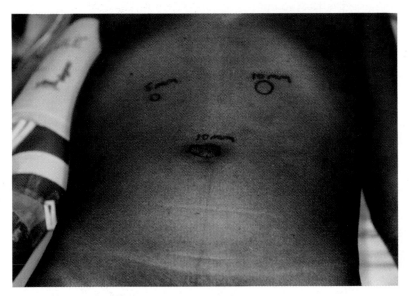

Figure 8.16 Trocar Sites—Cholecystectomy Trocar sites for a laparoscopic cholecystectomy are marked on the abdomen.

The abdomen is first inspected and the gallbladder is visualized and grasped at the fundus, using a grasper inserted into the right anterior axillary line cannula (Fig 8.17). The gallbladder is retracted cephalad and anterior to expose the porta hepatis.

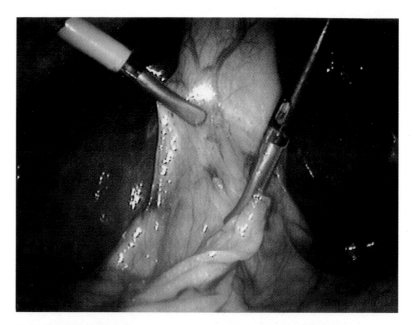

Figure 8.18 Adhesions are dissected from the gallbladder.

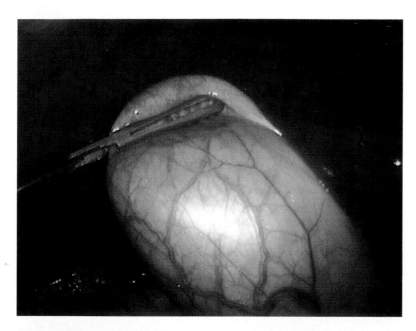

Figure 8.17 The gallbladder is visualized through the laparoscope. A grasper elevates the fundus of the gallbladder.

Using instruments passed through the two remaining cannulae, the surgeon dissects free any adhesions to the gallbladder and the peritoneum (Fig 8.18) until the cystic duct and the cystic artery can be seen (Fig 8.19). Clips are placed on the cystic artery (Fig 8.20), which is then divided (Fig 8.21). The junction of the cystic duct and the common bile duct is determined either by close inspection (Fig 8.22) or by a cholangiogram (Fig 8.23), after which the cystic duct is divided between clips (Fig 8.24). The gallbladder is then dissected free from the liver bed (Fig 8.25) and, once freed, can be removed via one of the cannulae or in an endoscopic pouch (Fig 8.26).

After the operative site is inspected to ensure hemostasis, the wounds are closed (Fig 8.27), and the patient is treated as described previously for an appendectomy.

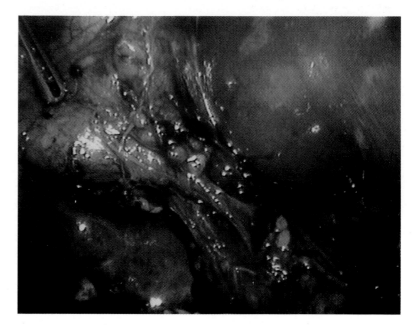

Figure 8.19 With the gallbladder retracted cephalad (a grasper can be seen in the upper left of the photograph), the cystic artery and the cystic duct can be seen.

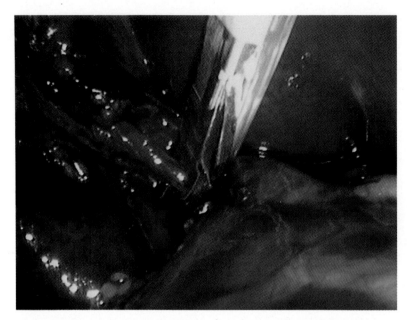

Figure 8.20 Endoscopic clips are being placed on the cystic artery.

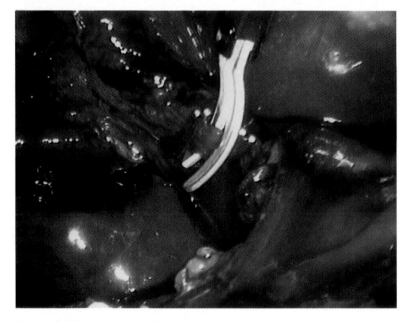

Figure 8.21 With the clips in place, the cystic artery is divided with a pair of endoscopic shears.

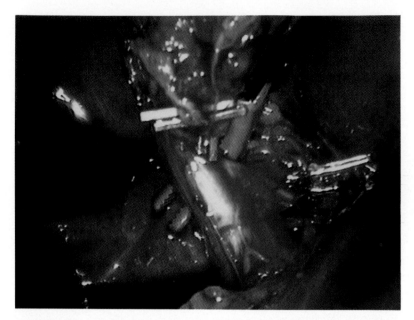

Figure 8.22 A dissector is inserted behind the cystic duct and is resting on the anterior wall of the common hepatic duct.

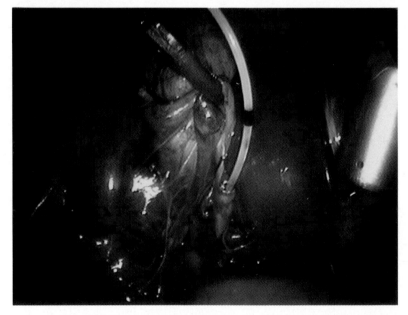

Figure 8.23 A balloon cholangiogram catheter has been placed via a percutaneous introducer and is inserted into an incision in the cystic duct in preparation for an operative cholangiogram.

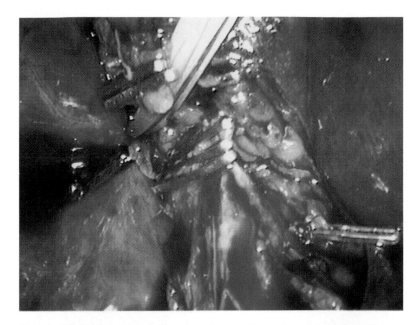

Figure 8.24 The cystic duct has been clipped and is being divided.

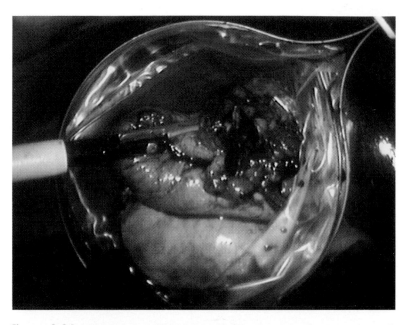

Figure 8.26 The freed gallbladder is placed inside the opening of an endoscopic pouch for removal.

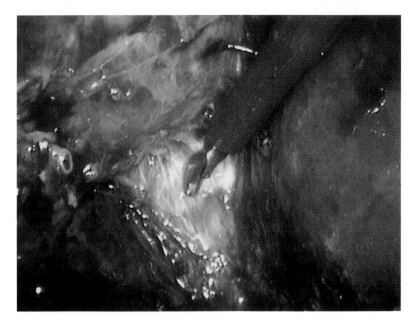

Figure 8.25 The gallbladder (upper left of photograph) is being dissected free from the liver bed with a Harmonic scalpel.

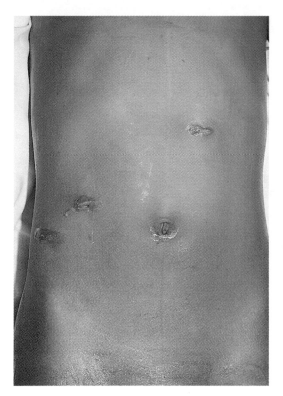

Figure 8.27 The midline fascia is closed at the umbilical laparoscope port. All the skin incisions are closed with subcuticular absorbable sutures, leaving minimally visible incisions.

Nissen Fundoplication, Gastrostomy, and Jejunostomy

A laparoscopic Nissen fundoplication can be performed quite easily by those familiar with endoscopic suturing techniques. The indications and preoperative preparation are identical to those for any antireflux procedure. With the patient anesthetized and the stomach emptied, cannulae are placed as follows: in the umbilicus (for the telescope), in the right and left midclavicular line below the costal margin (for suturing and dissecting), and in the left anterior axillary line (for dissecting and retracting). One additional cannula is for retraction of the liver and is placed either in the midline below the xyphoid (in the infant) or in the right anterior axillary line (in larger patients) (Fig 8.28).

With the liver retracted anteriorly to expose the esophageal hiatus, the esophagus is dissected circumferentially and is encircled with a short (6 cm) length of umbilical tape, which is then grasped firmly and held with a grasper placed through the left lateral port. The crura are exposed, and the hiatus is closed with 2-0 silk sutures. The fundus of the stomach is wrapped around the distal esophagus and is secured there with interrupted 2-0 silk sutures (Fig 8.29). These patients can be fed on the day of surgery and are on full diet and ready for discharge by 36 hours after surgery.

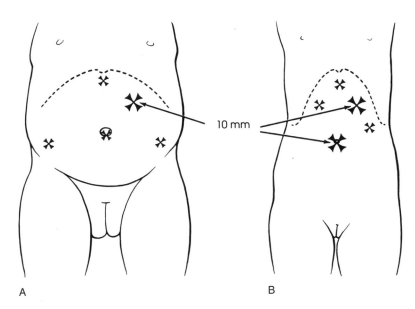

Figure 8.28 Trocar Sites—Fundoplication Trocar insertion sites are indicated for a laparoscopic fundoplication: **A** depicts the trocar sites for an infant; **B** depicts the trocar sites for the older patient. (Reprinted with permission from Lobe TE, Schropp KP [eds]: Pediatric Laparoscopy and Thoracoscopy. WB Saunders, Philadelphia, 1994, p 169.)

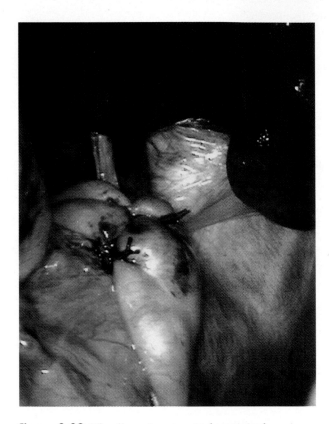

Figure 8-29 The liver is retracted anteriorly using a standard endoscopic grasper that has been passed via a right, subcostal, anterior axillary line cannula (upper left of photograph). It may be helpful to grasp the diaphragm with the shaft of the grasper to hold the liver away from the line of sight. Several sutures of the completed wrap can be seen in the center of the photograph.

A gastrostomy can also be performed, if indicated. The anterior wall of the stomach is held up to the abdominal wall with an endoscopic grasper (Fig 8.30) and is secured there with the use of percutaneous Brown-Mueller "T" fasteners (Fig 8.31). A Seldinger technique is then used: a needle is inserted through the abdominal wall into the stomach between the "T" fasteners; a guidewire is passed through the needle into the stomach; and serial dilators are passed over the guidewire until the opening in the stomach and abdominal wall is large enough for placement of the gastrostomy tube (Fig 8.32). The "T" fasteners then are pulled up to secure the stomach against the anterior abdomen.

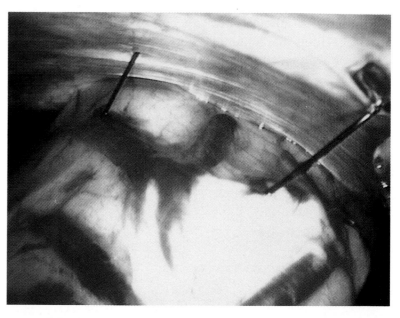

Figure 8.31 The stomach is secured to the anterior abdominal wall with four percutaneously placed "T" fasteners.

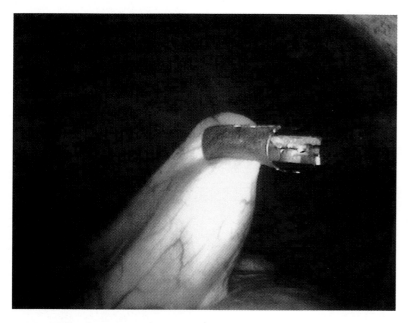

Figure 8.30 Gastrostomy The stomach is grasped with an endoscopic grasper.

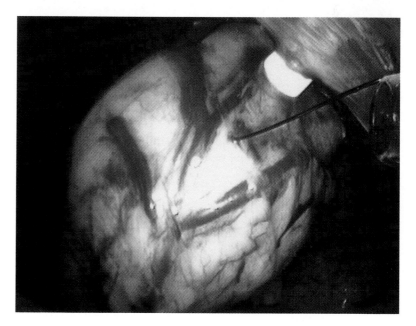

Figure 8.32 The percutaneous gastrostomy tube has been inserted under laparoscopic visualization, and the retention balloon has been inflated in the stomach. To facilitate placement of the gastrostomy tube, the wires of the "T" fasteners have not yet been secured.

Similarly, a jejunostomy can be created by selecting a proximal loop of jejunum (Fig 8.33) into which "T" fasteners are placed (Fig 8.34) in a diamond configuration (Fig 8.35). Percutaneous dilators are used to make the opening in the jejunum sufficiently large (Fig 8.36) to insert a #10 Fr jejunostomy tube, which is directed distally before the "T" fastener wires are secured (Fig 8.37).

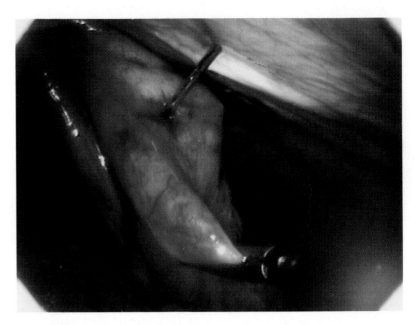

Figure 8.34 A "T" fastener is being inserted into the jejunum.

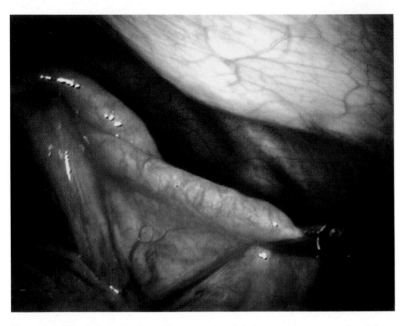

Figure 8.33 Jejunostomy The proximal jejunum is grasped with two instruments, the left one being medial and proximal.

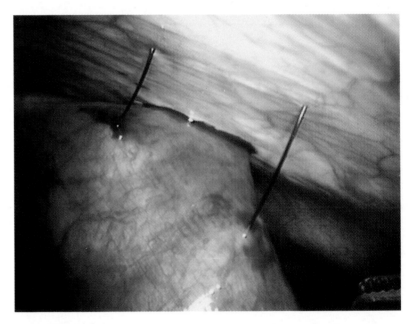

Figure 8.35 A diamond configuration of "T" fasteners has been inserted, in preparation for the percutaneous insertion of the jejunostomy tube.

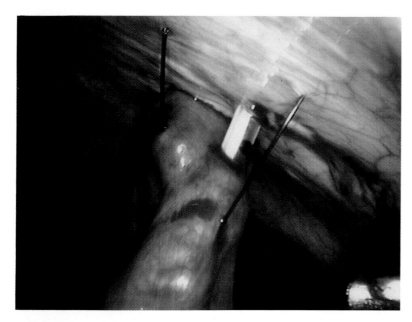

Figure 8.36 Dilators are used to enlarge the opening in the jejunum.

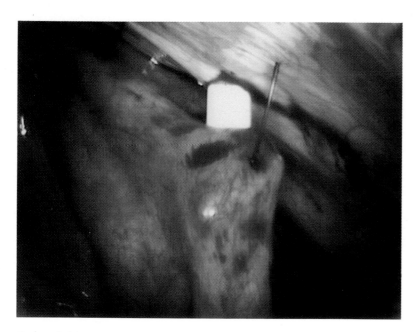

Figure 8.37 The jejunostomy tube is in place, and the "T" fasteners are being secured to the anterior abdominal wall.

Laparoscopic Splenectomy

The indications for a laparoscopic splenectomy are the same as those for an open splenectomy. The limiting factor is the size of the spleen relative to the endoscopic pouch that will be used to remove it.

With the patient under general endotracheal anesthesia, the stomach and bladder are emptied. Because the colon often gets in the way, we give the patient three doses of paregoric, 6 hours apart beginning the evening before surgery, to contract the colon and improve visualization. Cannulae are placed as follows: in the umbilicus for the telescope, in the left midclavicular line for inserting the stapler and pouch, below the right costal margin near the midline for dissection and retraction, and in the left anterior axillary line below the costal margin and above the iliac crest.

With the patient supine, the stomach is retracted to the right and the splenic hilum to the patient's left to splay out the short gastric vessels (Fig 8.38). These vessels are

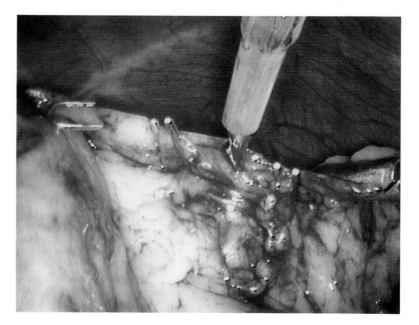

Figure 8.38 Splenectomy The stomach is retracted to the left of the photograph, and the splenic hilum is retracted to the right of the photograph. Clips have been applied to the first of several short gastric vessels, and a bipolar cautery is being used to divide these vessels.

divided with an endoscopic stapler or between clips. The patient is then turned in a full left lateral position so that the lateral attachments to the spleen can be divided (Fig 8.39). An endoscopic stapler is then applied across the splenic hilum to divide the splenic vessels en masse (Fig 8.40). The patient is returned to a supine position, and the spleen is inserted into an 8 × 10 cm endoscopic pouch. The neck of the pouch is brought out onto the abdominal wall and opened so that the spleen can be morcellated (Fig 8.41), with either a morcellator or a sponge forceps, and removed. The automatic morcellator is connected to suction to allow the tissue to be drawn into the blade for morcellation. When using the sponge forceps, it is helpful to use a suction cannula to perforate the spleen and to evacuate the liquid from the pouch, because the forceps removes only chunks of tissue.

Postoperatively, patients are treated as described earlier and are usually on a full diet and ready for discharge by 48 hours after surgery.

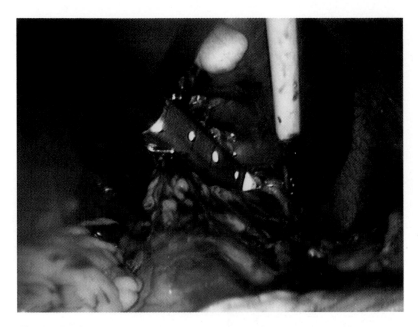

Figure 8.40 With the patient in a lateral position, the spleen is being supported posteriorly with an endoscopic grasper, and an endoscopic stapler is applied across the hilum in preparation for dividing the hilar structures en masse.

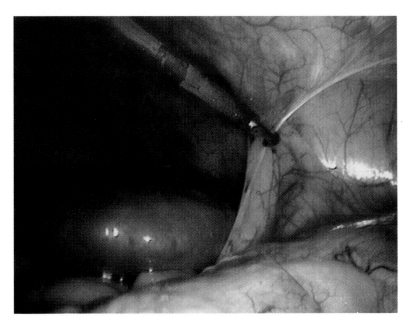

Figure 8.39 With the patient in a lateral position, the lateral attachments to the spleen are being divided using a Harmonic scalpel.

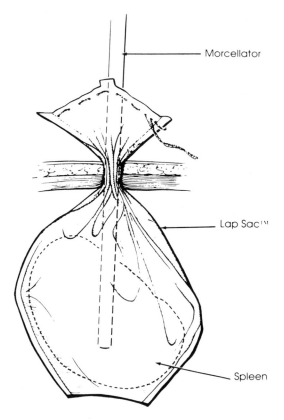

Figure 8.41 The spleen has been placed into a pouch, the neck of which has been extracted through a trocar site and opened. The tip of a morcellator has been inserted into the pouch to remove the spleen. (Reprinted with permission from Lobe TE, Schropp KP [eds]: Pediatric Laparoscopy and Thoracoscopy. WB Saunders, Philadelphia, 1994, p 193.)

Ovarian Cyst

Simple ovarian cysts (see Chapter 10) that develop, or continue to grow, after birth may be aspirated under laparoscopic visualization (Figs 8.42, 8.43). The cyst wall is then withdrawn out a port site and is resected (Fig 8.44).

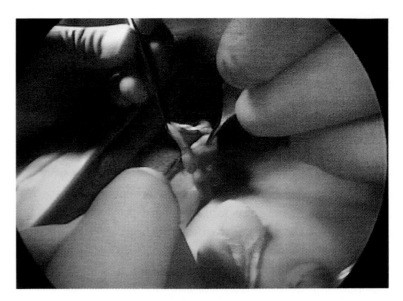

Figure 8.44 Pulled out through a trocar site, the wall of the cyst is opened and excised. (Courtesy of Steven Stylianos, M.D.)

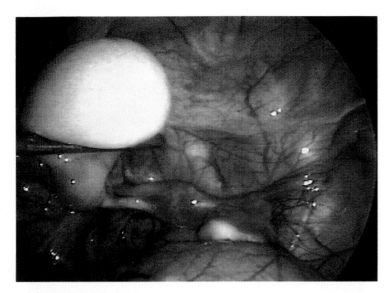

Figure 8.42 Ovarian Cyst This large ovarian cyst is visualized laparoscopically. It is a potential cause of torsion. (Courtesy of Steven Stylianos, M.D.)

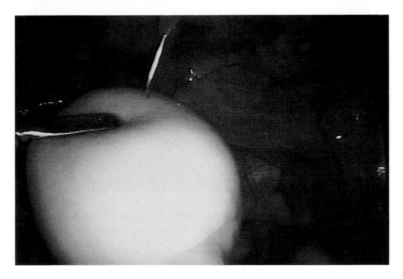

Figure 8.43 A needle is placed through the abdominal wall in the pelvis under direct vision, and the cyst contents are aspirated. (Courtesy of Steven Stylianos, M.D.)

Laparoscopic Pull-Through for Hirschsprung's Disease

A modification of the Soave procedure for Hirschsprung's disease can be performed in newborns and infants. The diagnosis must first be made on clinical grounds, supported with a contrast enema and a suction rectal biopsy showing the absence of ganglion cells and hypertrophy of the nerve fibers. A colostomy is not performed in these patients.

Patients under general anesthesia are placed at the end of a shortened operating table and are prepped circumferentially from the nipples to the midthighs. After insufflation of the abdomen, three 4- or 5-mm cannulae are placed: one in the right upper quadrant in the midclavicular line below the costal margin (for the telescope), and one lateral to each rectus muscle at or above the level of the umbilicus (Fig 8.45). A bladder catheter is inserted, and the lower abdomen is inspected (Fig 8.46). With the placement of a few towels underneath the patient's buttocks, a Trendelenburg position can be established. The colon is grasped and the transition zone is identified (Fig 8.47). The mesentery is opened by blunt dissection, and the retrorectal space is dissected (Fig 8.48). Mesocolic vessels distal to the transition zone are divided using bipolar cautery (Fig 8.49). These vessels can be divided over as long a segment of aganglionic bowel as necessary (one of our patients undergoing this procedure had total colonic Hirschsprung's disease). The endoscopic instruments are removed at this time, and the abdomen is deflated.

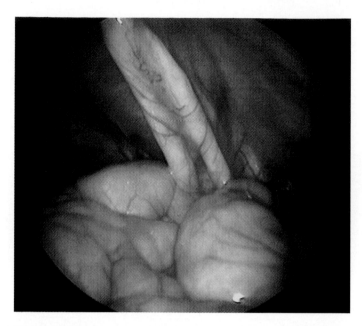

Figure 8.46 The umbilical ligaments and small bowel can be seen in the lower abdomen.

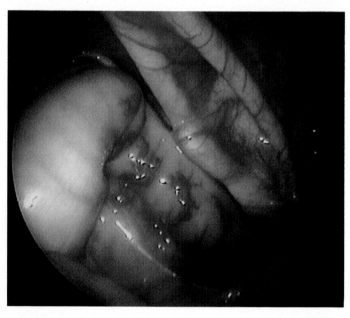

Figure 8.47 A grasper (upper left of center) is placed at the transition zone and forms the apex of a triangle, the right side of which is aganglionic bowel and the left side of which is presumed to be ganglionic.

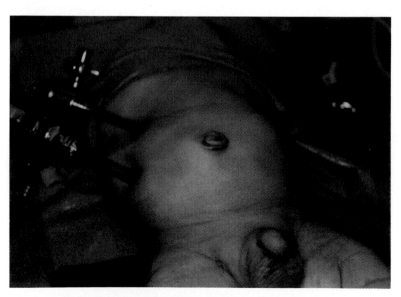

Figure 8.45 Pull-through for Hirschsprung's Disease The trocar placements are demonstrated.

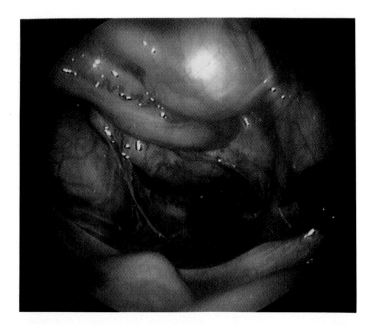

Figure 8.48 The retrorectal space is dissected to facilitate the pull-through.

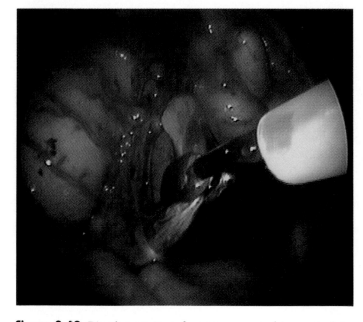

Figure 8.49 Bipolar cautery forceps are used to coagulate and divide any necessary mesocolic vessels.

Attention is then turned to the anus, where, with the patient's legs elevated over the abdomen, the rectum is everted with sutures (Fig 8.50). After the distal rectal submucosa is infiltrated with 1 : 200,000 epinephrine solution, a circumferential incision is made in the anal mucosa at the dentate line in the infiltrated area. A mucosal tube is then dissected from its muscular cuff proximally (Fig 8.51). After a short 1- to 2-cm dissection, the muscular cuff is divided posteriorly and the posterior rectal space is entered. The incision in the muscular cuff is then extended circumferentially. The rectum is dissected and freed proximally until the entire aganglionic colon and transition zone can been brought down through the anus (Fig 8.52). All of the dissection is carried out directly on the wall of the colon in a fashion similar to the mobilization of the rectum in a posterior-sagittal anorectoplasty performed for imperforate anus (see Chapter 7). Recently, we have been making our muscular cuff

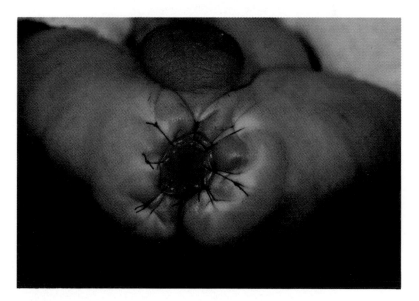

Figure 8.50 The rectum is everted with heavy sutures.

shorter and shorter, until the anastomosis may now resemble a Swenson procedure more than a Soave procedure. After a full-thickness biopsy confirms the presence of ganglion cells in the bowel proximal to the apparent transition zone, the muscular cuff is completely divided in the midline posteriorly; and a full-thickness anastomosis is then carried out between the distal normal ganglionated bowel and the rectum. The anastomosis is performed in quadrants, with interrupted 4-0 absorbable sutures (Fig 8.53), which are then cut to allow the anastomosis to retract into the anus (Fig 8.54).

These patients are fed on the day of surgery and can be discharged the following morning. We begin dilating the rectum of these patients at 2 weeks after surgery and continue dilatations as required.

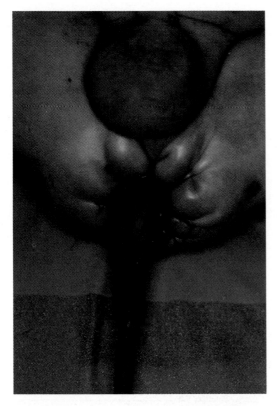

Figure 8.51 The mucosal tube is dissected from the muscular cuff.

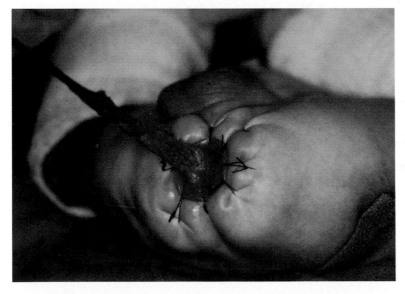

Figure 8.52 Dissection close to the wall of the bowel permits the internally freed bowel to come through the anus to the level of the presumed transition zone. A biopsy should be done just proximal to the transition zone to confirm the presence of ganglion cells.

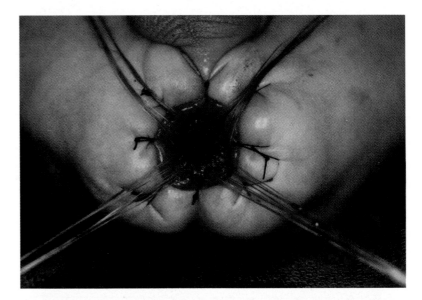

Figure 8.53 A full-thickness anastomosis is performed with absorbable sutures.

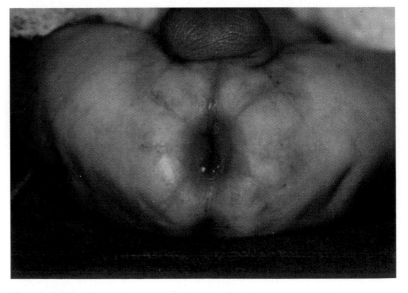

Figure 8.54 The anastomosis is completed.

Thoracoscopy

Evacuation of an Empyema

Loculated pleural effusions and empyemas can be easily treated using endoscopic techniques. Any patient in whom a loculated pleural fluid collection is documented by diagnostic images (usually a computed tomography [CT] scan), or by failure of thoracentesis to evacuate the fluid, should be considered as a candidate for thoracoscopic drainage of the fluid and placement of a thoracostomy tube.

Patients are positioned laterally as if for a thoracotomy, and selective intubation of the main bronchus of the contralateral lung is used to facilitate collapse of the lung on the operative side; in larger children, a double-lumen endotracheal tube can be placed. Initially, a cannula is inserted directly over the fluid collection through the lowest possible intercostal space, any apparent fluid is aspirated to facilitate visualization, and a telescope is inserted to inspect the pleural space. Adhesions can be taken down by using the telescope as a dissecting instrument (Fig 8.55), or, preferably, a second intercostal cannula can be inserted through which a suction/irrigation cannula can be inserted. Any exudate is stripped from the pleural surface. We find that a ring forceps inserted through one of the cannula sites (with the cannula removed) works well for this purpose. The entire entrapped lung is freed, and a chest tube is inserted through one of the two cannula sites (Fig 8.56). The chest tube is left in place until there is no significant drainage (usually 48–72 hours), and appropriate antibiotics are continued on an outpatient basis after the fever has defervesced.

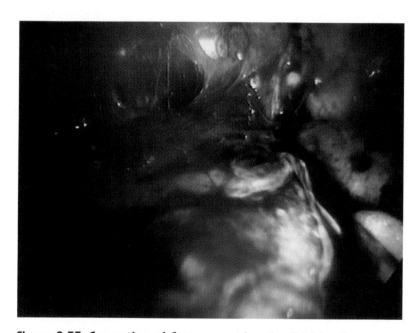

Figure 8.55 Evacuation of Empyema After the fluid has been evacuated, pleural adhesions can be seen readily and should be divided bluntly.

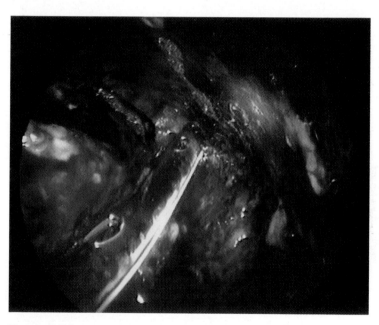

Figure 8.56 After all the lung has been freed, the exudate debrided, and all fluid evacuated, a chest tube is inserted through one of the trocar sites.

Recurrent Pneumothoraces

If pulmonary apical blebs can be demonstrated by CT scan, they may be resected (Figs 8.57, 8.58) with or without subsequent pleurodesis. Other patients with recurrent pneumothoraces or recurrent pleural effusions can be treated simply with a thoracoscopic pleurodesis. With the patient under general anesthesia and selective intubation, a thoracoscope is inserted through the chest tube site if a tube has already been inserted, or through a new cannula site if a chest tube has not been placed. A peanut gauze

sponge on a grasper may be used to abrade the visceral and parietal pleura to create adhesions. We prefer to use dry, sterile, USP pure talc, which is placed in the bulb of a disposable insufflation cannula; the cannula is inserted through either the operating port of a right-angle scope (Fig 8.59) or a separate cannula site (Fig 8.60), and the pleural surface is dusted with the talc. A chest tube is then inserted and placed on suction for 48 hours. These patients usually run a low-grade fever for a few days as a result of the inflammatory reaction to the talc.

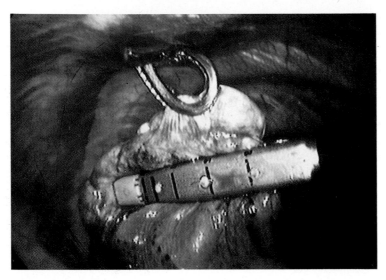

Figure 8.57 Pleural Blebs A ring forceps, placed directly through the intercostal incision of a cannula site, grasps the apex of the lung containing pleural blebs. (Courtesy of Steven Stylianos, M.D.)

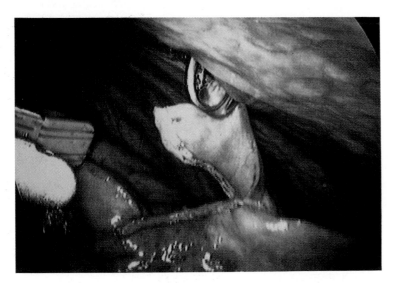

Figure 8.58 The endoscopic stapler has been placed across the apex and has been fired, leaving a fine row of staples. Sometimes more than one bite of the stapler is necessary to excise the entire specimen. It is being removed from the chest incision. (Courtesy of Steven Stylianos, M.D.)

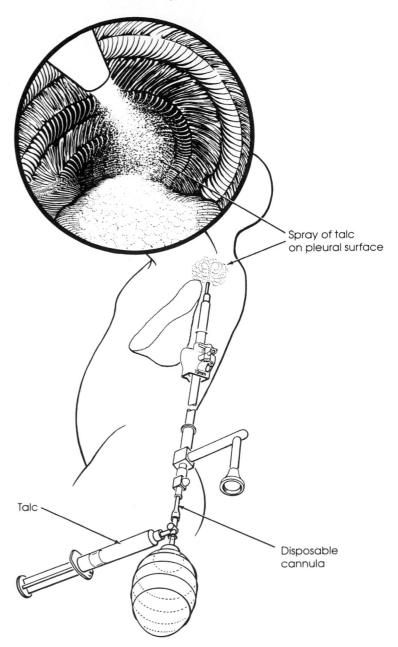

Spray of talc on pleural surface

Talc

Disposable cannula

Figure 8.59 Talc Poudrage Talc can be applied through a disposable plastic cannula. The talc is placed in a syringe, the plunger of which is advanced as the bulb is squeezed to blow the talc into the pleural cavity. (Reprinted with permission from Lobe TE, Schropp KP [eds]: Pediatric Laparoscopy and Thoracoscopy. WB Saunders, Philadelphia, 1994, p 233.)

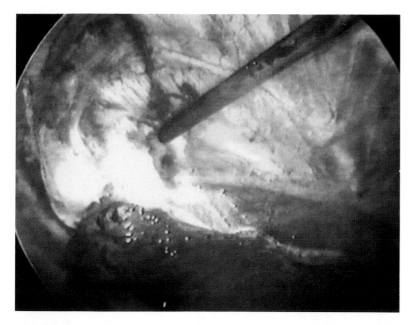

Figure 8.60 Alternatively, the talc can be placed directly into the rubber bulb (such as the bulb syringe used to suction newborns) and applied through a thoracoscopy cannula, as shown in this photograph.

Lung Biopsy

Endoscopic linear staplers make segmental biopsies a simple procedure in children. This procedure is best performed for focal, discrete lesions rather than for diffuse lung disease.

The patient is placed in a lateral position, and three cannulae are used. One of these is for the telescope, one is for a grasping device, and the other is for the stapler (Fig 8.61). The position of these cannulae depends on the location of the lesion. After the lesion for biopsy has been spotted with the telescope, the lung is grasped with a grasping forceps and the linear stapler is applied (Fig 8.62). Usually several applications (two or three) are necessary to complete the biopsy. The specimen is then removed via the largest cannula. We do not routinely insert a chest tube unless the patient has significant lung disease and may require positive pressure ventilation.

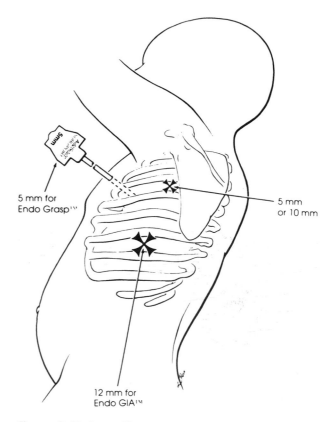

5 mm for Endo Grasp™

5 mm or 10 mm

12 mm for Endo GIA™

Figure 8.61 Lung Biopsy Trocar positions are illustrated for lung biopsy. (Reprinted with permission from Lobe TE, Schropp KP [eds]: Pediatric Laparoscopy and Thoracoscopy. WB Saunders, Philadelphia, 1994, p 251.)

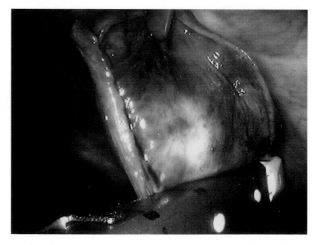

Figure 8.62 The tip of a grasping forceps can be seen in the upper center of the photograph. One staple line is seen on the left as the stapler is applied again, perpendicularly to the previous application.

Excision of Apical Tumor

Small tumors lend themselves well to excision using thoracoscopic techniques. The patients are placed under general anesthesia in a lateral position with selective intubation. Usually four cannulae are necessary: one for the telescope, and three others for dissection and retraction. To the extent possible, the cannulae should surround the lesion, with the lesion in the center.

First the apical lesion is visualized (Fig 8.63). Then, working around the periphery of the tumor, the surgeon dissects the lesion (Fig 8.64) until it is completely free (Fig 8.65). The tumor bed is inspected for hemostasis (Fig 8.66). The tumor is placed in a plastic pouch and is then removed by use of a morcellator (as with the spleen) or by extension of one of the trocar sites along an intercostal space creating a thoracotomy incision long enough to extract the tumor intact.

A chest tube is not necessary unless the lung has been entered in the course of dissection. Patients usually can go home the day after surgery.

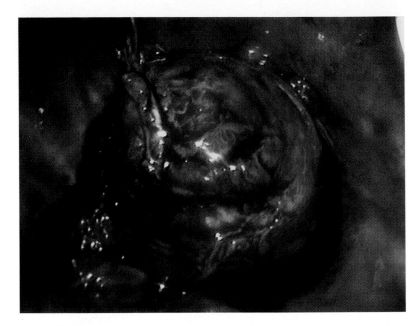

Figure 8.65 The tumor is completely freed.

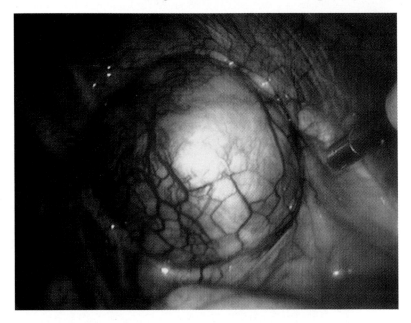

Figure 8.63 Apical Tumor A tumor (diagnosed after excision as a nerve sheath tumor) is first visualized in the apex of the pleural cavity of a teenage girl.

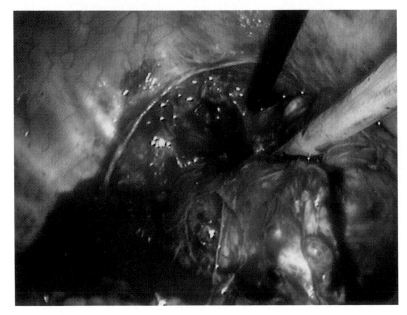

Figure 8.64 A Harmonic scalpel is used to dissect the tumor free from its bed.

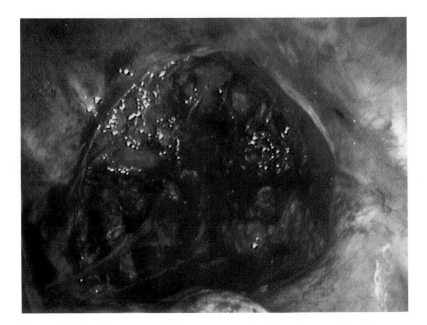

Figure 8.66 The tumor bed is inspected. There is no bleeding.

Chapter 9

Liver, Spleen, and Pancreas

Liver and Biliary Tract

Tumors, benign and malignant, and congenital and acquired liver and biliary tract abnormalities are the nontraumatic problems the surgeon must deal with in the right side of the upper abdomen. Liver trauma is discussed in Chapter 13.

Diagnosis of Liver Masses

Most intrahepatic masses are detected by palpation. The definition of their nature and extent relies on a variety of imaging studies. Plain radiographs of the abdomen may show the soft-tissue mass and displacement of adjacent structures (Fig 9.1). The lesion can be outlined by its impression on contrast-filled intestine (Fig 9.2). Sonography may distinguish cystic from solid lesions. Radionuclide scans (Figs 9.3, 9.4), selective angiography (Fig 9.5), and computed tomography (CT) (Fig 9.6) help delineate the intrahepatic extent of a mass. Magnetic resonance imaging (MRI) has been used for some lesions (Fig 9.7), but the tissue definition in the liver does not equal that of CT.

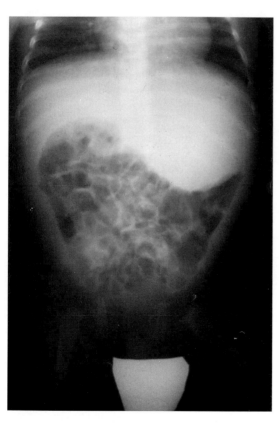

Figure 9.1 Liver Mass This large asymptomatic mass, in the left lobe of an infant's liver, displaces the intestine and is clearly visible.

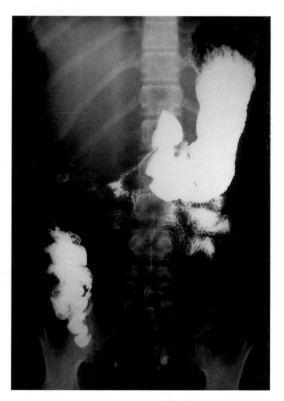

Figure 9.2 A large hamartomatous cyst of the right lobe of the liver compresses the barium-filled duodenum.

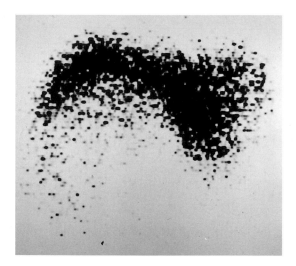

Figure 9.3 A radionuclide scan outlines the liver cyst seen in Figure 9.2.

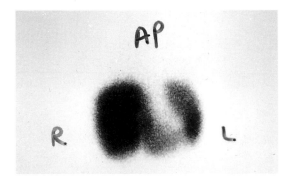

Figure 9.4 The "cold" area of this liver–spleen scan represents a large hepatoblastoma of the middle and left lobes.

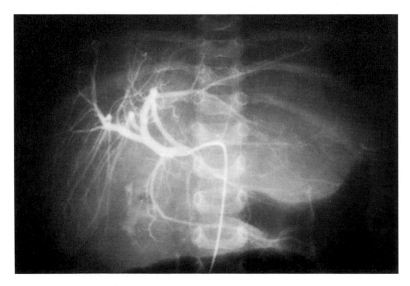

Figure 9.5 The hepatic arteries are splayed out over the malignant liver tumor in this selective hepatic arteriogram.

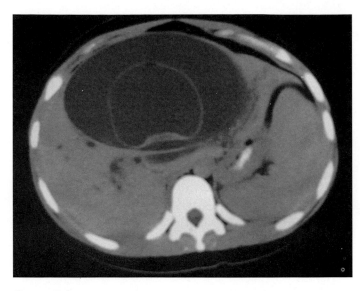

Figure 9.6 This abdominal CT scan of a 14-year-old girl demonstrates a huge cyst of the liver, with a contained daughter cyst characteristic of an echinococcus (hydatid) cyst.

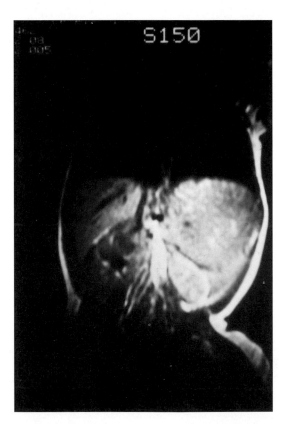

Figure 9.7 The mass in the left liver lobe shown in Figure 9.1 is seen here on magnetic resonance imaging (MRI). The lesion displaces, but does not invade, contiguous structures.

Cysts and Hamartomas

Congenital cysts of the liver are often palpable. They may also present because of pain, hemorrhage into the cyst, or infection. The content is usually serous fluid, unless there is a biliary communication or abscess.

Mesenchymal hamartoma is a benign malformation of the liver, usually cystic. It may be detected on abdominal examination (Fig 9.8), contrast radiographs (see Fig 9.2), ultrasonography, or liver scan (see Fig 9.3). Either excision or decompression of the cyst may be used, as suits the cyst size and location (Figs 9.9, 9.10).

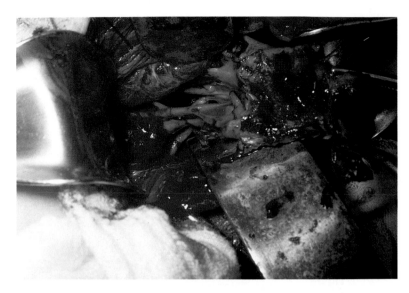

Figure 9.10 The cyst contains bile-stained connective tissue in a trabecular pattern.

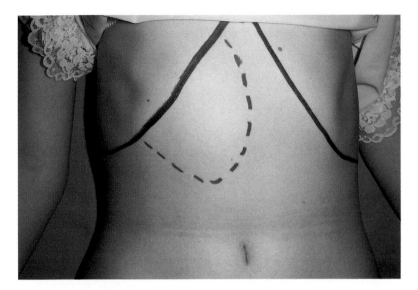

Figure 9.8 The large mass outlined in red is palpable in the right side of the upper abdomen of this asymptomatic 16-year-old girl.

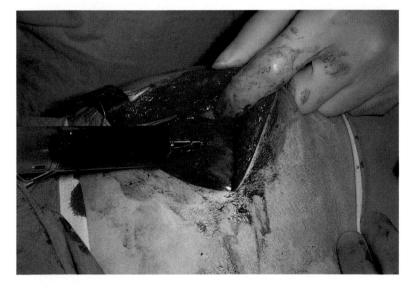

Figure 9.9 At exploration, bilious material is aspirated from the hamartomatous cyst.

Echinococcus (hydatid) cysts of the liver are found most often in children from South America and the Mediterranean area. The parasitic cysts may develop over many years and may achieve considerable size (Figs 9.11, 9.12). The presenting symptoms are those of fever, discomfort from compression of adjacent structures, and occasional toxicity. Sonography or CT shows the characteristic fluid-filled cyst containing multiple smaller daughter cysts (see Fig 9.6). The cysts are resected, after the contents are sterilized by irrigation with scolicidic solution or hypertonic saline to prevent intraabdominal dissemination from seeding (Fig 9.13).

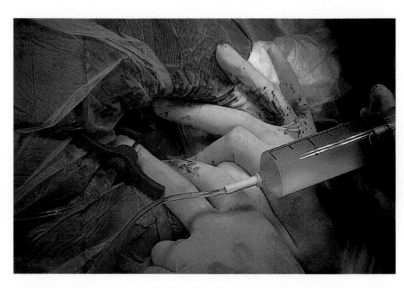

Figure 9.13 The cyst is irrigated with hypertonic (20%) saline to kill the scolices prior to resection of the cyst wall from the liver. A plastic drape over the operative field prevents intraabdominal contamination.

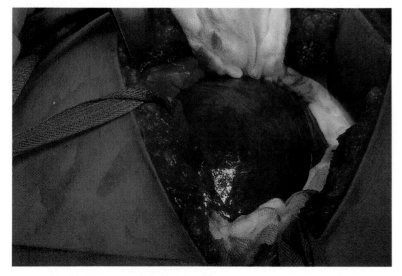

Figure 9.11 The massive distention of the upper abdomen of this 14-year-old girl represents an echinococcus cyst of the liver. The girl was born on a farm in Albania but has lived in the United States for 13 years.

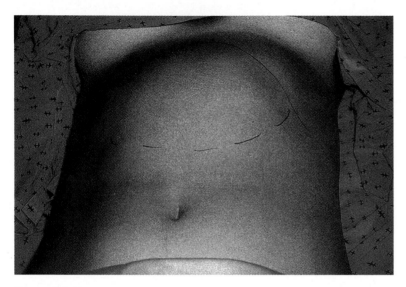

Figure 9.12 The huge cyst of the liver is seen at exploration.

Biliary Atresia

The neonate who presents with persistent direct hyper-bilirubinemia (> 3.0 mg/dL) and acholic stools must be studied as early as possible for biliary atresia. If radionuclide studies (technetium 99 [^{99}Tc] DISIDA scan, following phenobarbital stimulation) show failure of bile passage out of the liver into the duodenum, atresia is strongly suspected (Fig 9.18), and referral should be made for definitive correction. Atresia involving only the distal portion of the extrahepatic bile duct is amenable to choledochoenterostomy or cholecystoenterostomy, usually with a Roux-en-Y anastomosis to the jejunum.

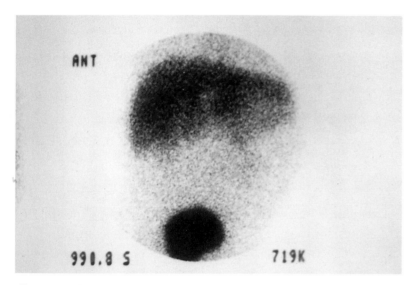

Figure 9.18 Biliary Atresia The DISIDA scan shows radionuclide in the liver and bladder, but none in the intestine, in this infant with biliary atresia. Phenobarbital is administered for 2–3 days before the study to enhance biliary excretion from the liver.

Atresia involving the proximal or the entire extrahepatic duct system was considered "noncorrectable" until Kasai described the operation of portoenterostomy; in that procedure, the atretic extrahepatic ducts are excised, and an anastomosis is performed by bringing an intestinal segment to the dissected liver hilum (Figs 9.19–9.22). It is expected that microscopic ducts, which can be demonstrated in the resection specimen of the liver hilum, will drain into the attached intestine. Lack of subsequent bile flow is the result of either inadequate dissection into the liver hilum prior to anastomosis or, more likely, an associated atresia of the intrahepatic ducts. The best chance for long-term success is afforded when the procedure is done within the first 4–6 weeks of life—before severe liver damage occurs.

Cholangitis, the common postoperative complication, occurs only in those patients with successful establishment of bile flow, in the author's experience. The likelihood of cholangitis is thought to be diminished by initial exteriorization of the efferent jejunal segment (see Fig 9.21), a procedure that also allows early assessment of bile flow from the portoenterostomy. After 3–12 months, the vented jejunum is closed; in patients who develop increased portal venous pressure as a result of cirrhosis, mucosal bleeding from the exteriorized jejunum may force earlier closure. All patients are given prolonged prophylactic antibiotic therapy (sulfamethoxazole-trimethoprim [Septra, Bactrim]) after portoenterostomy.

Initial enthusiasm for the Kasai procedure has been tempered by the generally poor long-term prognosis for those with progressive hepatic disease, half of the patients in some series. Only approximately 25% are now thought to have satisfactory survival. Liver transplantation is the only currently available alternative in those whose livers fail.

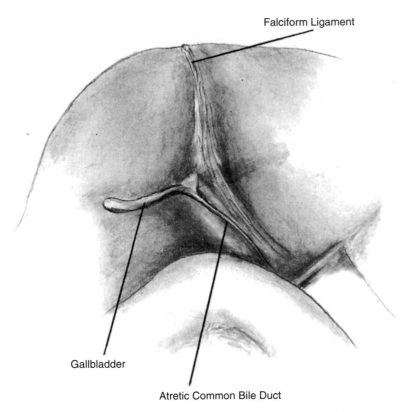

Falciform Ligament

Gallbladder

Atretic Common Bile Duct

Figure 9.19 The anatomy of the most common form of biliary atresia is illustrated, with cordlike, fibrotic extrahepatic ducts. In some cases, even these atretic ducts cannot be detected.

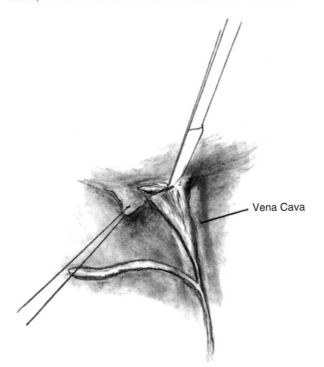

Vena Cava

Figure 9.20 The dissection of the porta hepatis is carried into the liver anterior to the inferior vena cava. Prior to anastomosis, existing fibrous tissue is surgically divided close to the liver in the porta hepatis.

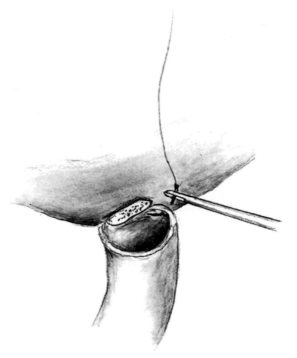

Figure 9.21 A segment of jejunum is brought to the porta and is sutured to the liver capsule around the dissected area; there is no true "anastomosis" of two visible hollow structures.

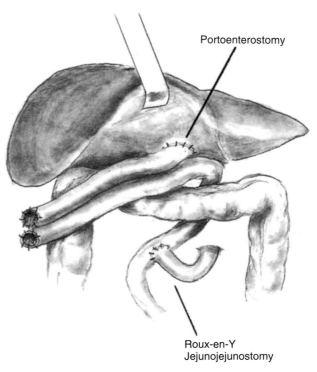

Portoenterostomy

Roux-en-Y Jejunojejunostomy

Figure 9.22 The author exteriorizes the efferent jejunal loop and completes the jejunojejunostomy, as shown.

Congenital Bile Duct Stenosis

Congenital stenosis of the extrahepatic bile duct is a very unusual condition. Most children present after infancy with recurrent pain in the gallbladder area, often with nausea and fullness. Sometimes an enlarged gallbladder is palpable.

Percutaneous or operative cholangiography provides the best definition of the problem (Fig 9.23). Frequently the pancreatic duct enters the common bile duct more proximally than is normal. Because of the possibility of an anomalous entrance of the pancreatic duct, proximal decompression by cholecystoenterostomy is recommended (Fig 9.24).

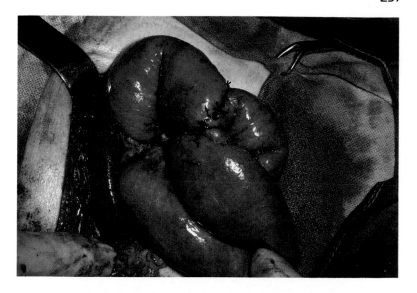

Figure 9.24 A Roux-en-Y cholecystojejunostomy is performed to decompress the biliary tract proximal to the narrowing.

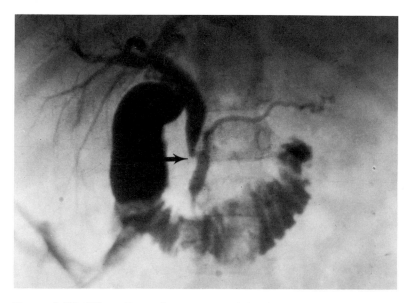

Figure 9.23 Biliary Stenosis Stenosis of the bile duct is seen in this operative cholangiogram of a 7-year-old with recurrent right-sided upper abdominal pain. The pancreatic duct enters proximally.

Choledochal Cysts

Choledochal cyst, a cystic dilatation of the extrahepatic bile duct, can present in early infancy with jaundice alone. In the newborn, choledochal cyst must be distinguished from biliary atresia. Past the age of 2 years, the classic findings are jaundice, pain, fever, and a palpable epigastric mass; a minority of patients actually present with all findings. Bile peritonitis, from acute perforation of the cyst or the proximal bile duct, may be the presenting problem (Fig 9.25).

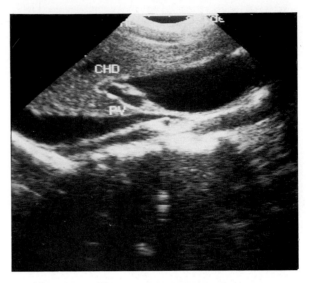

Figure 9.26 A large choledochal cyst is demonstrated in the upper right of this ultrasonogram. The common hepatic duct (CHD) and portal vein (PV) are seen to the left and below the cyst. (Courtesy of R. Peter Altman, M.D.)

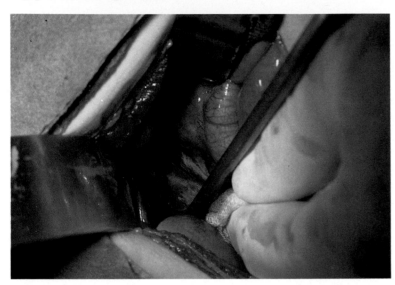

Figure 9.25 Choledochal Cyst This 4-year-old Japanese girl presented with massive bile peritonitis. A spontaneous perforation in the common hepatic bile duct is seen just above the tip of the instrument. Note the bile staining of adjacent structures.

The cause is thought to be a congenital abnormality of the wall of the bile duct combined with a distal obstruction. There may be associated cystic dilatation of the intrahepatic ducts. There is a 4:1 female predominance and a high incidence among the Japanese.

Ultrasonography is the primary diagnostic modality (Fig 9.26), although barium gastrointestinal series (Fig 9.27), computed tomography, intravenous and operative cholangiograms (Fig 9.28), and ^{99}Tc DISIDA scans have been used. Endoscopic retrograde choledochopancreatography (ERCP) and transhepatic cholangiography are used in some centers.

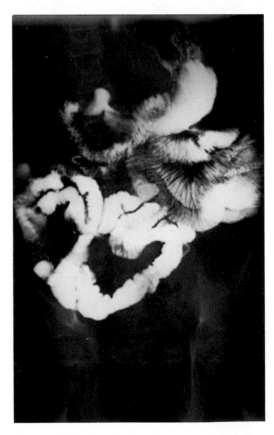

Figure 9.27 The impression of a large, round mass is seen at the lesser curvature of the barium-filled stomach of this jaundiced 13-year-old.

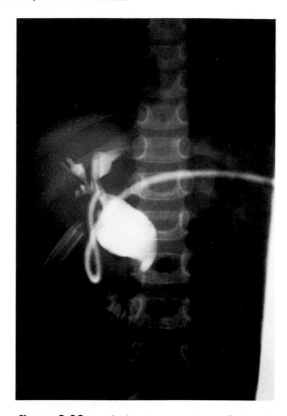

Figure 9.28 A cholangiogram is performed through the T-tube placed in the perforation of the common hepatic duct seen in Figure 9.25. There is cystic dilatation of the common bile duct and the right and left hepatic ducts; tight stenosis of the distal duct allows only a wisp of contrast into the duodenum.

In the treatment of choledochal cyst (Fig 9.29), the complications of anastomotic stricture and cholangitis following cyst-duodenostomy and cyst-enterostomy have led to abandonment of those procedures in favor of cyst excision and Roux-en-Y choledochojejunostomy or portoenterostomy (see Fig 9.21). If the inflamed cyst is adherent to the portal vein and hepatic artery posteriorly, the surgeon may choose to excise only the anterior cyst wall, leaving the posterior adherent portion from which the lining is then dissected (Figs 9.30, 9.31).

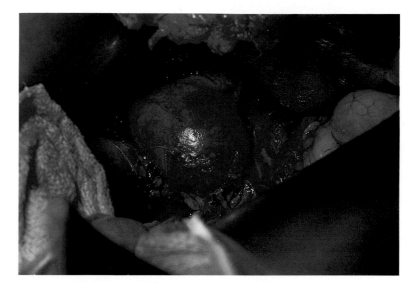

Figure 9.29 The choledochal cyst involves the common hepatic duct in this 12-year-old boy whose symptoms were recurrent pain and fever.

Gallbladder Disease

Cholelithiasis is common in children with hemolytic disease, such as spherocytosis, sickle cell disease, and thalassemia (Fig 9.32). In adolescents with right upper abdominal pain of gallbladder origin, there is a female predominance, an association with pregnancy, and a high incidence of cholesterol stones—as in the adult. Infants receiving total parenteral nutrition (TPN) may develop bilirubinate gallstones. The diagnosis of cholelithiasis may be confirmed by abdominal film (Fig 9.33), ultrasonography (Fig 9.34), oral cholecystography, or HIDA scan. The author currently performs laparoscopic cholecystectomy on most patients with cholelithiasis, except those undergoing abdominal surgery for another reason.

Noncalculous cholecystitis may result from bile stasis, dehydration, and infection, especially with salmonellae. The signs and symptoms are those of a right upper abdominal inflammatory process. Ultrasonography may be helpful in demonstrating edema and dilatation of the gallbladder. Initial therapy consists of nasogastric suction, intravenous fluids, and antibiotics. The decision for surgery is based on signs of increasing peritoneal irritation and distention of the gallbladder.

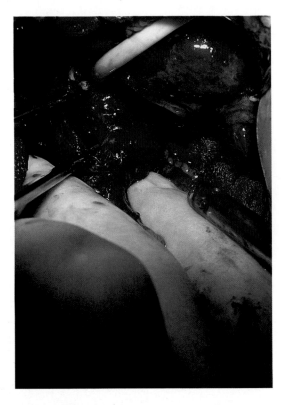

Figure 9.30 The choledochal cyst demonstrated in Figure 9.28 is seen at surgery. The T-tube is still in place. Forceps enter an incision in the anterior wall of the cyst.

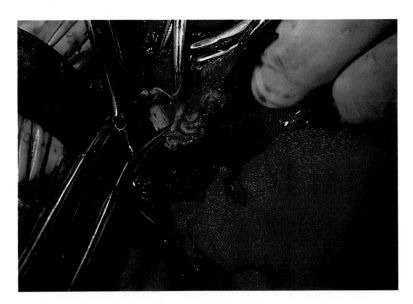

Figure 9.31 The anterior cyst wall is excised. The lining of the posterior wall is being dissected free, with hemostats at the edges. An incision is extended into the dilated portion of each main hepatic duct. They are both drained into the proximal jejunal segment of a Roux-en-Y anastomosis; the jejunal end is sutured to the liver capsule around the open ducts, as for a portoenterostomy.

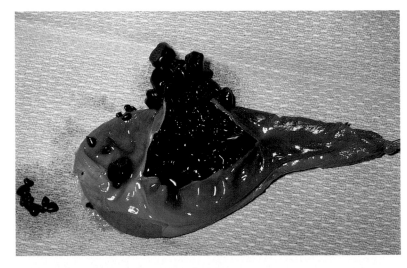

Figure 9.32 Bilirubinate stones fill the gallbladder of an adolescent boy with thalassemia major.

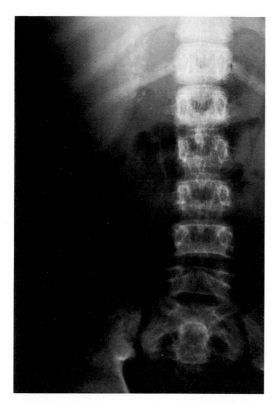

Figure 9.33 Small gallstones are seen on this plain radiograph of the abdomen of the same patient as in Figure 9.32.

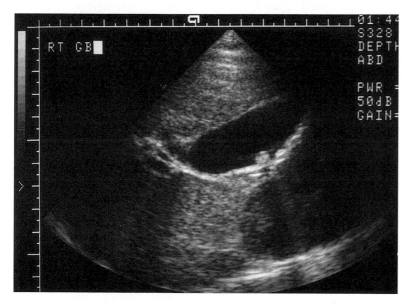

Figure 9.34 Sonography demonstrates a gallstone in this 13-year-old girl who had previously received chemotherapy for leukemia.

Portal Hypertension

In children, there are two common causes for portal hypertension: intrahepatic venous obstruction secondary to intrinsic liver disease, and extrahepatic obstruction resulting from venous thrombosis or cavernous transformation of the portal vein.

Neonatal hepatitis, biliary atresia, congenital hepatic fibrosis, glycogen storage disease, and cystic fibrosis all may lead to intrahepatic obstruction with development of increased portal venous pressure, hypersplenism, ascites, and esophageal varices.

Bleeding from such varices is complicated by the abnormal clotting factors and decreased ability to metabolize blood breakdown products in patients with liver disease. Endoscopy can help localize the bleeding site, and splenoportography (Fig 9.35) or angiography (Fig 9.36) demonstrates the portal venous channels and collaterals. With vessels of adequate size, portosystemic venous shunting is the procedure of choice for recurrent variceal hemorrhage (Figs 9.37, 9.38). Hepatic encephalopathy is much less a problem in children than in adults; the choice of shunt procedures is generally not limited by this consideration.

Cavernous transformation of the portal vein is thought to result from intrauterine or neonatal portal thrombosis and the development of alternate extrahepatic routes of venous return. Variceal bleeding may occur as early as the age of 2–5 years, when the small size of mesenteric and splenic vessels precludes a successful shunting procedure. Temporizing procedures must be used until the patient's veins are large enough to maintain patency after a shunt. Among these temporizing procedures are transthoracic ligation of esophageal varices, gastric division, selective venous ligation, and endoscopic variceal sclerosis. After the age of 8–10 years, mesocaval or splenorenal venous shunts may be performed, as determined by venous anatomy and patency (Figs 9.39, 9.40).

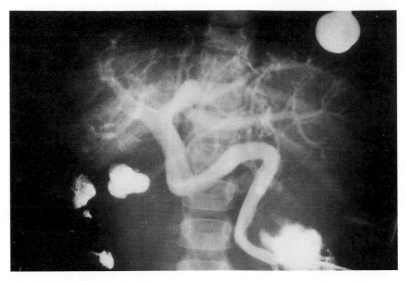

Figure 9.35 Portal Hypertension A dilated portal vein and small intrahepatic radicals are seen in this 7-year-old boy with recurrent upper gastrointestinal bleeding. He is thought to have had neonatal hepatitis.

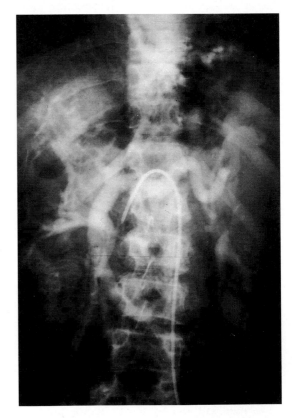

Figure 9.36 The venous phase of a selective angiogram shows dilated splenic and superior mesenteric veins but no portal flow directly into the liver. Contrast is seen in tortuous gastric and esophageal varices. Thrombosis of the portal vein in infancy is the presumed cause.

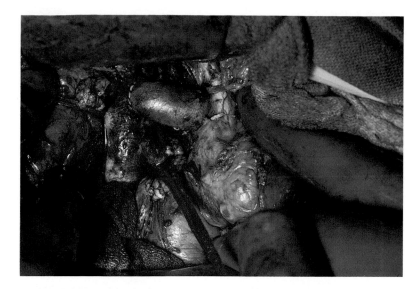

Figure 9.37 A completed end-to-side portacaval shunt is demonstrated in an 8-year-old girl with cirrhosis secondary to cystic fibrosis.

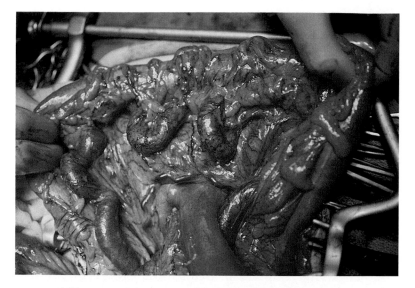

Figure 9.39 There is an unusually dilated marginal vein in the mesentery in this 12-year-old with portal hypertension.

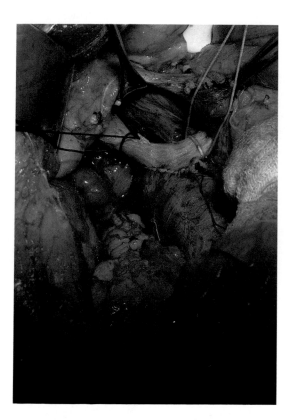

Figure 9.38 A side-to-side portacaval shunt is performed in this 14-year-old hemophiliac with hemosiderosis and portal hypertension following multiple transfusions.

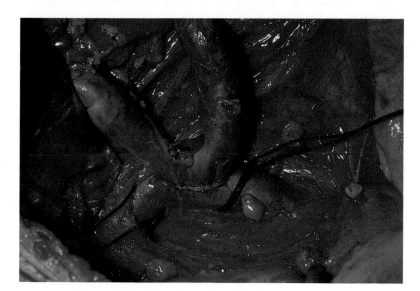

Figure 9.40 The dilated mesenteric vein is anastomosed to the inferior vena cava, with good flow and a measured decrease in portal pressure. This is *not* the standard mesocaval shunt.

Spleen

Splenic surgery in children is primarily for hematologic disease, hypersplenism, cysts, tumors, and trauma (see Chapter 13).

Hematologic Disease

Hereditary spherocytosis is characterized by chronic anemia; the abnormal red blood cells are easily trapped and destroyed in the spleen. There may be crises of rapid erythrocyte destruction, requiring immediate transfusion. Some patients have mild jaundice and gallstones. The spleen is enlarged and firm (Fig 9.41). Demonstration of increased osmotic fragility of the red cells confirms the diagnosis.

Splenectomy is performed for severe or recurrent anemia and is postponed as long as possible. At all surgery for hemolytic disease, accessory spleens must be sought in the lesser sac and mesentery and must be removed (Fig 9.42). Children are immunized with pneumococcal vaccine preoperatively, and they are given long-term antibiotic prophylaxis postoperatively, because of the threat of major sepsis. Parents of asplenic children must be warned about the need for immediate medical care of any acute febrile illness.

Thalassemia major often results in massive splenic enlargement, which interferes with normal physical activity (Figs 9.43, 9.44). Removal of the spleen decreases transfusion requirements.

Sickle-cell disease is an uncommon indication for splenectomy. However, when the spleen becomes the site for repeated episodes of thrombosis and segmental infarction during sickle cell crisis, splenectomy has been recommended. Preoperative preparation for children with sickle-cell disease is discussed in Chapter 1.

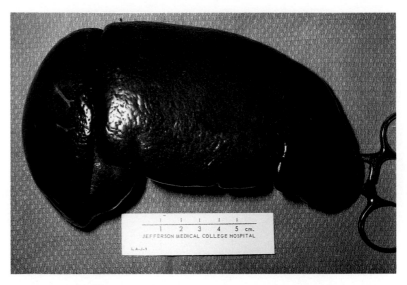

Figure 9.41 Hereditary Spherocytosis The enlarged, firm spleen is removed from an 11-year-old with anemia secondary to spherocytosis.

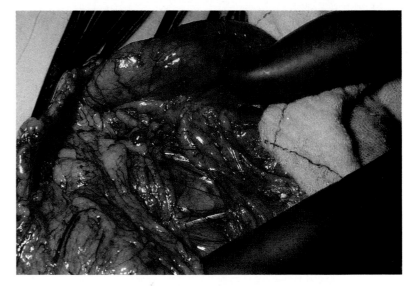

Figure 9.42 Accessory Spleen A small accessory spleen is found in the mesentery and is excised.

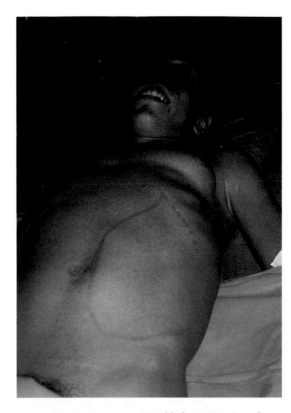

Figure 9.43 Thalassemia Major This boy has difficulty sitting and bending because of the massive splenic enlargement secondary to his hematologic disease.

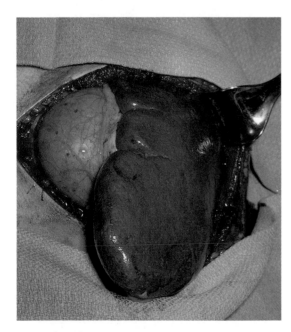

Figure 9.44 The huge spleen is seen at splenectomy. His stone-filled gallbladder (Figs 9.32, 9.33) is removed at the same time.

Idiopathic thrombocytopenic purpura (ITP) is an autoimmune disease (Fig 9.45) that requires splenectomy only when it becomes chronic and does not respond to steroid therapy. A persistent platelet count less than 50,000 is of concern. When splenectomy is planned, platelet transfusion is given 30 minutes before surgery to prevent bleeding.

Hypersplenism refers to the increased phagocytic activity of the enlarged spleen. Enlargement may be secondary to hemolytic disease, portal hypertension, or a storage disease such as Gaucher's disease. One, or all, of the formed elements of the blood may be depressed in number. Splenectomy is a last-resort procedure when medical therapy is of no avail. In a patient with hypersplenism and portal hypertension, a splenectomy should not be performed without consideration of a shunt procedure using the splenic vein (splenorenal shunt) at the same operation.

Tumor

Splenectomy is still considered part of the staging procedure to determine the presence and extent of intraabdominal involvement in Hodgkin's disease. However, with the availability of more accurate and sophisticated imaging modalities, operative staging is less often needed.

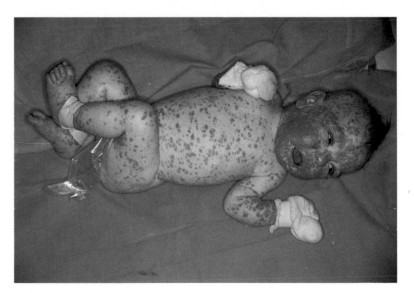

Figure 9.45 Thrombocytopenic Purpura This 6-month-old infant has the petechial rash of thrombocytopenic purpura.

Cysts

A splenic cyst may present with symptoms of abdominal pain and fullness or as a palpable mass. Ultrasonography (Fig 9.46), radionuclide scan, or computed tomography (Fig 9.47) will demonstrate the lesion. Excision of the cyst with preservation of splenic tissue is usually possible (Figs 9.48, 9.49).

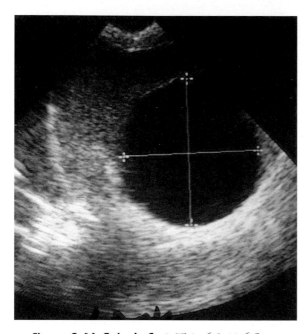

Figure 9.46 Splenic Cyst This 6.9 × 6.5 cm splenic cyst is seen on sonography of a 26-month-old with a palpable abdominal mass.

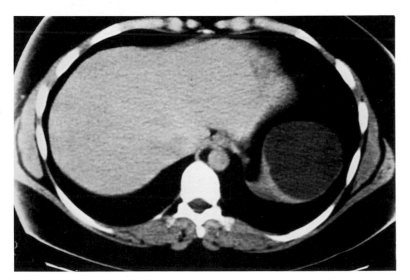

Figure 9.47 A palpable mass and left upper abdominal pain, in an older child, led to this computed tomography study, showing a large splenic cyst.

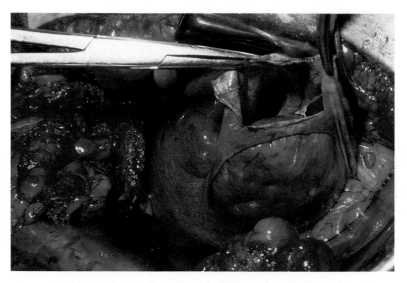

Figure 9.48 The open cyst of the entire lower pole of the spleen is seen at laparotomy.

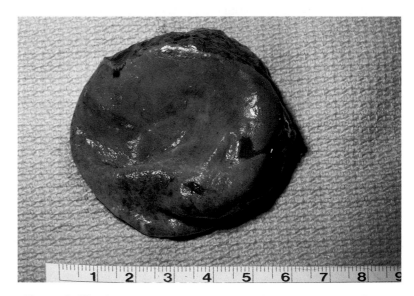

Figure 9.49 The resection specimen of the cyst is seen. The splenic margin is closed with carefully placed mattress sutures.

Pancreas

Annular Pancreas

The most common congenital abnormality of the pancreas is annular pancreas. It is formed during fetal development by an abnormality in rotation of the ventral pancreas prior to its fusion with the dorsal pancreas; a band of pancreatic tissue encircles the second portion of the duodenum. In a majority of cases, there is an associated duodenal atresia or stenosis (see Fig 6.34). At surgery, the annular pancreas is *not* divided; duodenojejunostomy is the safest procedure to bypass the obstruction.

Cysts and Pseudocysts

Simple pancreatic cysts are rare. Pancreatic pseudocysts are more frequent; in the pediatric age group, trauma is the principal cause. Presenting symptoms include epigastric pain, a bloated feeling, and occasional vomiting. Elevated serum and urinary amylase is the rule. A mass may be palpable or is demonstrated on ultrasonography, barium study (Fig 9.50), or computed tomography (Fig 9.51). Immediate surgery is to be avoided; the inflamed cyst wall is too thin and friable to hold sutures for internal drainage, and some pseudocysts resolve spontane-

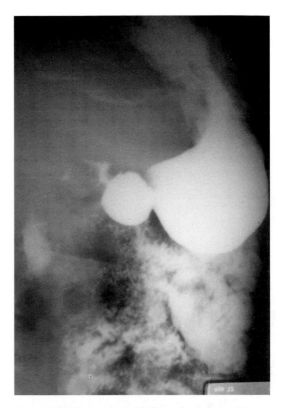

Figure 9.50 Pancreatic Pseudocyst A 12-year-old girl fell from her bicycle 3 weeks before this contrast study was done to evaluate persistent epigastric pain. The impression of a large mass on the lesser curvature of the stomach is seen.

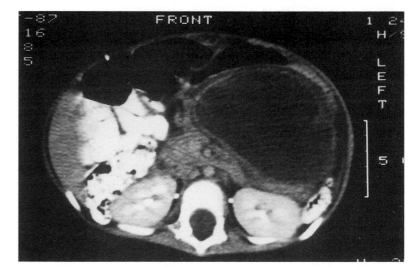

Figure 9.51 A large, palpable left upper abdominal mass is found in this 2-year-old who presents with pain, fever, and weight loss. There is no history of trauma. The computed tomography scan shows a cystic mass arising from the pancreas and displacing the stomach and intestine anteriorly.

ously. After 3–5 weeks, the cyst wall is mature, and resolution of the cyst is unlikely. A cyst-gastrostomy is performed to the posterior stomach for pseudocysts of the body of the pancreas (Figs 9.52, 9.53). Internal drainage into a Roux-en-Y jejunal segment is preferred for cysts of the head of the pancreas.

Hypoglycemia and Hyperinsulinism (Adenomas and Nesidioblastosis)

Insulin-producing islet cell adenomas of the pancreas present with symptoms of hypoglycemia shortly after birth. The babies are jittery and may have seizures. Blood glucose levels are less than 40 mg/dL. Endogenous insulin levels remain elevated during prolonged fasting and in response to the insulin suppression test. Imaging studies are rarely helpful in localizing the tumor.

Nesidioblastosis, in which islet cells remain attached to the ducts throughout the pancreas, presents with hyperinsulinism a little later in infancy. It cannot be distinguished clinically from an adenoma, and the treatment is the same.

Initial therapy, to counteract hypoglycemia, is administration of hypertonic glucose via a central venous line. When the infant's condition is stabilized, laparotomy is performed for pancreatic exploration. If an adenoma is seen or palpated, it is excised. If not, a 90% distal pancreatectomy is carried out, mobilizing the body and tail from the splenic vein and preserving the spleen (Figs 9.54, 9.55). Persistent hypoglycemia that is unresponsive to medical therapy may require total, or near-total, pancreatectomy.

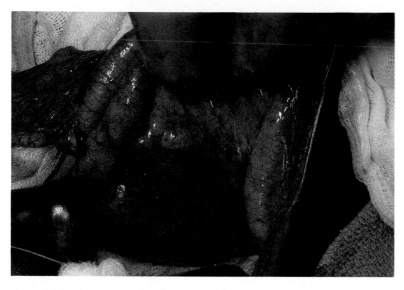

Figure 9.52 Elevation of the transverse colon reveals a large hemorrhagic pancreatic pseudocyst.

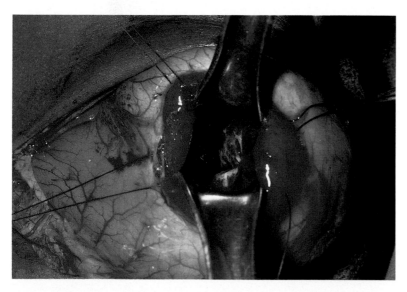

Figure 9.53 Exposure through an anterior gastrotomy allows entry into the mature wall of the pseudocyst through the posterior stomach. The inflamed lining of the pseudocyst is seen. Several interrupted sutures secure the cyst wall to the stomach, and the gastrotomy is closed in two layers.

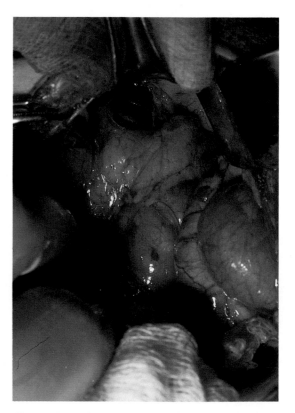

Figure 9.54 Nesidioblastosis A normal-appearing pancreas is seen in this infant with episodes of severe hypoglycemia. No adenoma is visible or palpable.

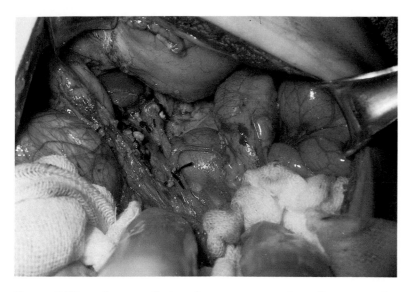

Figure 9.55 Only a small rim of pancreas remains adherent to the duodenum after a 90% pancreatectomy.

Tumors (Zollinger-Ellison Syndrome)

Zollinger-Ellison syndrome is characterized by peptic ulceration from acid hypersecretion, caused by a gastrin-secreting islet cell tumor. The diagnosis is made on the basis of high serum gastrin levels, either at rest or after infusion of calcium or secretin. Single tumors found at surgery are resected. If there is no demonstrable tumor, or if there are multiple tumors (Fig 9.56), total gastrectomy with esophagojejunostomy has been the surgical approach (see Chapter 6). Long-term treatment with a hydrogen ion–blocking agent (cimetidine) may become the preferred therapy.

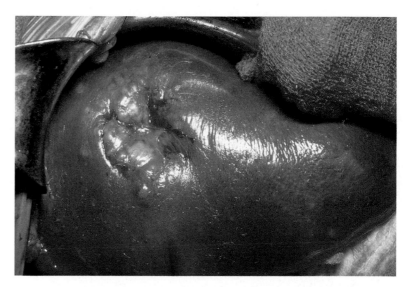

Figure 9.56 Zollinger-Ellison Syndrome Liver metastases of an islet cell tumor are seen in a 10-year-old boy with Zollinger-Ellison syndrome and no palpable pancreatic tumor. A total gastrectomy is performed (see Figs 6.25, 6.26).

Omental and Mesenteric Cysts

Omental and mesenteric cysts may be discovered because of abdominal distention, pain, intestinal obstruction, torsion of the cyst, or bleeding into the cyst. Most cysts are thought to be of congenital origin and are lined with endothelium, like lymphangiomas. They are generally unilocular and are filled with serous fluid or chyle. Plain radiographs show a gasless, fluid-filled abdomen (Fig 9.57). Ultrasonography or CT (Fig 9.58) will demonstrate a well-delineated cyst or multiple cysts.

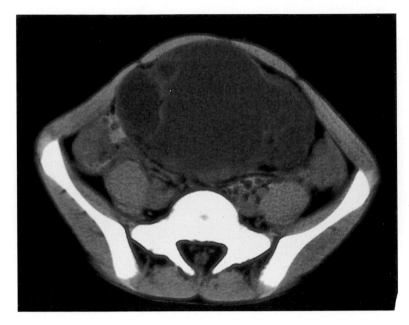

Figure 9.58 This computed tomography scan was performed for acute abdominal pain and vomiting in an 11-year-old boy with a palpable mass. A large cystic structure, with multiple septa and contents of uniform density, is seen.

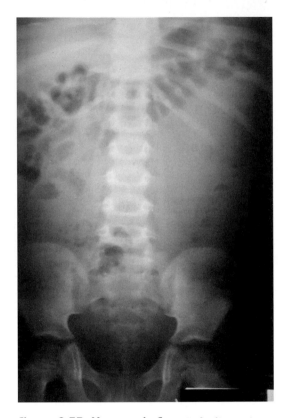

Figure 9.57 Mesenteric Cyst Soft distention of the abdomen led to this abdominal radiograph of a 5-year-old asymptomatic boy. The intestine is displaced laterally and cephalad by a mass of homogeneous density.

At surgery, the mesenteric cyst may be found adherent to the intestine, with excision requiring bowel resection. Others can be dissected carefully from the mesentery and surrounding structures (Figs 9.59, 9.60). A narrow base of attachment may allow torsion of the cyst (Figs 9.61, 9.62). Cysts with diffuse involvement of the mesentery may not be amenable to excision (Fig 9.63). The omental cyst has few intraabdominal attachments; ease of excision is influenced by the size of the cyst (Fig 9.64).

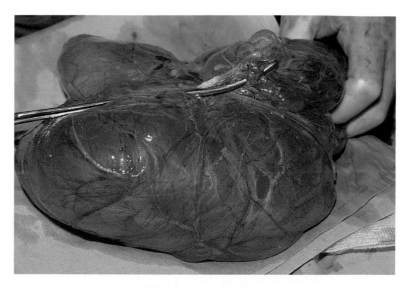

Figure 9.60 The cyst is removed intact. It measures approximately 18 × 12 cm.

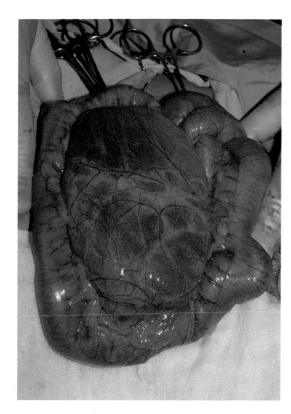

Figure 9.59 The mesenteric cyst of this 5-year-old occupies the entire midabdomen. It can be dissected easily from the mesentery without vascular damage, not the case with all such cysts.

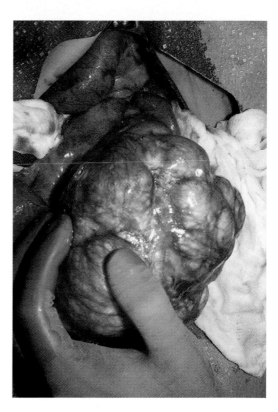

Figure 9.61 The mass visualized on abdominal CT in Figure 9.58 is a chylous mesenteric cyst; it can be seen to have twisted at its base, which is attached to the small bowel mesentery.

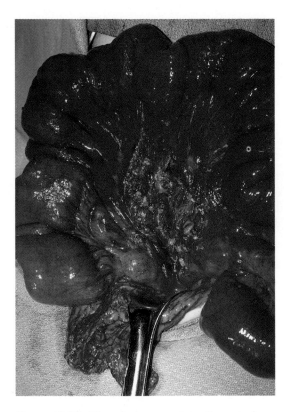

Figure 9.62 The chylous cyst is dissected from the mesentery without damage to the intestinal blood vessels at its point of origin.

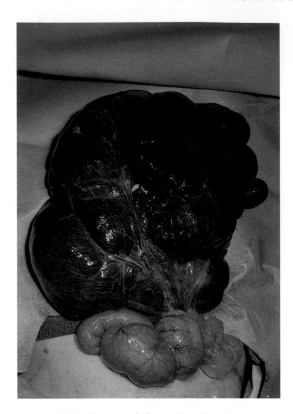

Figure 9.64 Omental Cyst Bleeding into a large omental cyst produced abdominal pain and a palpable mass in this 3-year-old girl. The attachment of the cyst to the transverse colon is seen.

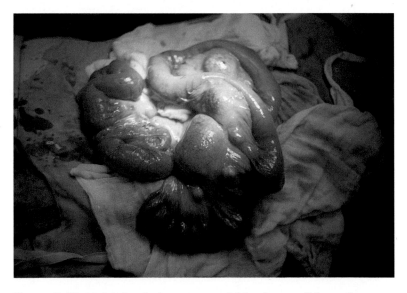

Figure 9.63 Multiple chylous cysts within the small bowel mesentery are seen in this patient. No resection is performed because of the diffuse involvement.

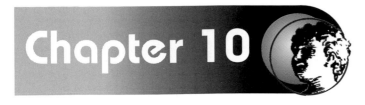

Chapter 10

Urinary Tract

Congenital abnormalities of the urinary tract are numerous. Correction, especially of obstructive lesions, may allow salvage of one or both kidneys or relief of chronic infection. Diagnosis and treatment of tumors are discussed in Chapter 12.

Kidney

Renal Cysts

A palpable kidney mass in a child is most often hydronephrosis, Wilms' tumor, or cystic disease—in that order of frequency. Ultrasonography is valuable as a screening study. Definitive evaluation often requires computed tomography with urinary contrast, voiding cystourethrogram (VCUG), renal scan, and (rarely) arteriography.

Cystic disease can be characterized as multicystic disease, polycystic disease, or solitary cysts. The multicystic kidney is a unilateral dysgenetic mass of large cysts without functioning parenchyma (Fig 10.1). There is no visualization on urography—or sometimes a negative shadow on total body opacification with intravenous contrast material. The multicystic kidney has frequently been removed for diagnosis, but some surgeons now feel that the accuracy of diagnostic imaging studies and absence of subsequent problems make excision unnecessary.

Infantile polycystic disease is an autosomal recessive congenital abnormality. It is bilateral and is associated with biliary duct ectasia or hepatic fibrosis, rarely liver cysts. The ultrasonographic appearance of the kidneys is one of increased medullary echogenicity, with small cysts in some cases (Fig 10.2). Polycystic disease of the autosomal dominant type presents infrequently in childhood and is associated with cysts of other organs. The gross appearance is that of small cysts on the surface and a honeycomb appearance on section. Progressive renal failure is the inevitable outcome of both types of polycystic disease, and dialysis and renal transplantation are the only available therapeutic solutions.

Solitary cysts (Figs 10.3, 10.4) may affect one or both kidneys and are significant only when they increase in size. Excision of the cyst wall suffices as treatment.

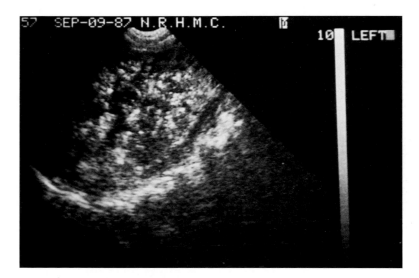

Figure 10.2 Polycystic Kidney Ultrasonography demonstrates the diffuse echogenicity of a poorly functioning polycystic kidney.

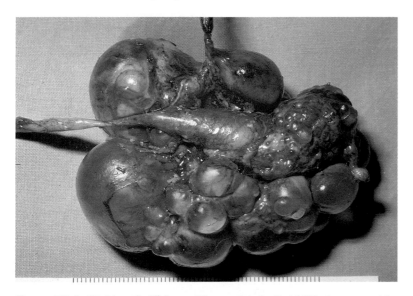

Figure 10.1 Multicystic Kidney The multiple fluid-filled cysts with no parenchyma represent the entire left kidney, which presented as a visible and palpable flank mass in a neonate.

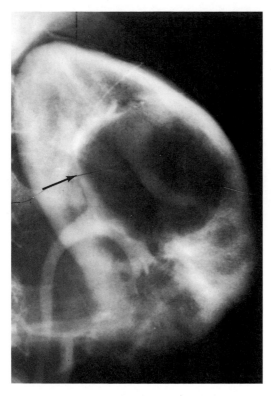

Figure 10.3 Solitary Renal Cyst The negative image of a renal cyst is seen on the venous phase of a selective angiogram of the left kidney.

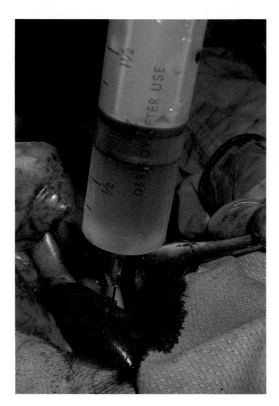

Figure 10.4 Aspiration of the cyst contents collapses this intrarenal cyst prior to its unroofing.

Hydronephrosis

Hydronephrosis is the result of chronic urinary tract infection, reflux, and/or obstruction at any level. In children, congenital obstruction is the most common cause, and hydronephrosis has been detected by ultrasonography of the fetus. There may be intrinsic narrowing of the ureter anywhere from the renal pelvis to the entrance to the bladder. Bladder neck obstruction and posterior urethral valves are lower obstructions. Relief of the obstruction must be accomplished early enough to preserve whatever kidney function is present. Fetal surgery, with drainage to relieve the obstruction, has been recommended for some forms of congenital urinary obstruction causing severe hydronephrosis of both kidneys.

Ureteropelvic Obstruction

Ureteropelvic junction obstruction leading to hydronephrosis may be detected in the newborn infant as a palpable enlarged kidney (Figs 10.5–10.7); in the toddler or older child, there is usually a history of recurrent infection or pain. Rarely, it may present as an asymptomatic palpable mass in an older child (Fig 10.8). Ultrasonography will confirm the hydronephrosis. Intravenous pyelography, or computed tomography with intravenous contrast material, allows visualization of the dilated pelvis, with

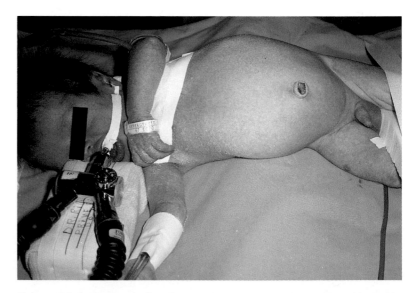

Figure 10.5 Hydronephrosis A large mass is seen in the left flank of this 9-day-old boy.

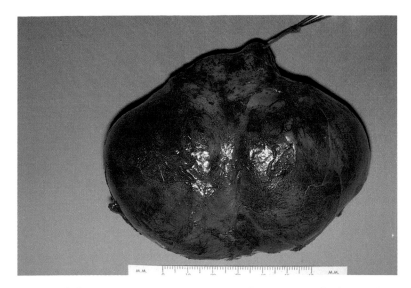

Figure 10.6 This massively dilated, nonfunctioning, hydronephrotic kidney is removed. The other kidney appears normal.

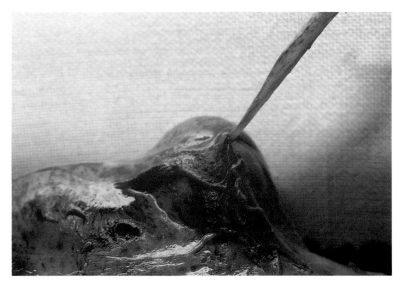

Figure 10.7 A close-up shows the marked narrowing of the ureteropelvic junction.

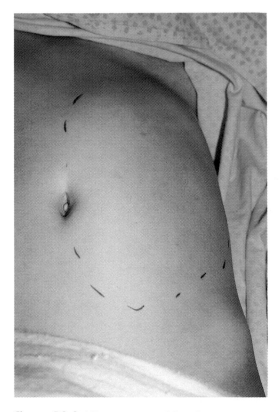

Figure 10.8 This 17-year-old girl presents with a visible and palpable left upper abdominal mass and no previous symptoms.

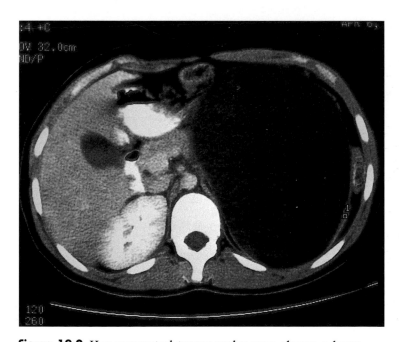

Figure 10.9 Her computed tomography scan shows a huge nonfunctioning hydronephrotic kidney.

late films to show the delayed emptying of ureteropelvic obstruction (Fig 10.9). Vesicoureteral reflux should be excluded by cystourethrography. A radionuclide renal scan, with furosemide washout, will help in the assessment of function, to decide whether the kidney can be salvaged. Massive hydronephrosis of many years' duration leaves only a nonsalvageable kidney with no functioning parenchyma (Figs 10.10, 10.11).

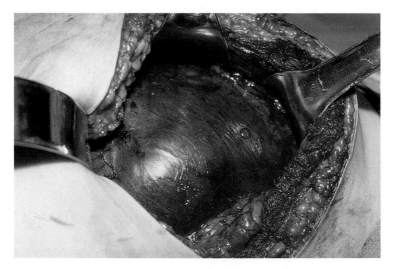

Figure 10.10 An intraoperative photograph shows the huge, fluid-filled hydronephrotic kidney, approached retroperitoneally. There is no visible renal parenchyma.

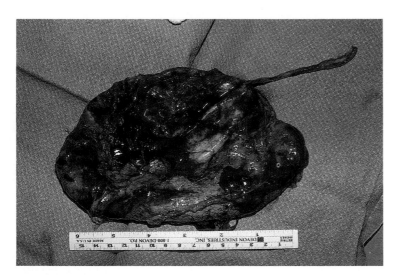

Figure 10.11 The kidney is removed after intraoperative trocar decompression. The residual capsule is seen, with marked ureteropelvic narrowing.

At surgery, the nature of the obstruction—intrinsic narrowing, external bands, or an aberrant vessel—is determined (Figs 10.12, 10.13). Extrinsic obstructions are resected when possible. Intrinsic narrowing requires ureteropyeloplasty.

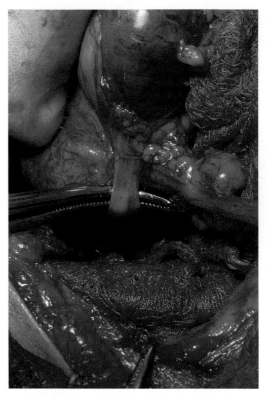

Figure 10.12 An anomalous renal vein crosses and partially obstructs the ureter, resulting in chronic pyelonephritis and hydronephrosis.

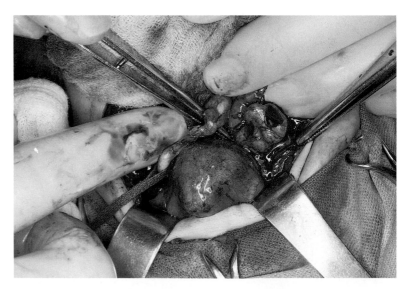

Figure 10.13 An intrinsic kinking and segmental narrowing of the distal right ureter is seen at the tip of the forceps. The 7-day-old patient presented with hydronephrosis.

Ureters

Vesicoureteral Reflux

Congenital or acquired abnormalities of the ureterovesical junction, with inadequate flap-valve mechanism, may lead to reflux of urine and subsequent infection and renal damage. In the child with recurrent urinary infections, performance of a voiding cystourethrogram confirms the diagnosis. Surgical correction, with reimplantation of the ureter into a bladder mucosal tunnel, is performed when urinary infections persist despite antibiotic prophylaxis, or when there is evidence of poor renal growth.

Duplication

Double ureters from the same kidney are commonly associated with vesicoureteral reflux and hydronephrosis of one pole or the entire kidney (Figs 10.14–10.17). Involvement of a pole can resemble a polar cyst on sonography. Ureteroceles are frequently found in association with duplication. A duplicate ureter may enter at, or below, the bladder neck, with uncontrolled dribbling of urine.

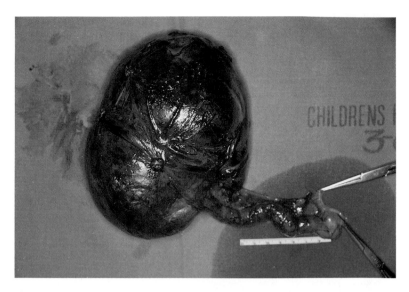

Figure 10.14 Double Ureters A duplex collecting system is seen from this kidney removed for massive hydronephrosis.

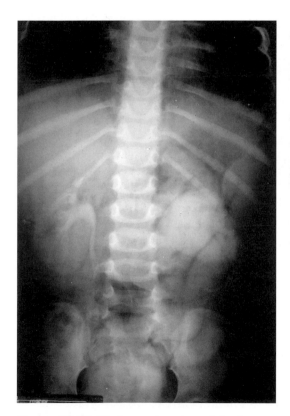

Figure 10.15 Hydronephrosis and hydroureters are seen on the patient's left in an infusion pyelogram.

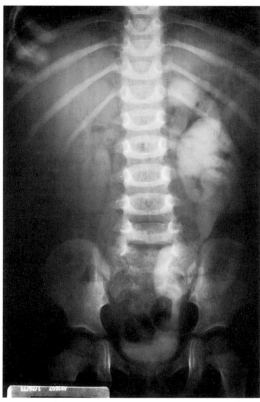

Figure 10.16 A delayed film shows the pelvicalyceal dilatation of the left kidney.

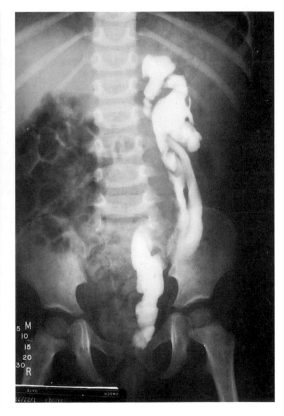

Figure 10.17 Retrograde urography demonstrates the double collecting system draining into the bladder neck.

Surgical correction involves either reimplantation of both ureters into the bladder, or end-to-side ureteroureteral anastomosis of the refluxing ureter into the normal ureter. Heminephrectomy is indicated for the nonfunctioning segment.

Ureterovesical Stricture

Congenital strictures may occur at the ureterovesical junction (Fig 10.18); however, the majority of strictures are secondary to bladder changes from distal obstruction. Ureteral reimplantation, occasionally combined with tapering of markedly dilated ureters, is performed after correction of the distal obstruction.

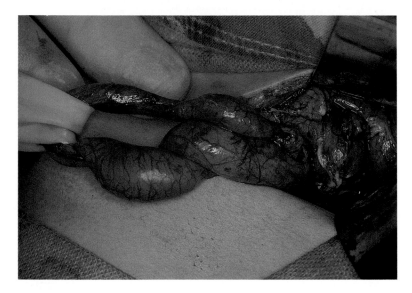

Figure 10.18 Ureterovesical Stricture The dilated, tortuous ureter is seen at exploration for bilateral congenital ureterovesical obstruction. The ureters are reimplanted into the bladder.

Ureterocele

Simple ureteroceles are much less common than those associated with ureteral duplication. Children may have symptoms of infection or bladder neck obstruction, with occasional prolapse through the urethra (Figs 10.19, 10.20). Cystourethrography confirms the diagnosis. The treatment of choice, especially in duplicated ureters with ectopic orifice, is excision of the ureterocele and reimplantation of the ureter, if renal function is satisfactory.

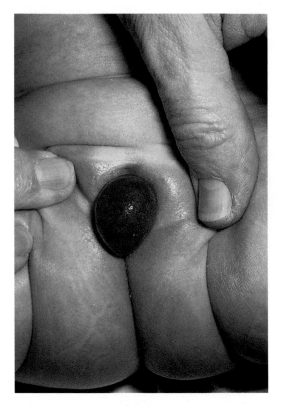

Figure 10.19 Ureterocele A prolapsed ureterocele appears suddenly when this infant girl tries unsuccessfully to urinate.

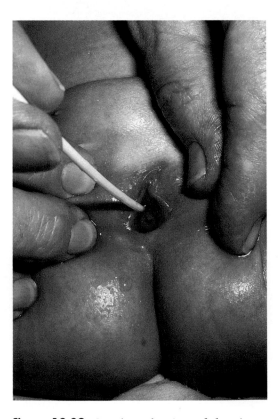

Figure 10.20 Gentle reduction of the simple ureterocele with a sterile cotton-tipped swab relieves the obstruction. Excision and ureteral reimplantation will be performed.

Megaureter

Megaureter, massive dilatation of the ureter, is usually the result of distal obstruction or severe vesicoureteral reflux. It is a frequent finding in children with absent abdominal musculature—prune-belly syndrome (Figs 10.21–10.23). The aim of surgery is to relieve the obstruction or reflux and to taper the ureter.

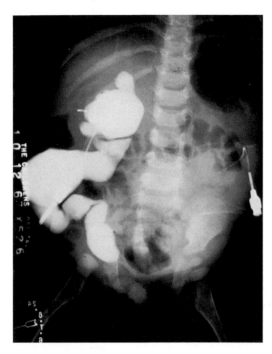

Figure 10.21 Megaureter Percutaneous pyelography gives this clear view of a huge dilated right ureter and pelvicalyceal system in this 17-month-old boy with absent abdominal musculature. The patient's abdomen is seen in Figure 5.74.

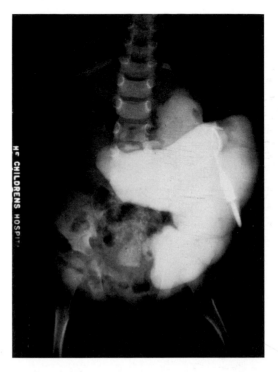

Figure 10.22 The left ureter of the same patient is so distended and tortuous that its outline cannot be seen clearly. The child had recurrent urinary infections.

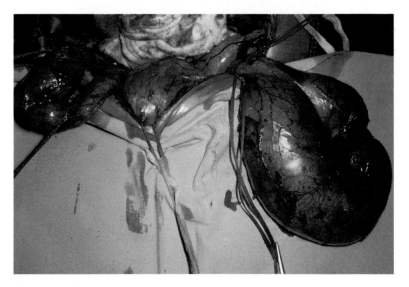

Figure 10.23 His massively dilated ureters (left and right umbilical tapes), as well as the patent urachus (middle tape) and abdominal undescended testes, are seen at surgery.

Bladder

Urachus

Remnants of the embryologic communication between the bladder and umbilical cord include (1) complete patent urachus, (2) urachal cyst, (3) umbilical remnant, and (4) urachal diverticulum of the bladder. Urinary drainage from the umbilical cord (Fig 10.24) characterizes the patent urachus. Contrast studies of the sinus demonstrate the bladder communication (Fig 10.25), and sonography or contrast radiographs may demonstrate other urinary abnormalities (Fig 10.26). Excision of the tract, with two-layer closure of the bladder, is recommended (Fig 10.27). Postoperative bladder decompression is not required if there is no distal obstruction.

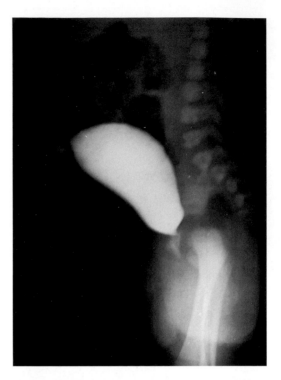

Figure 10.25 Contrast injected through the umbilical opening fills the bladder, confirming the diagnosis of patent urachus.

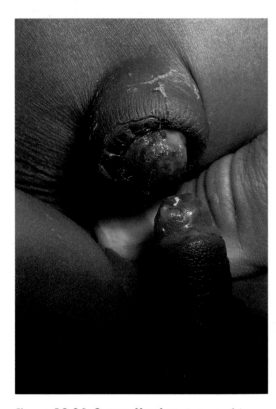

Figure 10.24 Patent Urachus Suprapubic compression produces urine from the umbilicus and the penis in this 5-day-old boy.

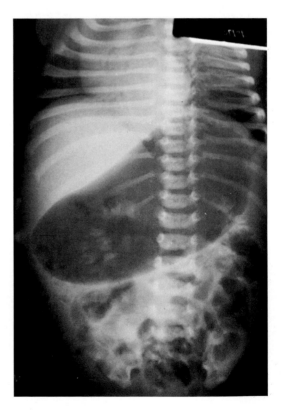

Figure 10.26 The same patient is shown to have mild hydronephrosis of the right kidney; the cause is ureteropelvic stenosis.

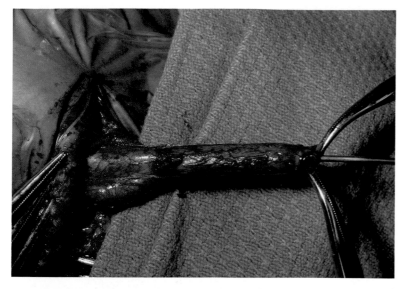

Figure 10.27 A probe passes into the bladder through the dissected urachal tract. The tract is excised at the bladder.

Urachal cysts are found when they become infected and present as red, tender masses in the mid-lower abdomen. An abscess may require immediate drainage; eventually the cyst must be excised.

Umbilical urachal remnants discharge clear material from the umbilicus. They, too, may become infected and should be excised.

A urachal diverticulum of the bladder may be found adherent to the underside of the umbilicus or to the wall of an omphalocele (Fig 10.28). It is resected at the bladder wall.

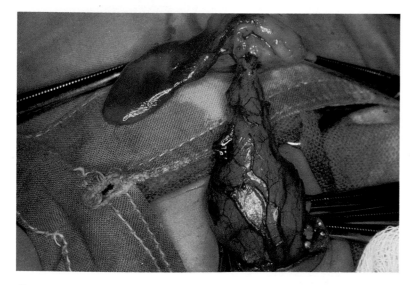

Figure 10.28 This urachal diverticulum is found adherent to the undersurface of a small omphalocele. It is resected.

Exstrophy of the Bladder

In exstrophy, the bladder lies completely open on the lower abdominal wall, the pubis is separated, and there is severe epispadias (Fig 10.29). The two surgical approaches have been (1) reconstruction of the bladder and (2) cystectomy with permanent urinary diversion. For reconstruction, most surgeons try to achieve early bladder turn-in with approximation of the pubic rami and closure of the abdominal wall. Subsequent surgery may involve reconstruction of the bladder neck to serve as a sphincter, reimplantation of the ureters to prevent reflux, bladder augmentation when necessary, lengthening of the penis in the male, and repair of the epispadias.

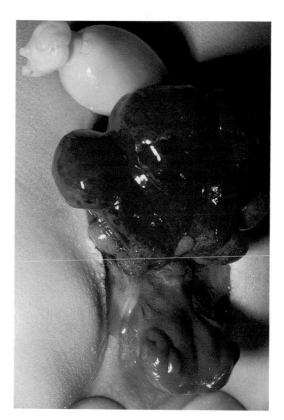

Figure 10.29 Exstrophy of the Bladder
The small bladder of this newborn boy lies open on the abdominal wall. Severe epispadias is seen.

Urethra

Posterior Urethral Valves

A cause of severe urinary obstruction in the neonate and infant, congenital posterior urethral valves may lead to vesicoureteral reflux, hydronephrosis, and even urinary ascites (Figs 10.30, 10.31). The diagnosis is made by cystourethrogram (Fig 10.32). Valves may be treated directly by endoscopic resection in the absence of infection. In some very sick infants, temporary urinary diversion is advised first (Fig 10.33). If reflux persists following resection of the valves, ureteral reimplantation may be necessary.

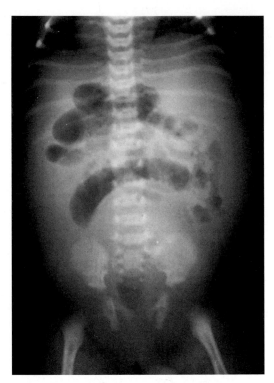

Figure 10.30 Posterior Urethral Valves
Urinary ascites and a distended bladder are shown in this abdominal film of a boy with abdominal distention and no passage of urine at birth.

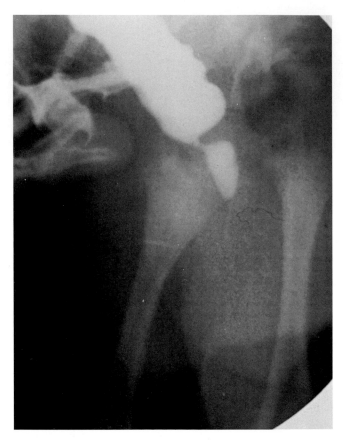

Figure 10.32 A cystourethrogram confirms the diagnosis of obstructing posterior urethral valves. Contrast can barely be seen distal to the obstruction.

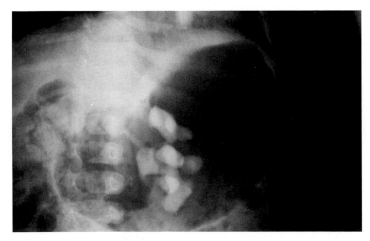

Figure 10.31 Hydronephrosis is demonstrated on intravenous pyelography in the same infant.

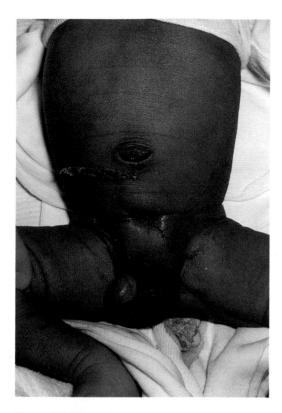

Figure 10.33 A cutaneous cystostomy is performed in this infant because of his clinical condition. After relief of the hydronephrosis and reversal of the bladder thickening, the valves will be excised.

Meatal Stenosis

Urinary and diaper irritation, with ulceration of the tip of the penis in the circumcised male infant, is thought to cause scarring and stenosis of the urethral meatus (Fig 10.34). Delayed bladder emptying and a fine urinary stream may be seen because of the pinpoint opening. A generous (4–5 mm) urethral meatoplasty, with interrupted 6-0 chromic gut to approximate the skin and mucosa, solves the problem (Fig 10.35). The application of sterile petrolatum or thick antibiotic ointment into the meatus with each diaper change for a week after surgery prevents recurrence and the need for dilatation or re-opening.

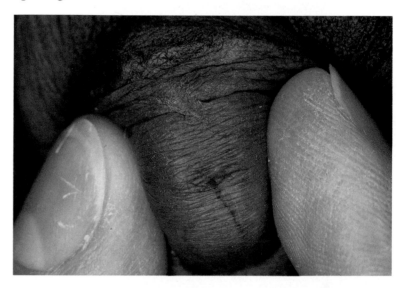

Figure 10.34 Urethral Meatal Stenosis A pinpoint opening in the urethral meatus is associated with urinary infection in this boy.

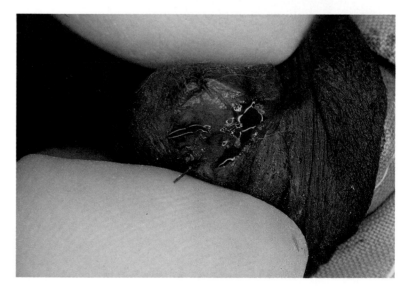

Figure 10.35 A 5-mm incision from the opening to the top of the penis is made. The skin and mucous membrane are then approximated with absorbable suture.

Hypospadias

The abnormally placed urethral opening in hypospadias may be coronal (Fig 10.36), subcoronal, distal or midshaft (Fig 10.37), penoscrotal, or perineal. Chordee (Fig 10.38), which is associated with hypospadias in many cases, must be released as part of any hypospadias repair. Most repairs are based on the creation of a new length of penile urethra by rolling in a flap of penile or preputial skin. It is, therefore, important to recognize the problem at birth and to avoid removing the prepuce by circumcision.

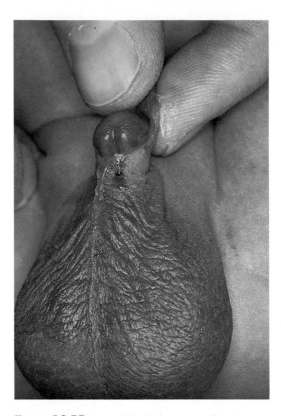

Figure 10.37 A midshaft hypospadias is demonstrated in this neonate, who also has an imperforate anus.

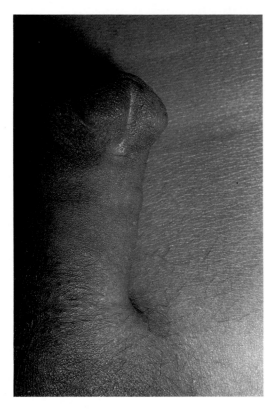

Figure 10.36 Hypospadias This coronal hypospadias does not interfere with urination. It will be repaired, however, at the time of relief of the associated chordee.

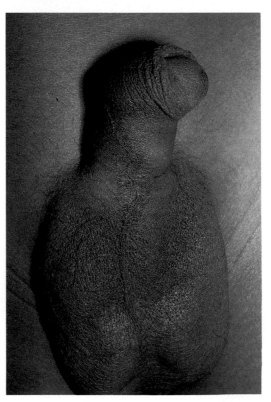

Figure 10.38 The ventral angulation of the penile shaft is a chordee, associated with a coronal hypospadias. It is thought to be the result of prenatal scarring of the ventral corpora.

Epispadias

A dorsal opening of the urethra, epispadias is most often associated with exstrophy of the bladder (see earlier). It may occur in either sex. In the male (see Fig 10.29), repair often requires penile lengthening as well as creation of a neo-urethra.

Adrenal

Pheochromocytoma

Tumors of the adrenal medulla may secrete epinephrine or norepinephrine, leading to hypertension, flushing, tremors, diaphoresis, tachycardia, weight loss, and increased appetite. The diagnosis of pheochromocytoma is made on the basis of imaging studies—ultrasonography, computed tomography, magnetic resonance imaging, and arteriography (Fig 10.39)—and is confirmed by measurement of catecholamines and their metabolites such as vanillylmandelic acid (VMA).

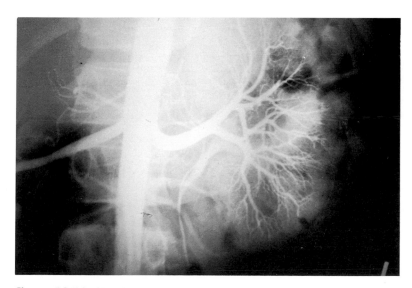

Figure 10.39 Pheochromocytoma A left adrenal tumor "lights up" on this arteriogram of a 14-year-old boy with intermittent flushing, tachycardia, and weight loss.

Alpha-adrenergic blockers such as phenoxybenzamine are administered to prevent hypertensive crises. Anesthetic management requires careful blood pressure regulation. Exploration must expose both adrenal glands and the sympathetic chain. Early control of the venous drainage of the tumor prevents the sudden release of catecholamines. The tumor is excised with the entire adrenal gland (Figs 10.40, 10.41). Prevention of hypotension is important in postoperative management.

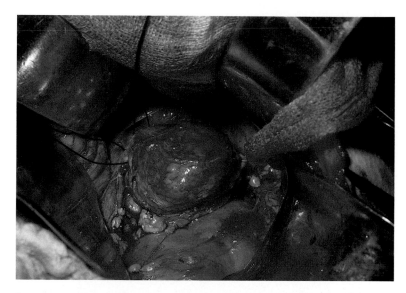

Figure 10.40 The tumor is seen at surgery. Early ligation of the venous drainage and gentle manipulation of the tumor are important to prevent intraoperative hypertension.

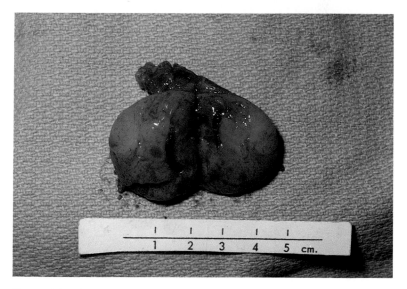

Figure 10.41 The sectioned tumor is almost all medullary tissue, with only a tiny rim of cortex.

Neuroblastoma

Neuroblastoma is the most frequent solid malignant tumor in childhood. The adrenal medulla is a common site of origin. It is discussed in Chapter 12.

Cushing's Syndrome

Cushing's syndrome, caused by adrenocortical hyperplasia or a functioning adenoma or carcinoma, is rare in childhood (Fig 10.42); it occurs most often in adolescents. Surgical exploration of the adrenal glands is indicated. Hyperplastic glands are removed bilaterally; adenomas are excised with their entire gland, and the opposite gland is biopsied; and wide excision is recommended for adrenal carcinoma.

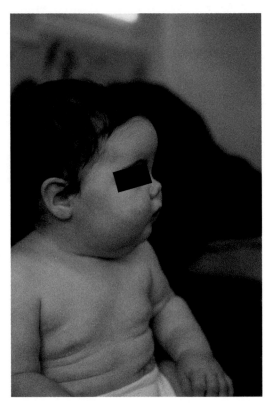

Figure 10.42 Cushing's Syndrome This infant girl has the moon face, ruddy cheeks, and "buffalo hump" characteristic of excess adrenocortical function. Adrenal hyperplasia is the cause.

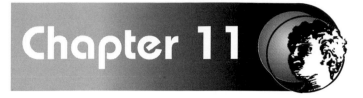

Chapter 11

Genitalia

Evaluation and correction of the congenital anomalies of the reproductive organs may be simple or quite complex. Benign tumors predominate over malignant ones. Torsion of the gonad is a true surgical emergency.

Ovaries

Cysts

Simple ovarian cyst is reported to be the most common palpable abdominal mass in the newborn girl (Figs 11.1, 11.2). In the older child, progressively increasing abdominal girth, urinary frequency, and/or constipation are presenting symptoms. Torsion of a cystic ovary results in acute pain and abdominal tenderness. In postmenarchal adolescents, corpus luteum cysts, when they rupture and bleed, may cause lower abdominal pain, simulating that of appendicitis.

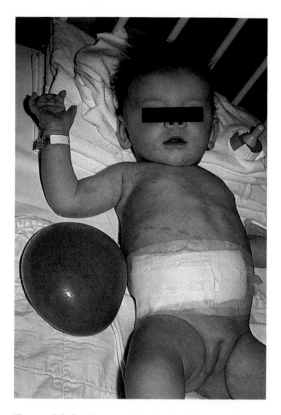

Figure 11.2 The excised cyst is seen next to the patient immediately after the operation.

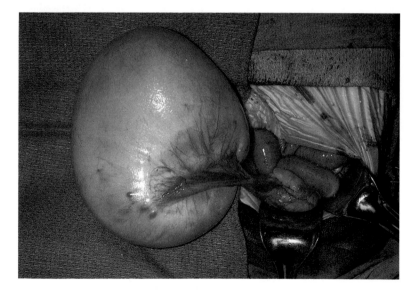

Figure 11.1 Ovarian Cyst A 3-month-old presented with a large, palpable right abdominal and flank mass. A simple ovarian cyst, with normal right tube, left ovary and tube, and uterus, is seen. The cyst is excised, with preservation of the right tube; there is no normal ovarian tissue on the right.

Some cysts are detectable on plain abdominal radiographs (Fig 11.3). Ultrasonography is the most helpful diagnostic study, showing the presence of an ovarian mass (Fig 11.4) or of pelvic fluid characteristic of a ruptured ovarian follicle. Some cysts may be detected antenatally. Of those present at birth, a few resolve spontaneously (Fig 11.5).

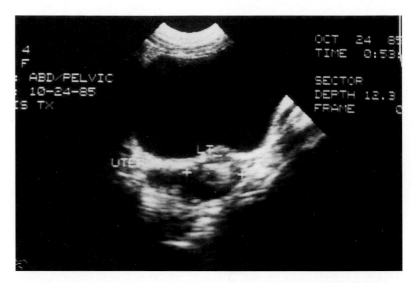

Figure 11.4 The cystic ovarian mass seen next to the uterus on this sonogram is a benign teratoma.

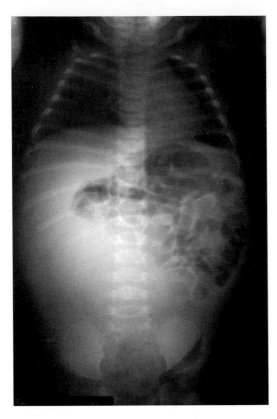

Figure 11.3 The radiograph shows a large mass (cyst) displacing abdominal contents from the right side of the abdomen.

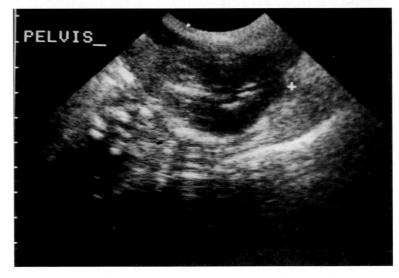

Figure 11.5 The ovarian cyst of a neonate, seen on this sonogram, was detected prenatally on maternal sonography. It could not be seen 1 month later on repeated sonography.

Ovarian cysts that do not involute in the infant, or sizable cysts presenting after infancy, should be removed. By doing so, one may excise a teratoma with its potential for malignant degeneration or reduce the chance for future torsion of a simple cyst. In many cases, a simple cyst can be excised with preservation of the ipsilateral tube and ovarian tissue (Figs 11.6–11.8). Laparoscopic visualization and decompression of an ovarian cyst are illustrated in Chapter 8.

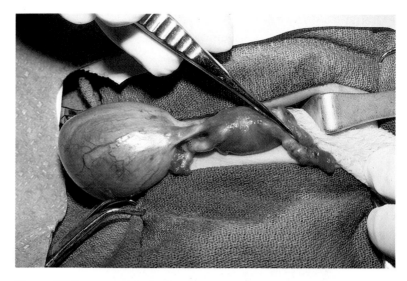

Figure 11.7 At exploration, a simple ovarian cyst is found, arising from the lateral part of the right ovary. The forceps point to a normal left tube and ovary.

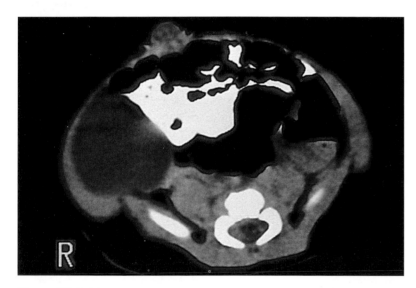

Figure 11.6 The right ovarian cyst, seen in this computed tomography scan of an infant, had been growing in size.

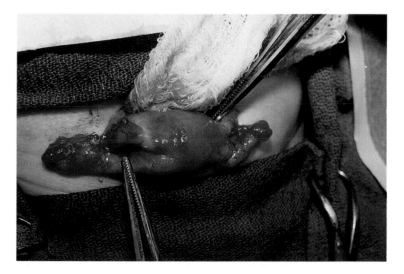

Figure 11.8 Careful dissection of the cyst preserves the right tube and normal ovarian tissue, seen at the tip of the forceps.

Tumors

Ovarian tumors represent only 1% of childhood neoplasms; the majority are benign. Symptoms include nonspecific abdominal pain, bloating or fullness, nausea, and urinary frequency. Pleural effusion (Fig 11.9) and ascites (Fig 11.10) may be associated with some malignant ovarian tumors.

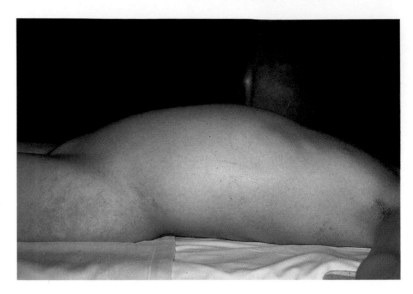

Figure 11.10 Malignant Ovarian Teratoma This 12-year-old has a large ovarian tumor that is difficult to palpate because of considerable ascites.

Teratomas are the most frequently found, accounting for approximately 30% of ovarian tumors in childhood. Composed of all three primary germ layers, they may contain foci of brain, bone, teeth, intestine, skin, and skin appendages like hair. The tumors may be cystic and/or solid, benign or malignant (Figs 11.11–11.15).

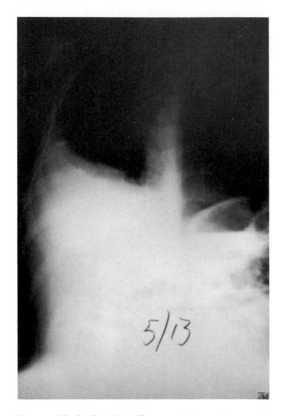

Figure 11.9 Ovarian Tumor The radiograph shows a pleural effusion that had developed during the 3 days prior to surgery in this 13-year-old with a malignant granulosa cell tumor of the ovary.

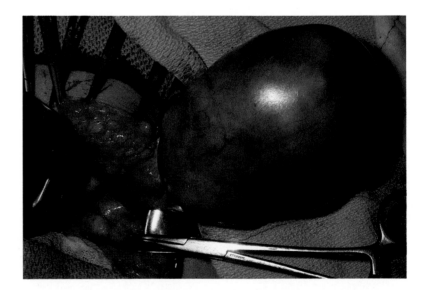

Figure 11.11 Benign Ovarian Teratoma This tumor of the left ovary is irregularly shaped, with prominent surface vessels and palpable cystic and solid areas. A normal-appearing right ovary contains no visible or palpable tumor.

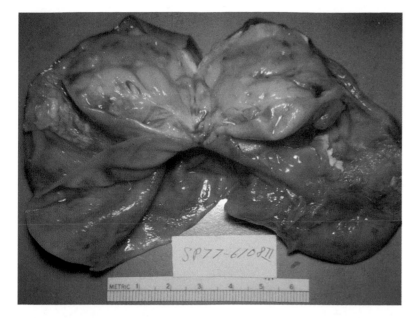

Figure 11.12 The sectioned benign tumor has numerous cysts, as well as a solid portion; on microscopic evaluation, all three germ layers were seen.

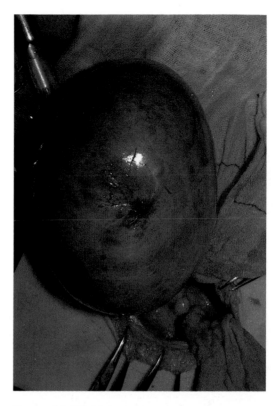

Figure 11.14 This malignant ovarian teratoma was the cause of ascites in the 12-year-old seen in Figure 11.10. It is solid, with a puckered central portion that represents an adhesion of malignant tissue to the abdominal wall.

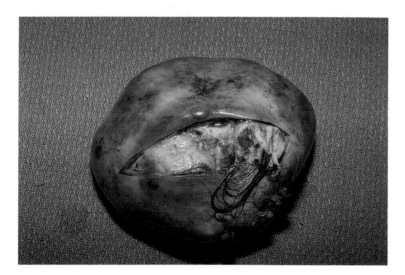

Figure 11.13 A benign ovarian teratoma was excised from a 15-year-old who presented with acute abdominal pain secondary to torsion. One of multiple cysts is unroofed, showing waxy sebaceous material and a growth of dark hair.

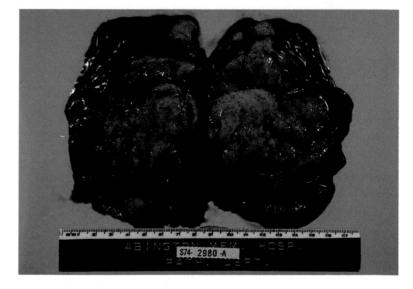

Figure 11.15 The solid malignant teratoma was sectioned. Following therapy, the patient is tumor-free 20 years later.

Epithelial tumors, such as serous or mucinous cystadenoma, constitute 10%–20% of pediatric ovarian tumors; the occurrence of malignancy in these is 10%–14%. At oophorectomy, the opposite ovary should be bivalved and examined carefully for tumor.

Dysgerminomas account for 10%–15% of ovarian tumors in children; 5%–10% are bilateral, and one third are malignant. Like seminomas in the male, they spread to retroperitoneal lymphatics and are highly responsive to radiotherapy.

Granulosa cell tumors constitute the majority of sex cord–stromal neoplasms. Most secrete estrogens and are diagnosed on the basis of precocious puberty (Fig 11.16). Fewer than 5% are malignant (Figs 11.17–11.20).

Rare tumors include gonadoblastoma, androblastoma, endodermal sinus tumor, and ovarian carcinoma and sarcoma.

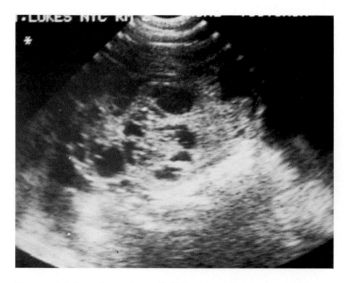

Figure 11.17 Granulosa Cell Tumor Ultrasonography shows the low abdominal mass to be primarily solid, with some cysts.

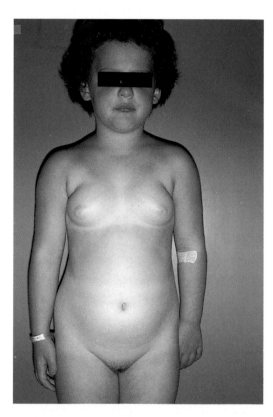

Figure 11.16 Precocious Puberty Pubic hair and breast development are apparent in this 4-year-old girl.

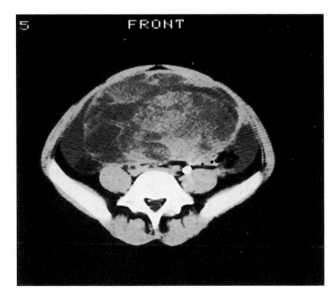

Figure 11.18 Computed tomography demonstrates the cystic and solid nature of this well-encapsulated intraperitoneal tumor.

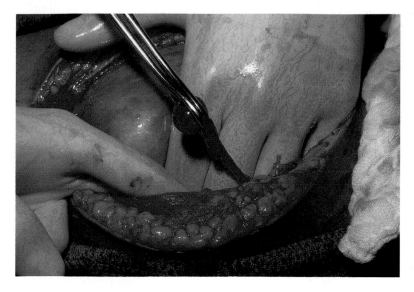

Figure 11.19 At surgery, gelatinous cysts are found adherent to the peritoneum. The large ovarian tumor is behind the surgeon's hand.

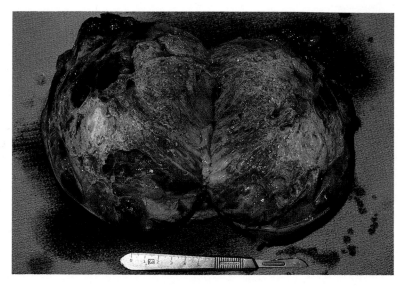

Figure 11.20 The malignant granulosa cell tumor is seen on cut section.

Torsion

Ovarian torsion is one of the problems that must be considered in the girl with acute lower abdominal pain. The etiology is uncertain, although a cyst or ovarian tumor predisposes to torsion. Pain of rapid onset, nausea and vomiting, and urinary frequency and dysuria are prominent symptoms. Tenderness is usually localized to the low abdomen, and a tender, enlarged ovary may be palpable on rectal or bimanual examination. Ultrasonography or computed tomography is sometimes helpful in confirming the diagnosis. Early surgical intervention and detorsion may save the ovary; often there is a gangrenous, hemorrhagic ovary that must be removed (Figs 11.21, 11.22). If possible, the tube on the side of the torsion should be saved. The opposite ovary must be examined, and sizable cysts should be opened to diminish the chance of torsion.

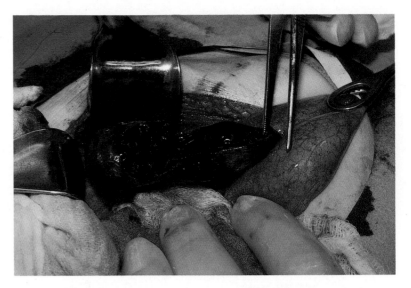

Figure 11.22 The hemorrhagic ovary ruptures easily with the slightest manipulation. It is excised, with preservation of the undamaged right tube.

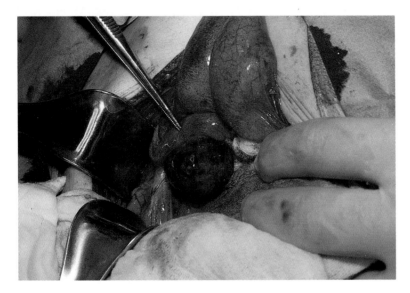

Figure 11.21 Ovarian Torsion An infarcted right ovary is seen at exploration of the abdomen of a 4-year-old with right lower quadrant pain and a tender mass felt on rectal examination.

Maternal sonography often demonstrates an ovarian cyst or mass in the female fetus. As mentioned previously, under "Cysts," some resorb spontaneously. However, those ovaries that have been subjected to intrauterine torsion (Figs 11.23, 11.24) will not diminish in size after birth, and the infant must undergo pelvic exploration by laparotomy or laparoscopy. Antenatal torsion usually results in a nonviable ovary, which should be removed.

Paraovarian cysts, in the broad ligament, may also result in adnexal torsion (Fig 11.25). The cyst should be excised (Fig 11.26), with preservation of the adjacent tube and ovary if they are viable.

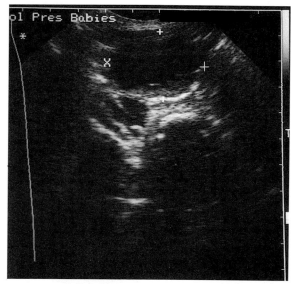

Figure 11.23 The ovarian "cyst" (2.58 × 3.66 cm) demonstrated on this sonogram of a 1-month-old girl was detected antenatally and grew in size from the time of birth.

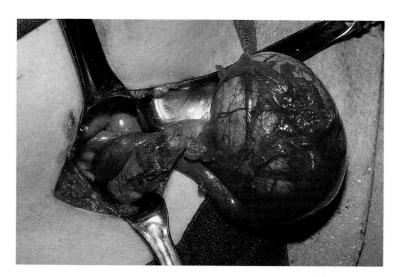

Figure 11.25 Paraovarian Cyst The torsion of this cystic structure intimately adherent to the fallopian tube was responsible for acute abdominal pain in a 16-year-old girl. It is a paraovarian cyst in the broad ligament.

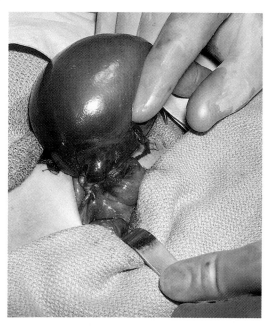

Figure 11.24 At laparotomy, it is seen to be an infarcted right ovary, with a 720° twist at the base.

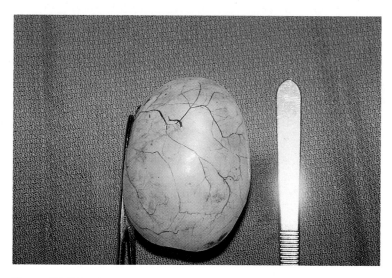

Figure 11.26 The entire cyst was removed, and the tube and ovary were preserved.

Fallopian Tube

Infection

Ascending infection through a patent cervical os is thought to be the rare cause of some tubal infections in the prepubertal girl. Most salpingitis is of venereal origin, reflecting sexual activity in the teenager or sexual abuse at any age, even infancy. In the sexually active adolescent, symptoms and physical signs of salpingitis may be indistinguishable from those of appendicitis. Clinical judgment should be weighted on the side of surgical exploration or diagnostic laparoscopy if there is serious doubt.

Torsion

Torsion of the fallopian tube alone is a rare phenomenon in children and adolescents (Fig 11.27). Symptoms are like those of ovarian torsion; early detorsion may save the tube from damage.

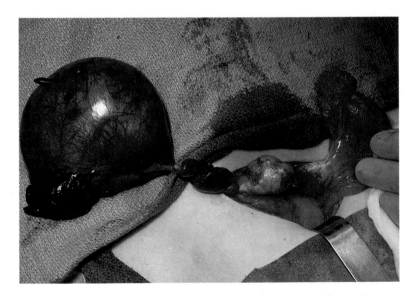

Figure 11.27 Isolated torsion of the right fallopian tube is found at exploration for appendicitis in this adolescent girl. The damaged tube is excised; the normal ovary is preserved.

Tubal Pregnancy

In adolescent girls presenting with acute lower abdominal pain, tubal pregnancy is a possible diagnosis. A serum level of human chorionic gonadotropin (hCG) should be obtained as part of the evaluation of these patients, even if they deny sexual activity.

Vagina

Atresia

Reported to occur once in 4000 female births, vaginal atresia may vary from a short atretic segment with proximal vaginal dilatation to absence of the entire vagina. Proximal vaginal cystic dilation may present as an abdominal mass in an infant at birth (Figs 11.28, 11.29) or in an adolescent at puberty. Urinary abnormalities are frequently associated. Evaluation should include ultrasonography, computed tomography, contrast urography, and chromosome studies.

Surgical correction is influenced by the nature of the abnormality. A dilated vagina is drained initially and may eventually be brought to the perineum (Figs 11.30–11.32). Absence of the vagina requires replacement with a skin graft on a stent (McIndoe procedure) or interposition of a segment of ileum or sigmoid colon.

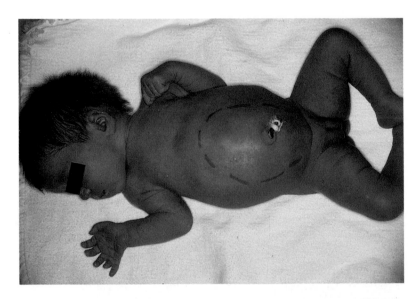

Figure 11.28 Vaginal Atresia A huge abdominal mass is outlined in this 5-day-old girl. There is no external vaginal opening. She has polydactyly, as do a number of her Pennsylvania Dutch relatives. A maternal aunt has a daughter with the same anomalies.

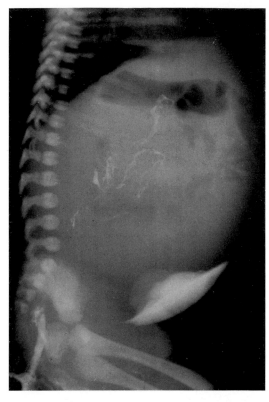

Figure 11.29 The contrast-filled bladder is compressed anteriorly, and the colon displaced superiorly, by the large pelvic mass.

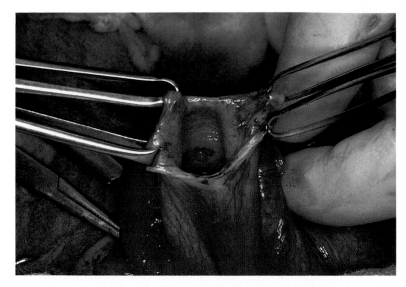

Figure 11.31 The posterior mass is opened and emptied of mucoid fluid. It is the proximal vagina; the cervix is seen. The surgeon's finger then is inserted into the vagina and pushes the distal end to the perineum for a perineal vaginoplasty.

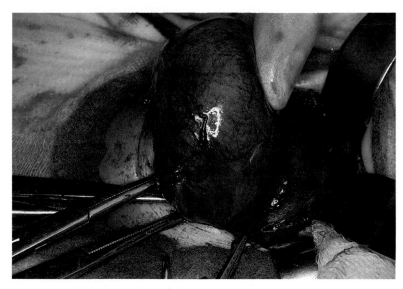

Figure 11.30 The surgeon's finger is on the distended, partially obstructed bladder. A large, posterior, fluid-filled mass is seen just to the right of the bladder in the photograph.

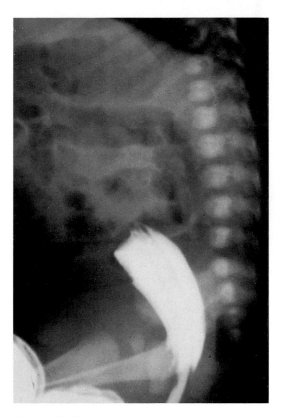

Figure 11.32 A vaginogram 3 months after surgery demonstrates a patent vaginal orifice and only moderate residual dilatation.

Septate Vagina

Associated with a two-horned (didelphic) or separated uterus, the vagina may be divided by a midline septum (Fig 11.33). Renal and other anomalies are often associated. The septum should be excised before puberty, with careful approximation of the mucosal edges. The resulting single vagina then has two cervices, one to each hemi-uterus. Future ability to sustain a pregnancy is in question.

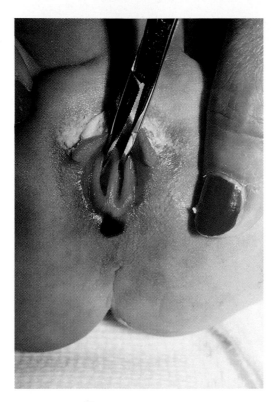

Figure 11.33 Septate Vagina This newborn girl has a septate vagina, imperforate anus with perineal fistula, and renal anomalies.

Imperforate Hymen

An imperforate hymen completely occluding the vaginal orifice may present shortly after birth as a hydrometrocolpos, or at puberty as hematocolpos. In the infant, the obstructing hymenal membrane bulges with mucoid material stimulated by maternal hormones (Fig 11.34). At puberty, the dark blood of menstrual origin fills the vagina behind the membrane (Fig 11.35). The fluid or blood is drained, the membrane is excised, and the cut edges of mucosa are approximated with fine absorbable sutures (Fig 11.36).

Trauma

Vaginal trauma is rarely accidental or self-induced. Sexual abuse must always be suspected (see Chapter 13).

Foreign Bodies

Crayons, candles, beads, safety pins, and other unusual objects may be inserted by a girl into her vagina. Any vaginal discharge in a child should be investigated, first by direct visualization, then by rectal examination, and finally by vaginoscopy under anesthesia if a foreign body is suspected. Smear and culture of the discharge is important, especially in cases of possible sexual abuse.

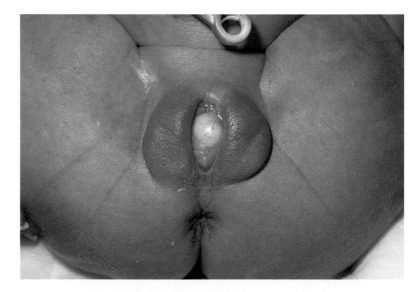

Figure 11.34 Imperforate Hymen The mucoid contents of the vagina are seen through the thin imperforate hymen of this neonate.

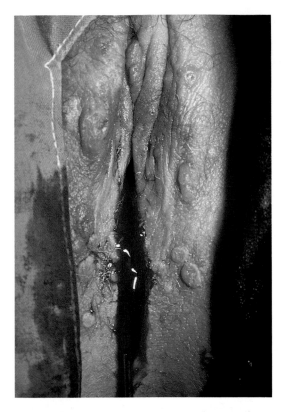

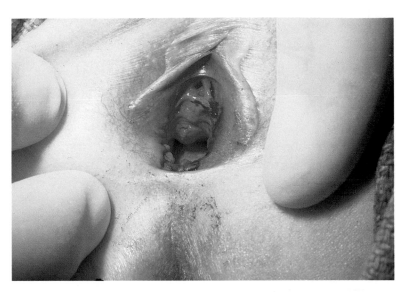

Figure 11.36 In another, infant patient with imperforate hymen, the hymenal membrane was excised, and the mucosal edges were approximated with fine, absorbable sutures.

Figure 11.35 The dark, bulging hymenal membrane in this pubertal girl's urogenital sinus is opened, with drainage of old menstrual blood.

Labia

Fusion

Labial fusion can occur as a congenital problem or may develop from irritation of the perineum. The labial adhesion may be partial or complete (Fig 11.37). Urinary pooling in the vagina and subsequent vulvovaginitis or urinary infection are the complications for which treatment is necessary. Local application of estrogen cream causes thickening of the labial skin and is effective in many cases. Some may require gentle separation or, rarely, surgical division. Application of petrolatum to the cut or separated edges for several days prevents recurrent adhesion.

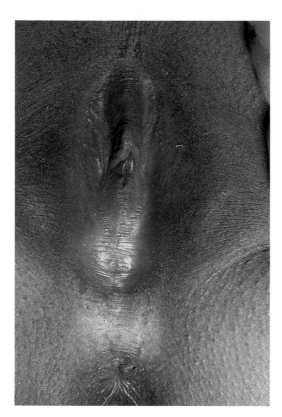

Figure 11.37 A complete labial fusion is seen in this 9-year-old. It did not respond to applications of estrogen cream and was divided surgically.

Trauma

Falls and bicycle accidents are the principal cause of labial trauma. The most common site of laceration is alongside the clitoris, where bleeding may be profuse. A large hematoma may occasionally require drainage for comfort (Fig 11.38). For psychological reasons, all surgical procedures on the external genitalia in girls are best conducted under a light general anesthesia.

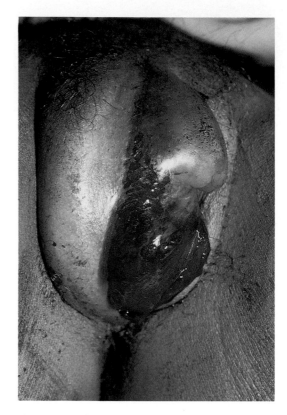

Figure 11.38 A 12-year-old girl suffered this labial hematoma in a bicycle accident. It was drained surgically to relieve pain.

Condylomata

Labial condylomata in a child (Fig 11.39) should raise the question of possible sexual abuse, although they are not invariably the result of abuse. The lesions are removed under general anesthesia with electrocautery or laser.

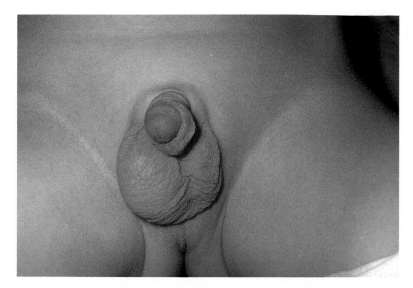

Figure 11.40 Undescended Testis The flattened left hemiscrotum of this 14-month-old is empty. The testis is palpable high in the inguinal canal.

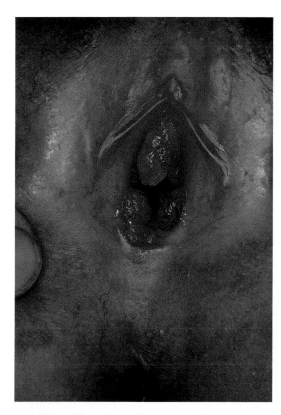

Figure 11.39 The labia and vaginal orifice of a 7-year-old are seen to have multiple condylomata. A venereal cause is suspected.

Testes

Undescended Testis

The boy with an empty hemiscrotum (Fig 11.40) has a testis that is undescended, ectopic, retractile, or absent. The right side is more commonly affected, as the left testis descends first during fetal development. Occasionally both sides are affected (Fig 11.41). Undescended testes are found at birth in 2%–3% of full-term and up to 10% of premature infant boys. By 1 year of age, the testes have descended spontaneously into the scrotum in half of the premature and three quarters of full-term infants. Up to 85% of undescended testes have an associated inguinal hernia; most are found at orchidopexy, but a few present as inguinal bulges in early infancy and require repair at that time.

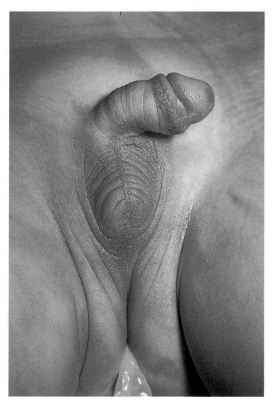

Figure 11.41 The "ironed-out" flat appearance of the entire scrotum is characteristic of bilateral undescended testes.

The true undescended testis is found along the normal line of migration from the retroperitoneal genital ridge adjacent to the kidney to the low inguinal canal (Fig 11.42). When palpable in the inguinal canal, it cannot be manipulated into the midscrotum, thereby distinguishing it from a retractile testis.

An ectopic testis has taken a ''detour'' during descent, placing it outside the scrotum in a suprapubic, perineal, or femoral site (Figs 11.43, 11.44).

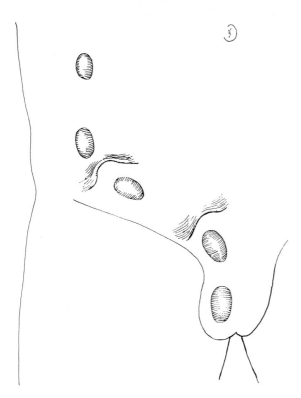

Figure 11.42 The true undescended testis may lie anywhere along the line of embryologic descent, from the abdominal retroperitoneum to the low inguinal canal. The normal position is in the midscrotum.

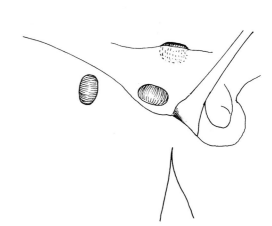

Figure 11.43 The ectopic testis migrates during descent into a femoral or perineal position, where it is palpable, or into a site deep to the pubic ramus (suprapubic), where it may not be detectable.

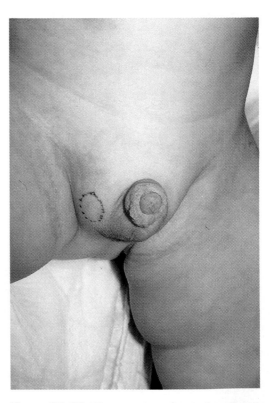

Figure 11.44 The testis in this infant lies in the perineum, lateral to the scrotum. It will never get into the scrotum without surgical assistance.

Placement of the testis in the scrotum should take place before age 2 to achieve optimal growth and function. Orchidopexy is indicated for true undescended testes and all ectopic testes (Figs 11.45–11.52). The inguinal hernia associated with undescended testis is repaired at the same time; separation of the cord structures from the adherent hernia sac is essential to give adequate length of the vessels and vas to allow scrotal placement of the testis. The author has found no benefit in dividing the internal ring and epigastric vessels, as suggested by some to achieve additional cord length.

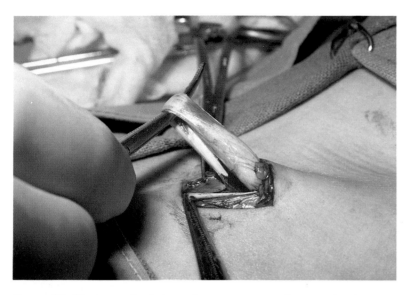

Figure 11.45 A standard 3- to 4-cm transverse herniorrhaphy incision is made at the level of the internal inguinal ring. The external oblique fascia is opened through the external ring, and the cord structures are elevated gently from the incision.

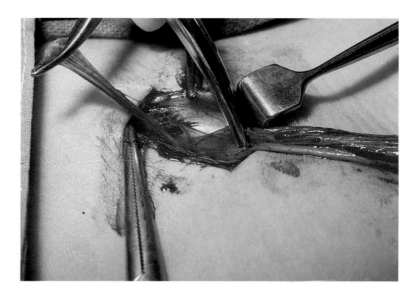

Figure 11.47 When the sac is completely separated from the cord structures, it is divided and the proximal sac grasped with a single hemostat. The vessels and vas are then teased from the hernia sac up to, and beyond, the internal ring; this maneuver is essential to give enough length to bring the testis into the scrotum without tension.

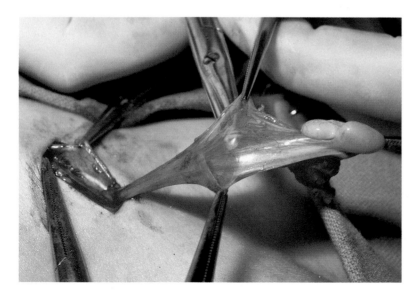

Figure 11.46 The testis is identified, and its distal attachments are divided. The "typical" undescended testis has a redundant vas and epididymis, which may extend distally beyond the testis; great care must be taken *not* to divide it. The thin hernia sac is opened and is dissected carefully from the vessels and vas under direct vision.

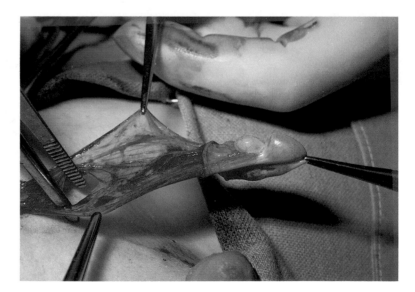

Figure 11.48 If the length of the cord structures is still inadequate, the investing connective tissue of the vessels and vas is carefully thinned, as shown.

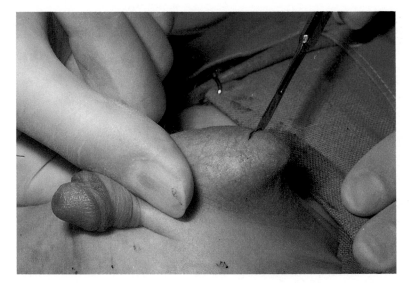

Figure 11.49 After adequate freeing of the vessels allows the testis to reach the scrotum, a new tract is dissected by the surgeon's finger from the inguinal canal into the bottom of the scrotum. An incision in the scrotal skin and blunt dissection between the skin and underlying dartos fascia create a dartos pouch in which the testis will lie.

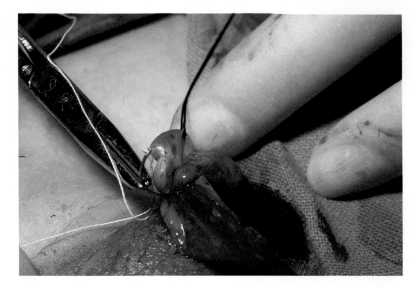

Figure 11.51 The testis is withdrawn down the new tract into the scrotum, care being taken to avoid twisting the cord structures. The defect in the dartos fascia is closed loosely with an absorbable suture, as shown, to help retain the testis in the dartos pouch.

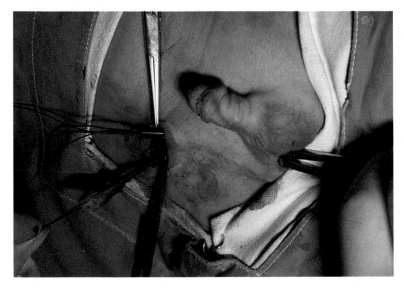

Figure 11.50 A large curved Kelly hemostat follows the tip of the surgeon's finger up the inguinal canal, perforates the inverted dartos fascia, and grasps the silk suture that has been placed through the body of the testis.

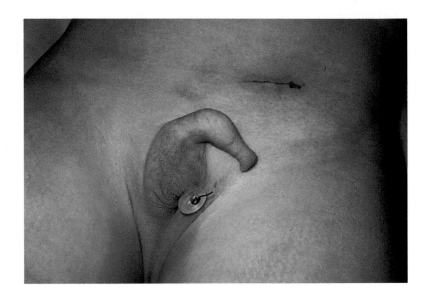

Figure 11.52 The testicular retention suture is passed through the skin of the dartos pouch at the bottom of the scrotum, and is subsequently tied loosely around a sterile button. The inguinal incision is closed in layers, as for a hernia, and both skin incisions are closed with absorbable subcuticular sutures.

The very high testis, just at the internal inguinal ring or in the abdominal retroperitoneum, may need a two-stage procedure or the Fowler-Stephens operation to achieve normal scrotal position. In the staged procedure, the testis is first freed and fixed by sutures at the most distal position to which it can be brought without tension; in 4–6 months, it is dissected from its attachment and brought the rest of the way into the scrotum. In the Fowler-Stephens procedure, length for orchidopexy is achieved by division of the abnormally short testicular artery; the vessels along the long-loop vas then support testicular circulation. In treating a boy with an impalpable testis, many pediatric surgeons now use laparoscopy to confirm the presence and location of the testis. If indicated, the testicular vessels can be clipped and divided, and the abdominal retroperitoneal testis can be mobilized laparoscopically for a Fowler-Stephens orchidopexy (see Chapter 8).

Retractile Testis

Retractile testes are those that are normally descended, but lie in the inguinal canal at the time of examination because of a hyperactive cremaster muscle. Gentle manipulation in a relaxed child can usually bring the testis into the midscrotum. Other boys may need to be observed in a warm bath or when asleep—at a time when the cremaster muscle is relaxed. No therapy of any kind is indicated, and normal enlargement of the testis at puberty keeps it in the scrotum.

Atrophic or Absent Testis

Occlusion of the blood supply of the developing testis, as occurs in prenatal torsion, results in an atrophic testis. In rare instances, the testis may not have been formed at all. Exploration is always indicated when the testis cannot be palpated (Fig 11.53). Any clearly abnormal testis should be removed as a potential source of future malignancy. The appearance of the scrotum can be made normal by placement of a Silastic testicular prosthesis, preferably at puberty (Fig 11.54).

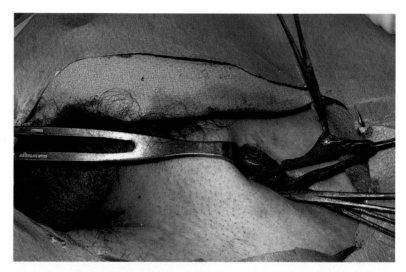

Figure 11.53 This adolescent, with an empty left hemiscrotum since birth, has a tiny nubbin of scar tissue at the end of normal-appearing cord structures. The atrophic testis was excised.

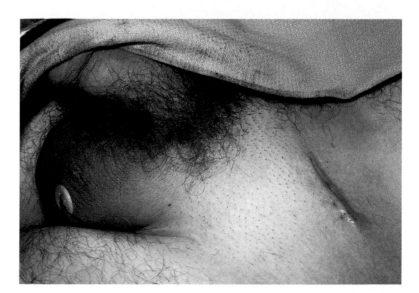

Figure 11.54 A Silastic gel-filled testicular prosthesis of adult size is placed into a newly dissected scrotal pouch and is temporarily retained by a single scrotal suture tied around a button.

Tumors

Tumors of the testis in childhood include endodermal sinus (yolk sac) tumors, teratoma, and paratesticular sarcomas—primarily rhabdomyosarcoma. The majority of these patients are younger than 6 years of age and present with a painless testicular mass (Fig 11.55).

Exploration for diagnosis is carried out through an inguinal incision. If the tumor is confirmed to be malignant, radical orchiectomy is performed, with ligation and division of the cord at the internal ring. Retroperitoneal lymph node dissection is carried out routinely in some centers, and by others only if enlarged nodes are detected on computed tomography or on sonography. Radiotherapy and chemotherapy are recommended for metastatic disease.

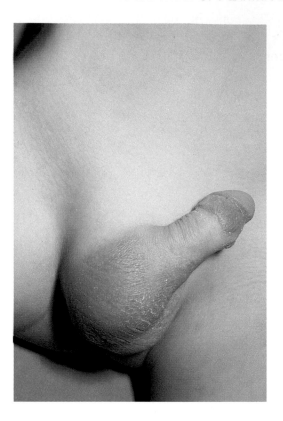

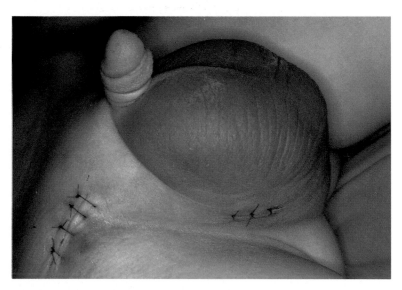

Figure 11.55 Testis Tumor This 4-year-old was referred for definitive care after a biopsy of a paratesticular mass and inguinal nodes revealed reticulum cell sarcoma.

Testicular Torsion

Testicular torsion is a true surgical emergency. If the testis is to survive and function, there must be prompt diagnosis and surgical reduction. The possibility of testicular torsion should always be considered when there is a sudden development of scrotal swelling, pain, and erythema (Fig 11.56). Epididymitis, orchitis, trauma, and torsion of the appendix testis are the alternative diagnoses. Radioisotope scan of the scrotum is the best study if the diagnosis is in doubt (Fig 11.57); but it is not 100% accurate, and the decision for exploration must sometimes be made on clinical grounds alone.

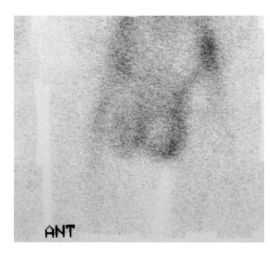

Figure 11.57 A technetium pertechnetate scan in this 14-year-old confirms the suspicion of testicular torsion. The right testis is perfused; there is a "cold" area of diminished perfusion in the left side of the scrotum.

Torsion occurs in one of two forms, extravaginal (axial) or intravaginal. In extravaginal torsion, the entire scrotal contents rotate with the cord (Fig 11.58). Prenatal torsion of this type results in testicular infarction and atrophy (Figs 11.59, 11.60). Intravaginal torsion is based on an inadequate attachment of the testis to the tunica vaginalis—the ''bell-clapper'' testis. The intravaginal suspension of the testis only from the vessels and vas predisposes to a twist of the testis and epididymis within the tunica (Figs 11.61, 11.62). Because this anatomic abnormality is frequently present bilaterally, suture fixation of both testes is advisable at the time of reduction of an intravaginal torsion; fixation of the opposite testis may be transseptal (Fig 11.63) or through a separate scrotal incision.

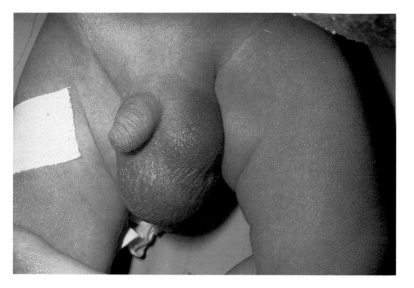

Figure 11.59 A dark, hard mass is seen in the left hemiscrotum of this asymptomatic newborn.

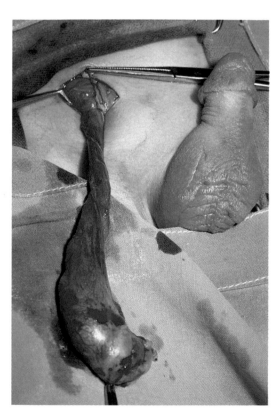

Figure 11.58 An extravaginal (axial) torsion of the entire cord was found in the patient seen in Figure 11.56; it was then untwisted. The testis was found to be viable and was replaced in the scrotum with a retention suture.

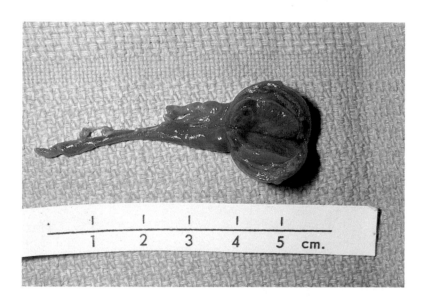

Figure 11.60 A necrotic testis found at inguinoscrotal exploration was removed with the attached cord structures. The cause was most likely a prenatal torsion.

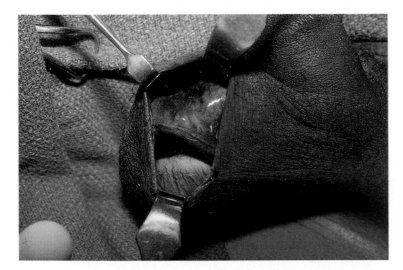

Figure 11.61 This 13-year-old with sudden left scrotal pain and tenderness had a radionuclide scan confirmatory of torsion. Exploration of the scrotum shows an intravaginal torsion, with the veins on the surface of the testis engorged from vascular obstruction. The testis is supported only by its cord structures and has no attachment to the tunica vaginalis testis.

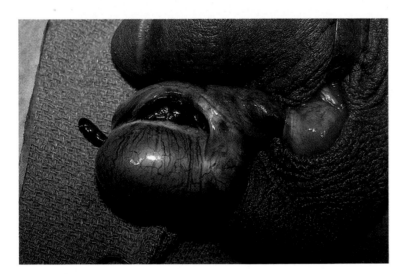

Figure 11.62 The testis is delivered from the scrotum. The intravaginal torsion is clearly visible, with a twist seen at the junction of the cord and the testis. There is no fixation of the testis to the scrotal wall.

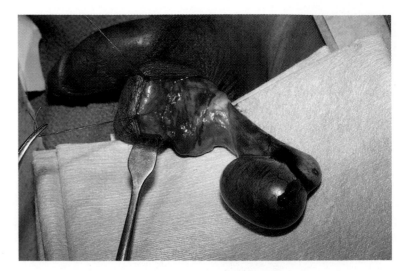

Figure 11.63 The testis still appears dark immediately after detorsion but improved in appearance under observation. It was assumed that the opposite testis also had a "bell-clapper" configuration. A transseptal pexy of the opposite testis was performed with two interrupted sutures (seen here) to prevent future torsion. The left testis was also pexed to prevent recurrence.

Torsion of the Appendix Testis

The appendix testis is a mullerian duct remnant normally attached to the upper pole of the testis. When it undergoes spontaneous torsion, the symptoms are similar to those of testicular torsion. Tenderness is more localized, and the necrotic appendix may often be seen through the skin as a dark spot—the "blue dot" sign. Scrotal exploration and excision of the remnant are indicated only when the diagnosis is uncertain or when pain and swelling persist (Fig 11.64).

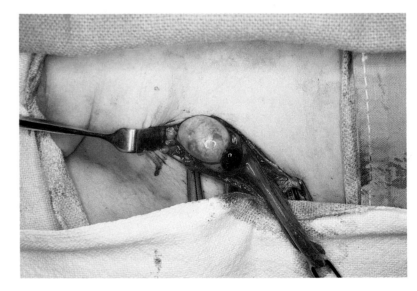

Figure 11.64 Torsion of Appendix Testis A dark, necrotic appendix testis is found at exploration in this 6-year-old who presented with sudden severe pain, swelling, tenderness, and erythema of the scrotum. The appendix testis was removed.

Penis

Phimosis, Paraphimosis, and Balanitis

Phimosis is an abnormally tight foreskin that cannot be retracted over the glans for proper hygiene (Fig 11.65); in the extreme case, the foreskin balloons with urine during voiding. The foreskin in paraphimosis is too tight to be drawn forward again once it has been retracted over the glans, and an emergency dorsal slit may be necessary to alleviate distal edema. Balanitis is an inflammation of the prepuce (Fig 11.66). Circumcision is indicated for all these conditions.

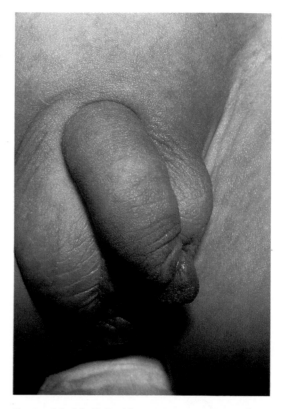

Figure 11.66 Balanitis Redness and swelling are seen only at the tip of the prepuce in this 3-year-old with a healing balanitis. The inflammation had been more extensive; in some boys, it may involve the entire penile shaft.

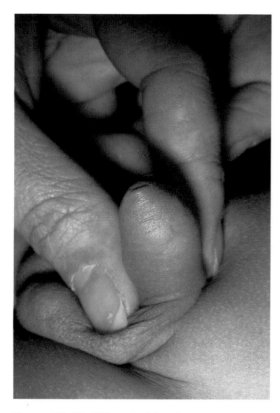

Figure 11.65 Phimosis The foreskin of this 5-year-old is so tight that it cannot be retracted over the glans at all and balloons with urine during voiding.

Micropenis

Micropenis is a rare anomaly, often associated with other congenital anomalies (Fig 11.67). Most cases are not amenable to satisfactory surgical lengthening.

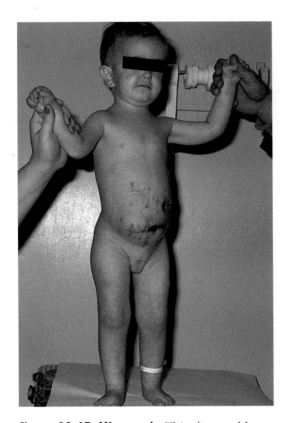

Figure 11.67 Micropenis This 4-year-old boy has a tiny, underdeveloped penis, imperforate anus, Hirschsprung's disease, and growth failure.

Ambiguous Genitalia

Ambiguous genitalia may result from a chromosome abnormality, endogenous or exogenous endocrine abnormality, or tissue unresponsiveness to hormonal stimulation.

Adrenogenital Syndrome

Female pseudohermaphrodism results from adrenocortical hyperplasia, with excessive androgen and mineralocorticoid production. Infant girls with the adrenogenital syndrome may present with an enlarged clitoris resembling a penis (Fig 11.68) and labioscrotal fusion. In salt-losing patients, the hyponatremia and hyperkalemia can prove fatal unless treated with intravenous saline and steroids. Reconstruction of the external genitalia, with clitoral recession and vaginoplasty, is performed before 6 months of age.

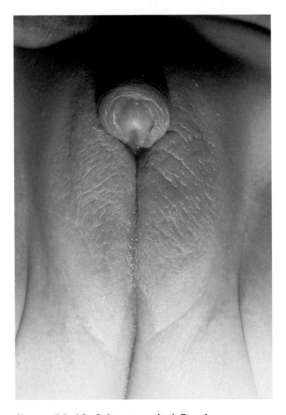

Figure 11.68 Adrenogenital Syndrome The enlarged clitoris and fused scrotolabial folds in this infant girl are the result of adrenocortical hyperplasia. She was admitted at 5 months of age to undergo surgical repair.

Testicular Feminization

Testicular feminization, or male pseudohermaphrodism, occurs in a genetic male (XY) who forms female external genitalia because of a failure of tissue response to testosterone during fetal development. There is a female phenotype (Fig 11.69), with inguinal, intraabdominal (Fig 11.70), or absent testes. The children are raised as girls, perineal reconstruction is performed if indicated, female hormones are administered at puberty, and the testes are removed.

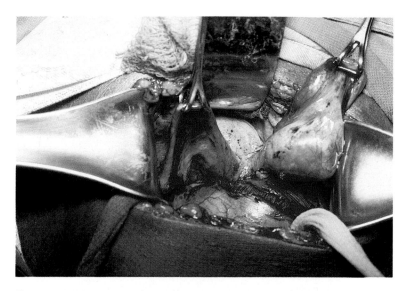

Figure 11.70 At abdominal exploration, no uterus or fallopian tubes are found, and testes are seen attached to the broad ligament. They were removed, and female hormones were administered.

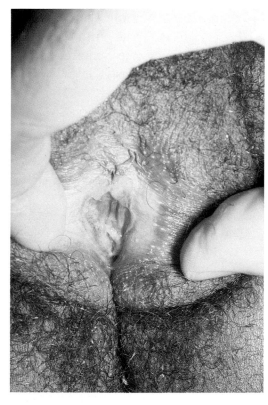

Figure 11.69 Testicular Feminization This genetic male (XY) is seen at puberty with normal female external genitalia.

Gonadal Dysgenesis

Gonadal dysgenesis, as seen in Turner's syndrome (XO syndrome), requires removal of the abnormal gonads because of their malignant potential. Most patients are raised as females, with repair of the external genitalia and hormone administration at puberty.

True Hermaphrodism

True hermaphrodism is extremely rare and may be associated with XX, XY, or a mosaic XX/XY sex chromosome arrangement. These children have both ovarian and testicular tissue, phalluses of varying size, and internal genitalia with both wolffian and mullerian remnants (Fig 11.71). Sex assignment depends on assessment of the external genitalia.

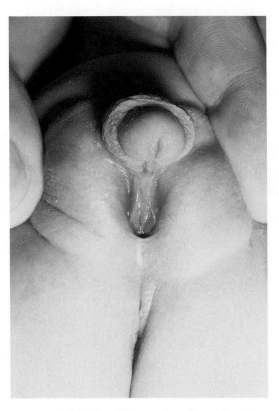

Figure 11.71 True Hermaphrodism This infant, with a boy's name, has a small penis with a normal urethra, a narrow vagina, a uterus and fallopian tubes, and intraabdominal gonads that are ovotestes.

Chapter 12

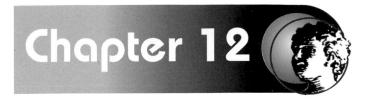

Solid Tumors

Malignant tumors are the second most common cause of childhood deaths in the United States, exceeded only by accidents (see Chapter 13). Hematologic malignancies predominate, followed by the pediatric solid tumors—Wilms' tumor, neuroblastoma, rhabdomyosarcoma, and teratoma. Prognosis varies widely, depending on tumor type, tissue type, patient age, and tumor stage (extent of spread).

Wilms' Tumor

Wilms' tumor is an embryonal malignancy of the kidney, without clear etiology. It is rarely familial and has been seen in association with aniridia, hemihypertrophy, and genitourinary abnormalities.

Presentation is almost always as an easily palpable and visible asymptomatic flank mass (Figs 12.1, 12.2). Fever, pain, and hematuria may also be found, as well as hypertension. The tumor occurs more frequently on the left, and 5%–10% of cases are bilateral (Fig 12.3).

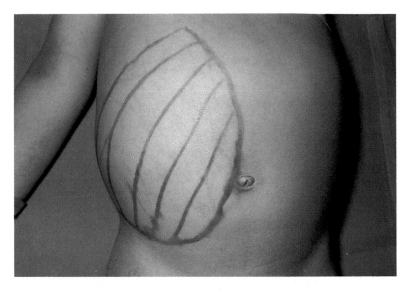

Figure 12.2 The mass of a right-sided Wilms' tumor occupies almost half of the abdomen in this 23-month-old boy.

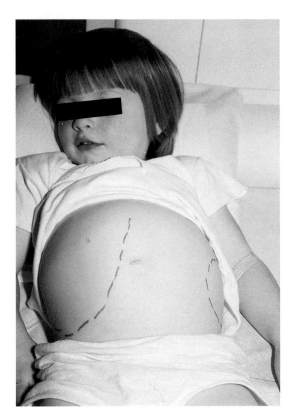

Figure 12.3 The finding of a huge right-flank mass led to referral of this 4-year-old girl. At the time of admission, a left-sided mass is also felt.

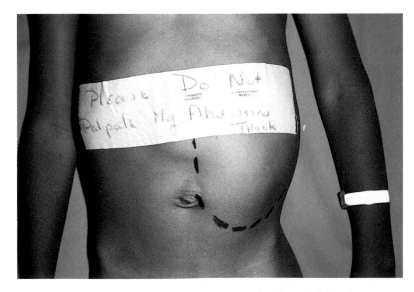

Figure 12.1 Wilms' Tumor The margins of a firm left flank mass are outlined on the abdomen of this 3½-year-old. Repeated palpation of the mass is discouraged, because the tumor capsule may be ruptured or malignant cells may be shed into the circulation.

Histologically, Wilms' tumor has round, hyperchromatic, undifferentiated cells with incomplete formation of tubules and glomeruli (Fig 12.4). Extreme undifferentiation (anaplasia) and sarcomatous changes are characteristics of the unfavorable histology that carries a significantly poorer prognosis.

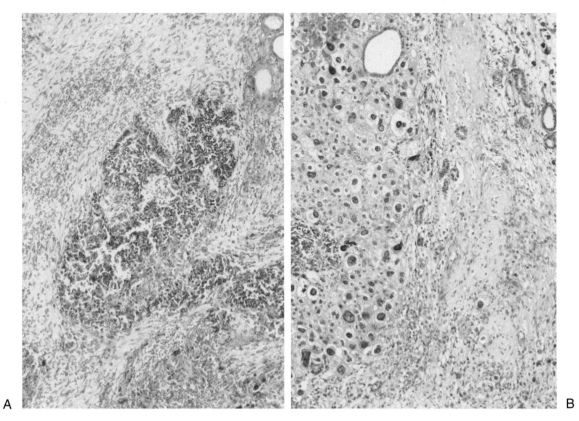

A   B

Figure 12.4 These photomicrographs show **(A)** a moderately well differentiated Wilms' tumor and **(B)** tubule formation within the tumor.

Diagnostic Procedures

Intravenous pyelography (IVP) was once the primary diagnostic procedure (Fig 12.5), with inferior venacaval contrast to detect venous tumor thrombus, enlarged retroperitoneal nodes, and retroperitoneal tumor extension (Figs 12.6, 12.7). Selective angiography has been useful in some bilateral tumors to help determine resectability (Figs 12.8, 12.9). Currently, ultrasonography (Fig 12.10) and computed tomography (CT) with intravenous contrast (Fig 12.11) yield the most information about the location and extent of the primary tumor and the presence of metastases (Fig 12.12). Lymph nodes, lung (Fig 12.13), liver, and brain are the most frequent sites of metastatic Wilms' tumor.

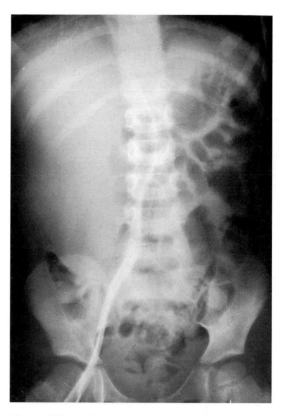

Figure 12.6 The presence of a tumor thrombus was suspected on the basis of this inferior venacavogram; the column of contrast is narrowed just above the entrance of the renal veins. There is a large Wilms' tumor of the right kidney.

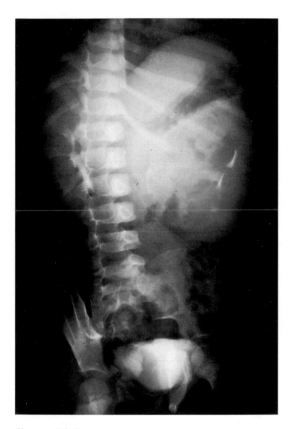

Figure 12.5 This intravenous pyelogram of the patient shown in Figure 12.1 demonstrates the distortion of the pelvicalyceal system that is characteristic of Wilms' tumor.

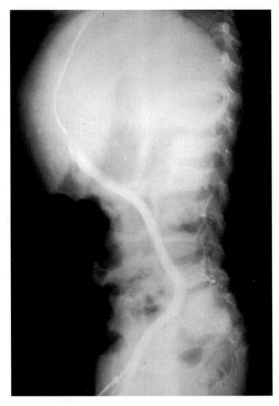

Figure 12.7 A lateral venacavogram of another child shows marked anterior displacement by a large retrocaval Wilms' tumor.

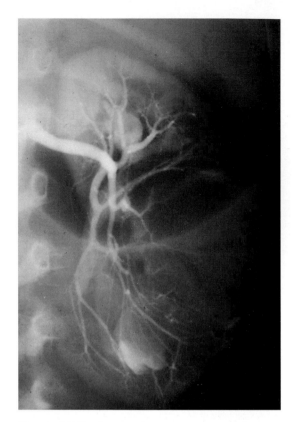

Figure 12.9 The left kidney, in the same child, has a baseball-sized mass displacing vessels in the midcortex. It is a salvageable kidney.

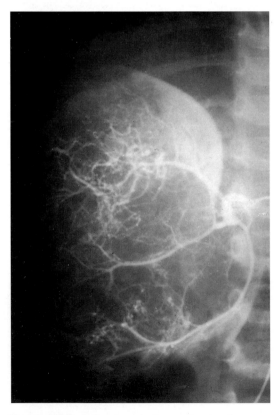

Figure 12.8 Selective angiography in the patient seen in Figure 12.3 shows the right kidney to be almost entirely replaced by tumor.

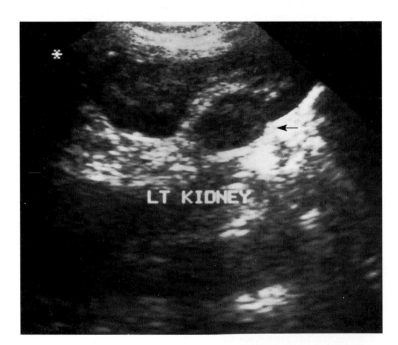

Figure 12.10 Ultrasonography demonstrates a 2.5-cm mass of the lower pole *(arrow)* of the left kidney in this 2-year-old.

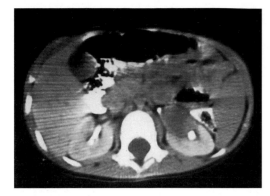

Figure 12.11 A computed tomography scan of the same patient in Figure 12.10 after administration of intravenous contrast confirms the presence of the mass, which is a small Wilms' tumor. Nephrectomy is curative.

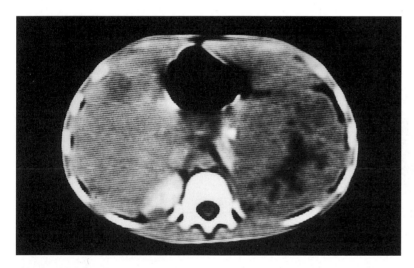

Figure 12.12 This computed tomography study shows a huge left Wilms' tumor, a small tumor in the posterior right kidney, and a metastatic nodule of tumor in the anterior liver. The child is alive and tumor-free 13 years after surgical resection of all detectable tumor and a course of chemotherapy.

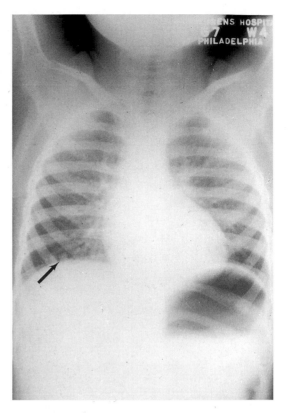

Figure 12.13 Metastases to the right lower lobe of the lung *(arrow)* are seen in this chest radiograph of a 4-year-old girl with a right-sided Wilms' tumor (see Fig 12.6).

Treatment of Wilms' Tumor

For this tumor with a generally good prognosis, the presence of known metastatic disease does not deter surgical removal of the primary. Excision of the primary tumor is carried out promptly, unless the tumor is so large as to make surgery hazardous, there is a large tumor thrombus, or there is extensive bilateral renal involvement. In those cases, pretreatment of the tumor(s) with chemotherapy may shrink the tumor mass, making excision safer.

Surgery

A generous transverse abdominal or thoracoabdominal incision is used for surgical exposure (Fig 12.14). Although many surgeons still evaluate the contralateral kidney by direct visualization (Fig 12.15), mobilization, and palpation, the accuracy of current imaging modalities in detecting even small renal tumors (see Fig 12.10) makes these maneuvers unnecessary in most cases. In the approach to the affected kidney, care is taken to mobilize the overlying structures: the hepatic flexure and duodenum on the right and the splenic flexure, spleen, and pancreas on the left.

Because the tumor may rupture, or tumor cells may be shed into the venous circulation during manipulation, handling of the mass should be minimal—prior to, and during, surgery. To prevent tumor embolism to the lungs, early visualization and ligation of the renal vessels is desirable, but this is not always technically feasible (Fig 12.16). When tumor is found growing into the renal vein and vena cava, a reasonable attempt is made to remove the tumor thrombus (Figs 12.17, 12.18), unless it is so large that removal would be dangerous or require cardiopulmonary bypass. A preoperative course of chemotherapy will often shrink the large tumor thrombus, making its removal easier. Primary tumor that extends directly into adjacent structures, such as liver and diaphragm, is to be resected when possible (Figs 12.19, 12.20). Hilar and periaortic lymph nodes, and any that may contain tumor, are identified and removed.

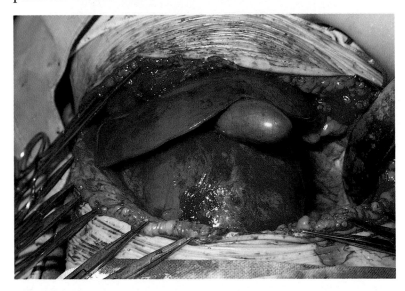

Figure 12.14 A thoracoabdominal incision is needed to expose the Wilms' tumor of the right kidney demonstrated in Figure 12.6. The liver and gallbladder are seen superiorly.

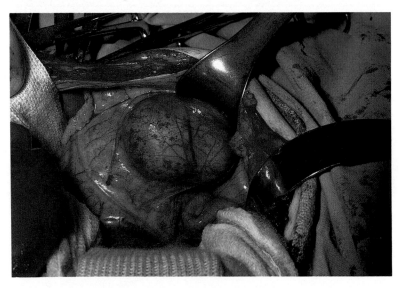

Figure 12.15 At exploration of the left retroperitoneum, before removal of a right-sided Wilms' tumor, the tumor mass in the left kidney (see Fig 12.9) is examined and marked with clips for subsequent radiotherapy.

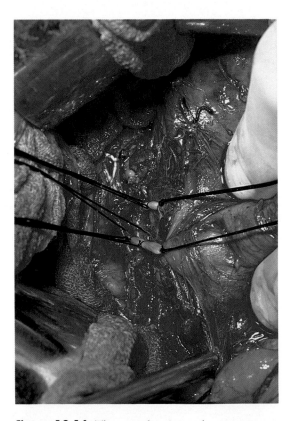

Figure 12.16 The renal vein and artery are ligated prior to dissection and manipulation of this Wilms' tumor of the left kidney (patient in Fig 12.1). Lymph nodes, like the one at the tip of the metal aspirator, are removed for microscopic examination; the lymph node pictured here contains no tumor.

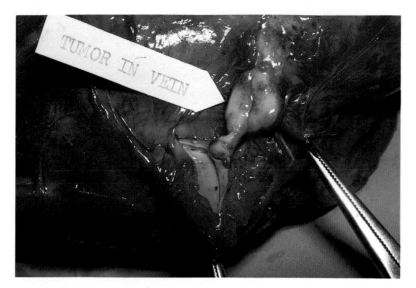

Figure 12.17 Inspection of this excised Wilms' tumor shows tumor thrombus in the renal vein.

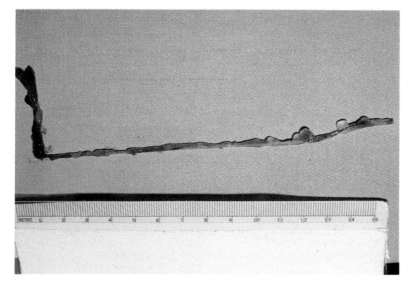

Figure 12.18 After nephrectomy, this long tumor thrombus is removed from the renal vein stump and vena cava; its presence explains the lung metastases seen in Figure 12.13.

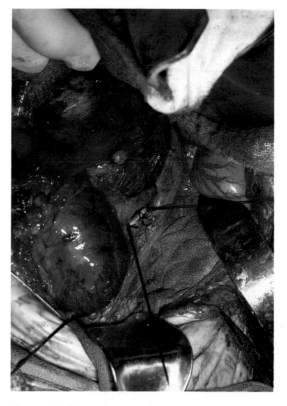

Figure 12.19 The large right-sided Wilms' tumor, as seen in Figure 12.7, displaces the vena cava anteriorly and extends into the liver. The vessels have been ligated prior to major tumor dissection.

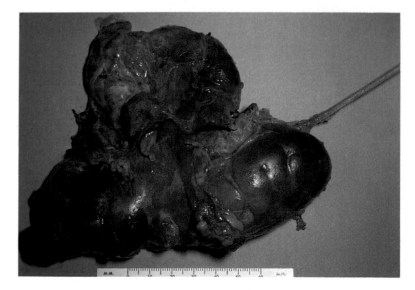

Figure 12.20 The kidney, with its superior-pole tumor, is excised with a margin of adjacent liver.

Tumor Staging

Wilms' tumor is staged as follows:

Stage I: tumor only in kidney and excised without spillage.

Stage II: tumor beyond the kidney that is completely excised, or local tumor spillage.

Stage III: residual tumor, confined to the abdomen.

Stage IV: hematogenous metastases.

Bilateral Wilms' has been termed *Stage V,* but therapeutic decisions are based on the extent of spread, by the above criteria.

Tumor Therapy

Widely accepted protocols, such as those of the National Wilms' Tumor Study Group, provide the basis for current therapy. Actinomycin D and vincristine are the first-line chemotherapeutic agents for Wilms' tumor. Others, such as cyclophosphamide and Adriamycin (doxorubicin), are added for stage IV and unfavorable-histology tumors. Radiotherapy is generally used for tumor spread, tumor recurrence, and unfavorable histology. With favorable histology, the 2-year survival rate for stages I–III is 85%–95%, and for stage IV, 65%–75%.

Mesoblastic Nephroma

Once thought to be a variant of Wilms' tumor, mesoblastic nephroma presents most often in early infancy as an abdominal mass and has been detected by prenatal sonography. Imaging studies reveal a solid mass in the kidney that cannot be distinguished from the appearance of a Wilms' tumor (Fig 12.21). Surgical excision is the treatment of choice and is definitive in most cases (Figs 12.22, 12.23). The microscopic appearance is that of spindle-shaped cells with hyperchromatic nuclei; cysts, lined by mesenchymal cells of the tumor, may be seen. There may be areas of necrosis and hemorrhage. The majority of these tumors are benign in behavior; atypical nephromas (less than 5%) may recur locally or metastasize, requiring chemotherapy.

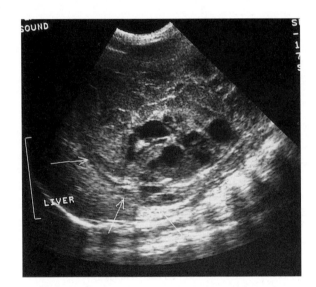

Figure 12.21 Mesoblastic Nephroma The abdominal sonogram of a 7-month-old girl shows a large tumor of the right kidney. The inferior edge of the liver is identified.

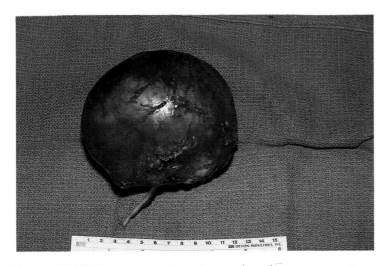

Figure 12.22 The resected renal mass has the gross appearance of a Wilms' tumor.

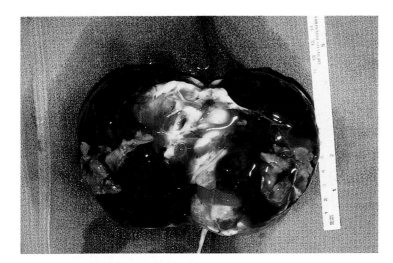

Figure 12.23 There is old hemorrhage into the tumor, seen on section of the specimen.

Neuroblastoma

Neuroblastoma is a tumor of neural-crest origin, arising from the adrenal medulla or any location along the sympathetic ganglion chain. The incidence is reported to be 1 in 10,000–12,000 children, slightly higher than for Wilms' tumor. There are reported familial occurrences and association with other neural crest abnormalities, such as Hirschsprung's disease, and with fetal alcohol syndrome.

The tumor originates from the abdominal retroperitoneum (adrenal or sympathetic chain) in 75%, posterior mediastinum in 20%, and neck or pelvis in approximately 5% of cases. The clinical presentation is generally as a mass (Fig 12.24). Symptoms include pain, fever, weight loss, and results of compression of adjacent structures. Proptosis and orbital ecchymosis (Fig 12.25) and extremity pain and swelling (Figs 12.26, 12.27) are manifestations of bone metastases. Paraspinal tumors may grow into the intervertebral foramina as "dumbbell" lesions, causing symptoms of spinal cord compression. Hypertension, when present, is related to the production of catecholamines by the tumor, and infants may have diarrhea from tumors that secrete vasoactive intestinal polypeptide (VIP). Cerebellar ataxia is a rare and unexplained manifestation of neuroblastoma; it usually resolves after tumor excision.

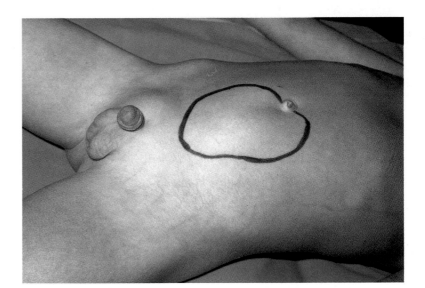

Figure 12.24 Neuroblastoma This large, firm, palpable mass is found on examination of a 5-year-old boy referred for repair of a right inguinal hernia. It is a neuroblastoma, originating from the abdominal sympathetic ganglia.

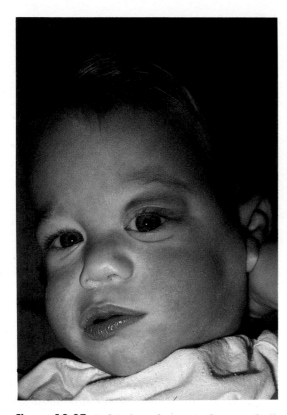

Figure 12.25 Orbital ecchymosis from a skull metastasis is the first sign of neuroblastoma in this 14-month-old.

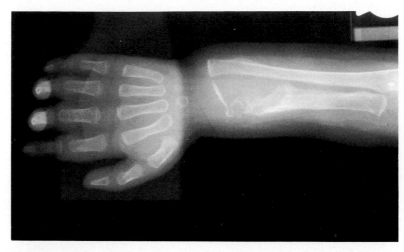

Figure 12.27 A radiograph of the wrist demonstrates a lytic metastasis in the distal radius.

Although the tumor mass may be visualized on chest or abdominal radiographs (Figs 12.28, 12.29) and may be seen to displace the kidney on IVP (Fig 12.30), CT with intravenous contrast is the current standard diagnostic modality (Figs 12.31, 12.32). It may be supplemented by magnetic resonance imaging (MRI) for visualizing the spinal cord. Occasionally, selective angiography has been helpful in distinguishing an invasive adrenal neuroblastoma from a Wilms' tumor (Figs 12.33, 12.34). A radiographic skeletal survey (Fig 12.35), skull films (Fig 12.36), and a bone scan—as well as a bone marrow aspirate (Fig 12.37)—identify metastatic disease. An elevated level of vanillylmandelic acid (VMA), a product of catecholamine metabolism, indicates a secreting tumor; a reappearance of elevated VMA levels postoperatively is an early sign of tumor recurrence. Elevated levels of serum ferritin and neuron-specific enolase, as well as an elevated number of copies of the N-*myc* oncogene and the ploidy of the tumor chromosomes, have prognostic significance.

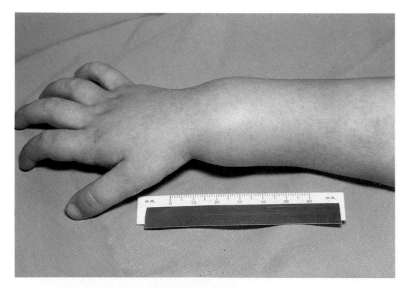

Figure 12.26 Painful swelling of the wrist is the presenting sign of neuroblastoma in this child.

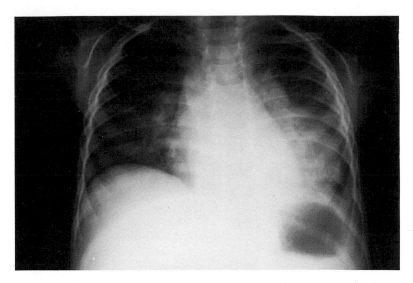

Figure 12.28 A large left mediastinal mass is shown on this chest radiograph of a 14-month-old with abdominal distention, weight loss, and fever.

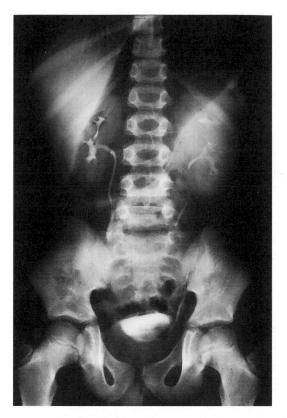

Figure 12.30 Intravenous pyelography in the patient depicted in Figure 12.29 shows caudal displacement of the left kidney by a mass in the adrenal.

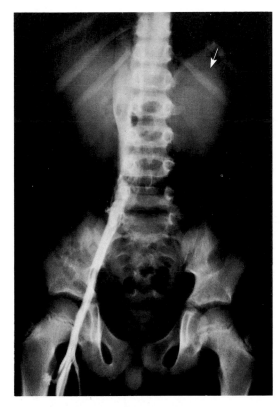

Figure 12.29 Fine calcification is seen in a left flank mass *(arrow)* on this initial film of an inferior venacavogram.

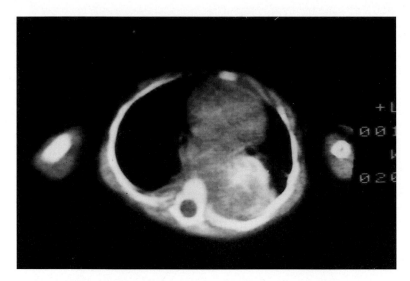

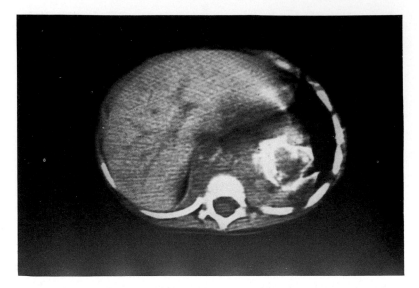

Figure 12.31 Computed tomography of the patient seen in Figure 12.28 shows the large, calcified mediastinal mass to be adherent to the aorta and vertebrae. **Figure 12.32** Lower cuts of the same computed tomography scan demonstrate extension of the tumor into the abdominal retroperitoneum.

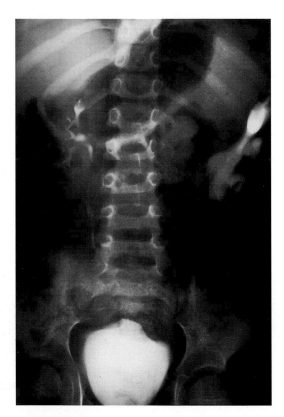

Figure 12.33 Distortion and displacement of the left pelvicalyceal system are seen on intravenous pyelography of a 5-year-old with a flank mass.

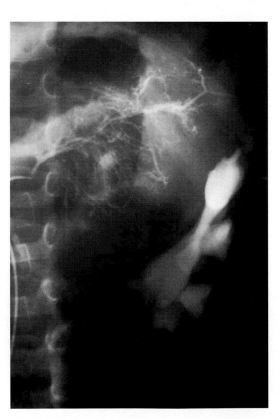

Figure 12.34 To differentiate between Wilms' tumor and neuroblastoma, a selective adrenal angiogram is performed. Tumor vessels are seen in the adrenal mass, which invades the adjacent kidney.

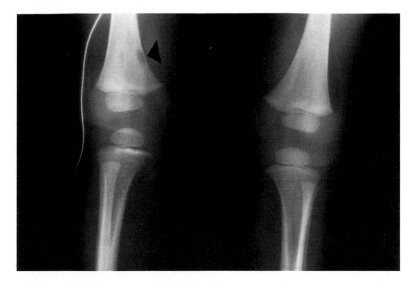

Figure 12.35 The metaphysis of long bones is a common site for metastatic neuroblastoma, seen here in the distal femur.

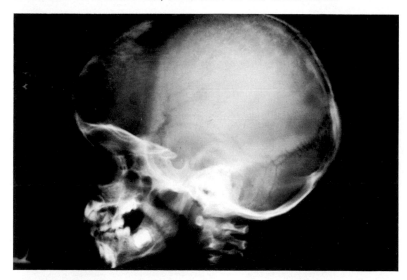

Figure 12.36 Widening of the sutures is demonstrated on the skull film of this child with metastatic neuroblastoma.

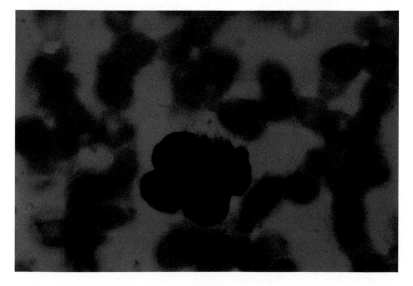

Figure 12.37 Neuroblastoma cells found in bone marrow aspirate.

Surgery

The role of surgery in neuroblastoma depends on the extent of disease. In stage I lesions, confined to a single organ, resection alone may be curative (Figs 12.38, 12.39). Stage II tumors, which extend beyond the organ of origin but do not cross the midline, are excised (Figs 12.40, 12.41); small amounts of residual tumor may re-

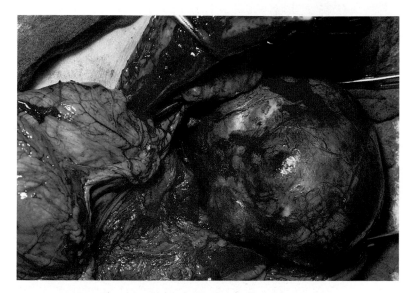

Figure 12.38 A transverse upper abdominal incision exposes a left adrenal neuroblastoma, which has been dissected from the kidney. The tumor is limited to the adrenal, a stage I lesion.

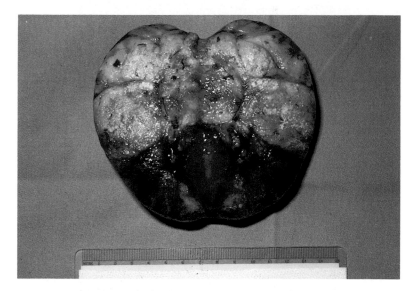

Figure 12.39 Hemorrhage and medullary tumor tissue are seen on the cut section of this adrenal neuroblastoma.

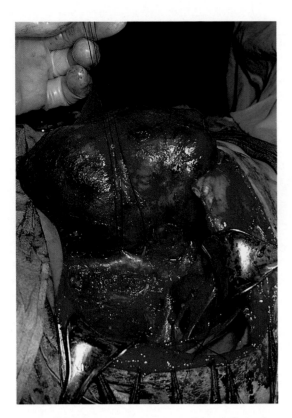

Figure 12.40 Local invasion of the kidney by the adrenal neuroblastoma, as demonstrated in Figure 12.34, necessitates removal of both the adrenal and kidney on the left. There are ligatures around the adrenal and renal arteries; the adrenal artery is almost as large as the renal. With no distant spread, it is a stage II tumor.

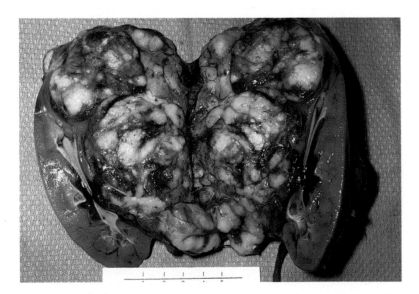

Figure 12.41 Section of the tumor specimen shows invasion of two thirds of the kidney by neuroblastoma, explaining the radiographic appearance in Figures 12.33 and 12.34.

ceive low-dose radiotherapy (Figs 12.42, 12.43). Laminectomy is necessary to relieve cord compression of a dumbbell tumor. Large tumors, extending beyond the midline, are classified as stage III and are often unresectable by virtue of size and location; removal of a large portion of the tumor (debulking) is thought to improve the response to aggressive chemotherapy and radiotherapy (Figs 12.44, 12.45) and provides tumor for histologic diagnosis (Fig 12.46). The tumor may shrink in response

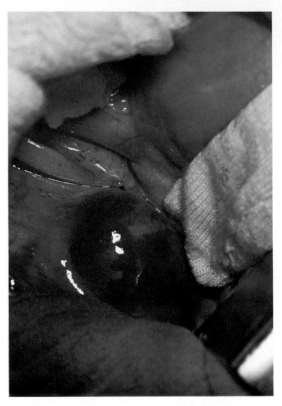

Figure 12.42 This small right-sided thoracic neuroblastoma is seen at thoracotomy. It was discovered on the chest radiograph of this 14-month-old girl admitted for cerebellar ataxia.

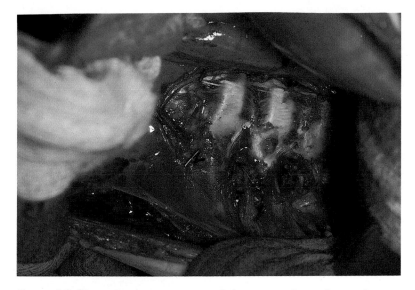

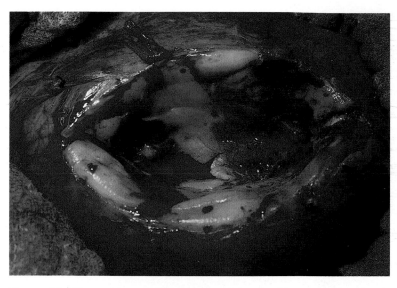

Figure 12.43 Following excision of the tumor from the surface of the vertebral bodies, small extensions of residual tumor are seen entering the intervertebral foramina. A small (600-rad) dose of radiotherapy to the local area was the only treatment. The cerebellar ataxia resolved after surgery. The patient is well and tumor-free 23 years later.

Figure 12.45 The mass pictured in Figure 12.44 is not resectable; debulking removes more than a third of the tumor mass, as shown.

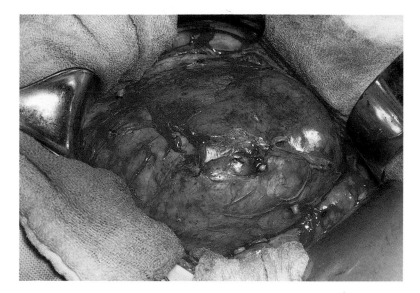

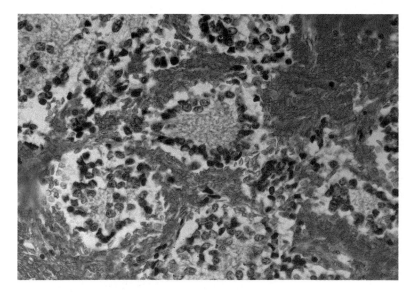

Figure 12.44 The mass outlined in Figure 12.24, a large neuroblastoma of sympathetic-chain origin, straddles the midline, displacing both ureters laterally. It is a stage III tumor.

Figure 12.46 Typical rosettes of tumor cells characterize the microscopic appearance of neuroblastoma.

to therapy, allowing subsequent complete excision (Figs 12.47–12.50). Stage IV disease is metastatic to distant sites, including bone, bone marrow, liver (Fig 12.51), soft tissues, and lymph nodes. Debulking of the primary tumor may increase the effectiveness of multimodal chemotherapy or may be followed by very rare spontaneous regression; however, in most stage IV disease, the prognosis is very poor.

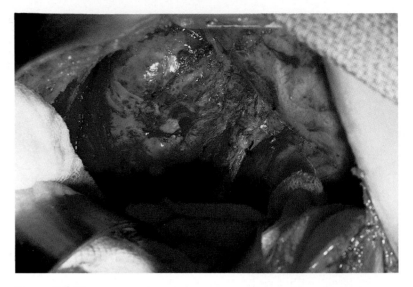

Figure 12.49 Following a short course of intensive chemotherapy, the mediastinal mass is smaller and is resectable. The abdominal extension is gone, leaving only calcified retroperitoneal lymph nodes, free of tumor.

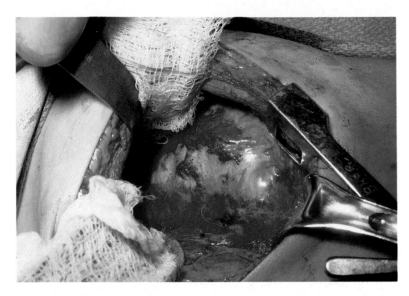

Figure 12.47 This stage III mediastinal neuroblastoma crosses the midline in the chest and extends below the diaphragm. It is the tumor demonstrated in the radiographs of Figures 12.28, 12.31, and 12.32. Only local nodes are involved with tumor; bone and bone marrow are clear.

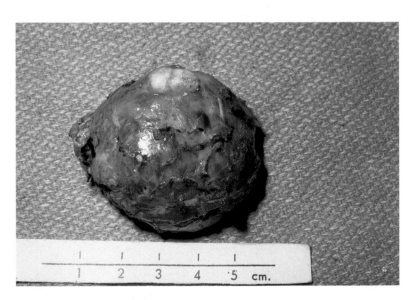

Figure 12.50 The entire resected specimen is seen; there are still tumor cells in the specimen. There is no recurrence in a 9-year follow-up.

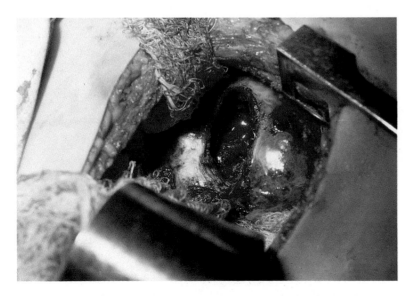

Figure 12.48 Initial surgery is limited to a large incisional biopsy, or debulking, of the intrathoracic tumor.

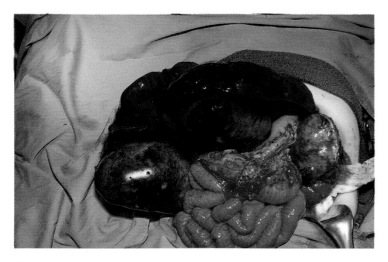

Figure 12.51 There are massive metastases in the liver of this 6-month-old with a visible primary neuroblastoma of the left adrenal. Although originally thought to be a stage IV-S tumor, it had unfavorable prognostic markers and failed to respond to therapy.

Stage IV-S

An unusual manifestation of metastatic neuroblastoma, classified as stage IV-S, is found in some infants younger than 1 year of age and carries an especially favorable prognosis. The metastases are confined to liver, skin, or bone marrow—with none in cortical bone. Congenital neuroblastomatosis (Figs 12.52–12.55) is an example of a stage IV-S tumor.

The 2-year survival rate with stages I, II, and IV-S is more than 75% in most series, as is the case with all patients younger than the age of 1 year. The prognosis also seems better for children with tumors arising in the chest, neck, and pelvis than with those of abdominal origin.

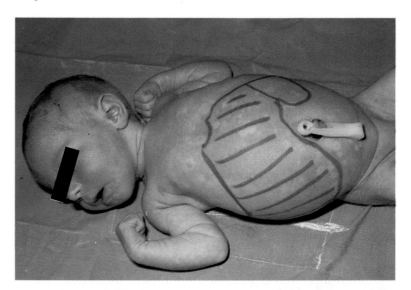

Figure 12.52 Congenital Neuroblastomatosis This newborn infant has multiple subcutaneous nodules of neuroblastoma and a massively enlarged liver.

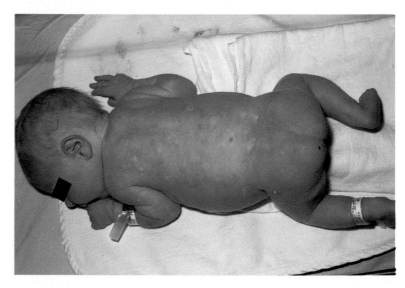

Figure 12.53 The blue tumor nodules have white halos, evidence of local vasoconstriction from catecholamine secretion.

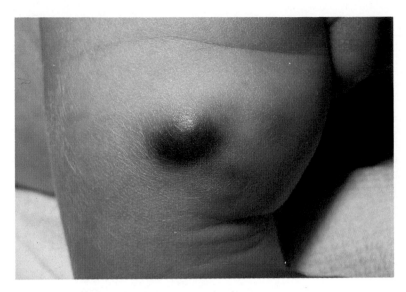

Figure 12.54 A close-up shows the subcutaneous nodules of the left thigh.

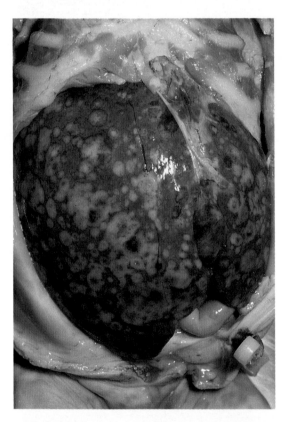

Figure 12.55 The child died of an unrelated cardiac anomaly. The liver is seen studded with neuroblastoma at postmortem examination.

Rhabdomyosarcoma

Arising from primitive mesenchymal tissue, rhabdomyosarcoma constitutes 5%–15% of all malignant solid tumors in patients younger than the age of 15 years. Common sites of origin include the orbit, head and neck, trunk, extremities, genitourinary tract, and perineum. Tumors of the bladder, prostate, vagina, and head and neck occur more often in infants and toddlers and are more likely to be of the favorable embryonal-cell type.

The majority of children with rhabdomyosarcoma have the embryonal type. Sarcoma botryoides is the polypoid embryonal tumor found protruding from the nasopharynx, bile ducts, bladder, and vagina (Figs 12.56, 12.57). The alveolar type is most common in the striated muscles of the limbs and trunk; it has a worse prognosis because of a higher recurrence rate after therapy. Some childhood tumors are mixed embryonal and alveolar. Rare in childhood is the pleomorphic type of rhabdomyosarcoma.

Clinical presentation is as a mass, visible under the skin or involving, or protruding into, a hollow viscus (Figs 12.58, 12.59).

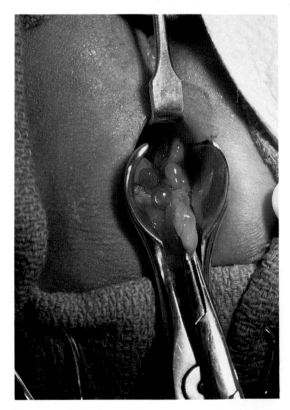

Figure 12.56 Rhabdomyosarcoma There is a grapelike cluster of tumor nodules in the vagina of this 2-year-old who presents with minimal vaginal bleeding.

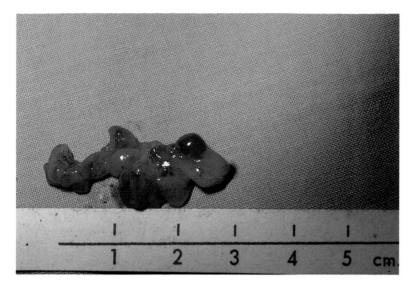

Figure 12.57 The excised tumor has the typical appearance of sarcoma botryoides.

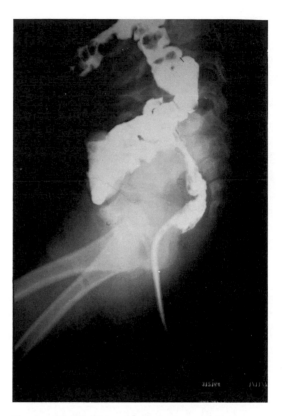

Figure 12.59 The prostatic tumor displaces the barium-filled rectum posteriorly. The parents of this boy refused major ablative surgery; local radiotherapy alone causes the tumor to shrink, with no recurrence during 5 years of known follow-up.

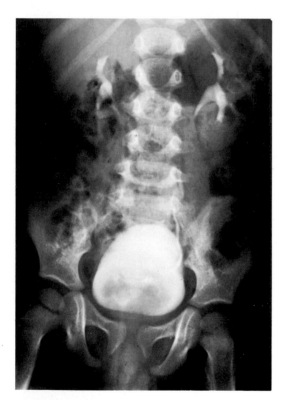

Figure 12.58 A rhabdomyosarcoma of prostatic origin appears as a large negative image in the contrast-filled bladder of this 2-year-old.

Management of Rhabdomyosarcoma

Wide total excision is the surgical goal in rhabdomyosarcoma. This goal must be balanced against functional loss, especially for lesions of the extremities and head and neck. For the extremities, wide local excision is generally preferred to amputation. Improved chemotherapy and localized radiotherapy have increased survival for those with pelvic and head and neck involvement, avoiding radical surgery (Figs 12.60–12.63). Paratesticular rhabdomyosarcomas are best treated by orchiectomy and node dissection; radiotherapy and chemotherapy are given if the nodes are positive.

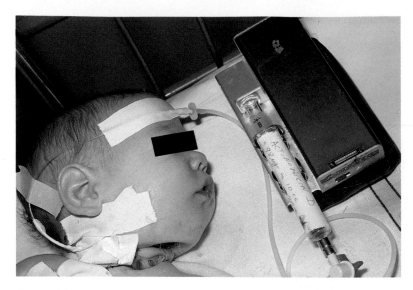

Figure 12.61 An infusion of actinomycin D through an external carotid artery catheter is continued for 5 days.

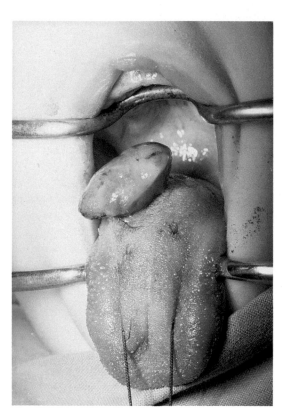

Figure 12.60 A mass in the posterior tongue of a 3-month-old boy is seen at the time of excisional biopsy. It is an embryonal rhabdomyosarcoma. (Reprinted with permission from Liebert PS, Stool SE: Rhabdomyosarcoma of the tongue in an infant; response to combined therapy. Annals of Surgery 178:62–66, 1973.)

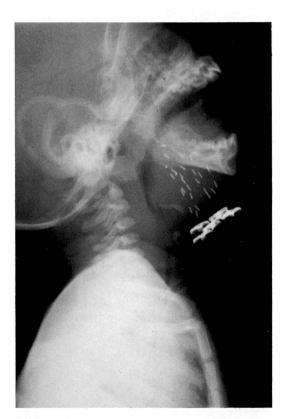

Figure 12.62 At the same time, radioactive iridium seeds are placed in the base of the tongue, as seen on this lateral radiograph of the neck. They are left in place for 10 days.

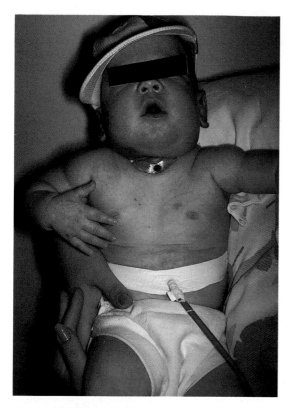

Figure 12.63 One month later, the child has considerable swelling of the neck and pharynx. The tracheostomy and feeding gastrostomy are removed in 2 months. Twenty-six years later, he is still free of tumor.

Teratoma

Teratomas are congenital tumors composed of cells derived from all three primary germ layers—ectoderm, mesoderm, and endoderm. They may be benign or malignant at the time of diagnosis. Teratomas have been found in the brain, the mouth, the neck, the mediastinum, the abdomen, the presacral and sacrococcygeal areas, the ovary, and the testis.

Clinical presentation of a huge posterior sacrococcygeal teratoma is most dramatic, with a mass protruding between the coccyx and rectum of a newborn infant (Fig 12.64). There may be great variation in size and shape of

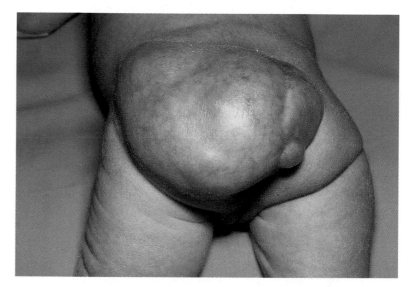

Figure 12.64 Sacrococcygeal Teratoma This infant girl is born with a huge cystic mass growing between the coccyx and the anus.

the teratoma and association with other anatomic abnormalities (Fig 12.65). Diagnosis by antenatal sonography is now common. The teratoma should not be mistaken for a myelomeningocele (Fig 12.66) or lipomeningocele (Fig 12.67). Abdominal and rectal examination and CT with intravenous contrast are performed to determine any presacral extent of the tumor. Those that are located only in the presacral space are often not detected until they produce bowel or bladder obstruction by their growth (Figs 12.68, 12.69).

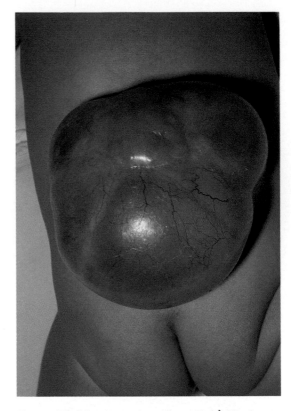

Figure 12.66 This transparent fluid-filled membrane is a myelomeningocele, which arises from the spinal canal and protrudes through a defect in the lumbosacral vertebrae.

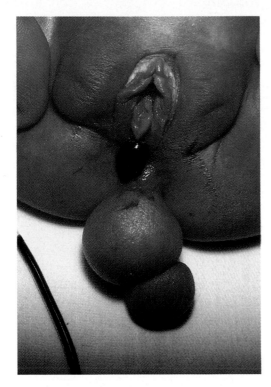

Figure 12.65 A small bilobed mass protrudes from the perineum of this newborn girl with imperforate anus and a fourchette fistula, from which meconium is being passed. The mass, excised at the time of perineal anoplasty, is a benign teratoma with no internal extension.

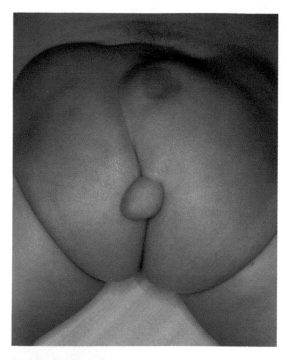

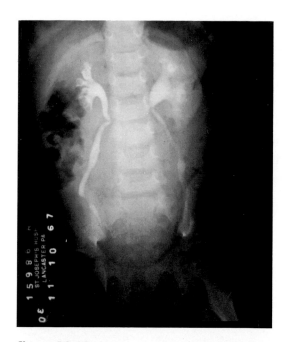

Figure 12.67 The fatty mass over the sacral vertebrae is a lipomeningocele, which extends into the spinal canal next to the cauda equina. A laminectomy is necessary for complete excision. There is frequently an associated tethered cord, which should be released.

Figure 12.69 An intravenous pyelogram of the same child shows the bladder distention and lateral displacement of both ureters.

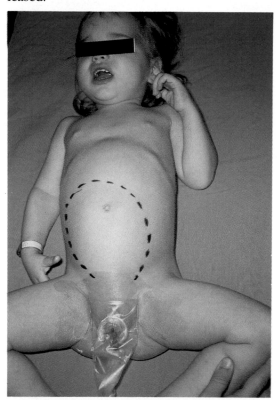

Figure 12.68 An anterior sacral tumor obstructs the bladder outlet in this 22-month-old. The outline on the abdomen is that of a distended bladder.

Surgery

Complete surgical excision of the tumor and adherent coccyx can usually be carried out through a posterior chevron (inverted V) incision (Figs 12.70–12.74). Occasionally a transabdominal approach is needed to free a pelvic retroperitoneal extension of the tumor. Long-term follow-up is important, as even benign teratomas can have local recurrence, which should be excised.

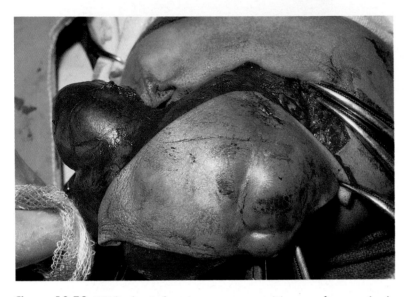

Figure 12.70 With the infant in a prone position, a chevron incision is made over the superior and inferior borders of the sacrococcygeal teratoma. The teratoma is dissected from the surrounding soft tissue structures.

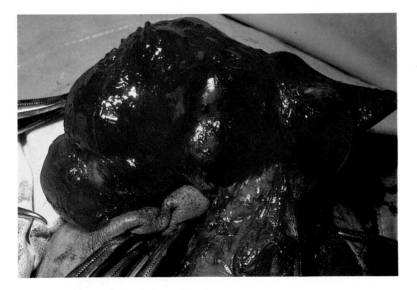

Figure 12.71 The multilocular cystic nature of this teratoma is seen at the dissection. The coccyx is excised with the tumor.

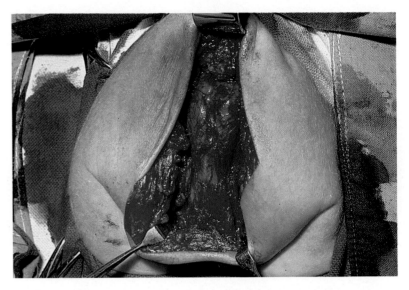

Figure 12.72 The teratoma is dissected from the entire length of the rectum.

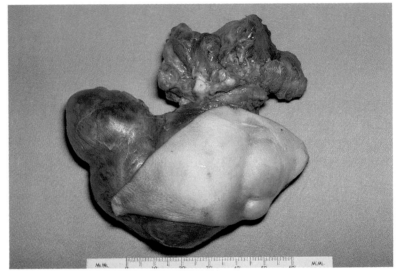

Figure 12.73 The specimen of resected teratoma is seen. It is found to be benign on microscopic evaluation.

Malignant sacrococcygeal teratomas have been found in the neonate but are more common in the older child (Fig 12.75). The type of malignancy depends on the tissue of origin and may be carcinoma or sarcoma. Despite aggressive radiotherapy and chemotherapy, the overall prognosis is poor (Figs 12.76–12.79).

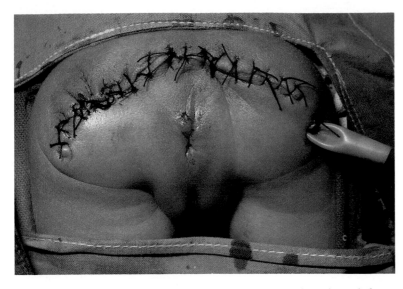

Figure 12.74 The incision is closed in layers, with a drain left in the extensive dissection area for several days. The cosmetic and functional result is excellent.

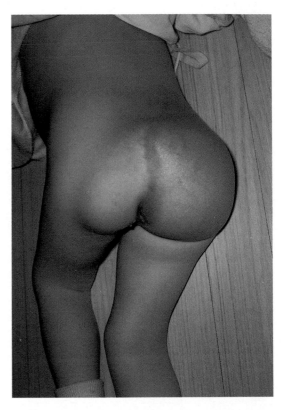

Figure 12.75 Rapid enlargement of the right buttock and difficulty with defecation bring this 2-year-old child to surgical evaluation.

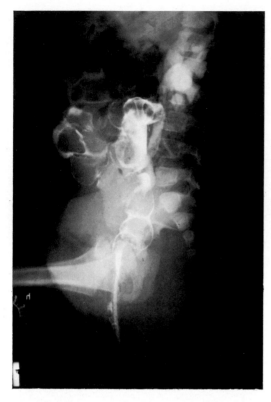

Figure 12.76 A barium enema shows the rectum to be displaced anteriorly by the presacral tumor mass.

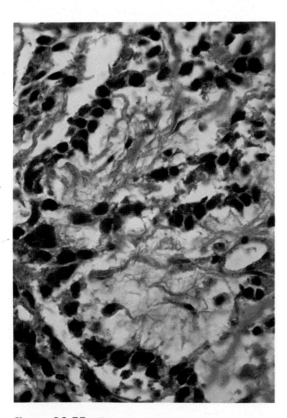

Figure 12.77 The photomicrograph is of the biopsy specimen of this unresectable anterior sacral teratoma. The malignant tumor is embryonal carcinoma.

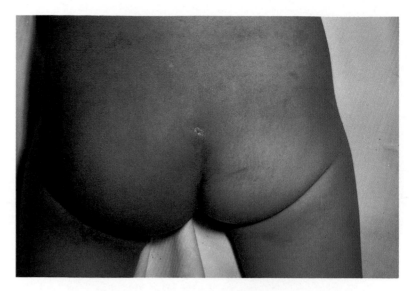

Figure 12.78 After 2 months of chemotherapy and radiotherapy, the primary tumor is no longer visible or palpable.

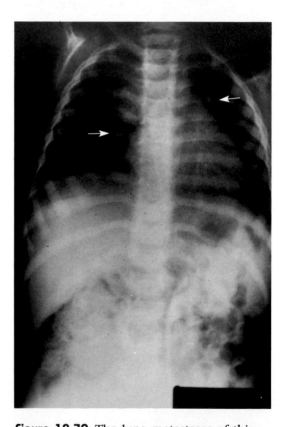

Figure 12.79 The lung metastases of this tumor do not respond to therapy, and the tumor is eventually fatal.

Cervical teratoma presents in the newborn as a large neck mass, sometimes producing respiratory impairment (see Figs 3.13, 3.14). Retroperitoneal abdominal teratomas become apparent as a result of size or compression of nearby structures (Figs 12.80, 12.81). They are treated by surgical excision (Figs 12.82, 12.83), with full postoperative chemotherapy for the small percentage that prove histologically malignant.

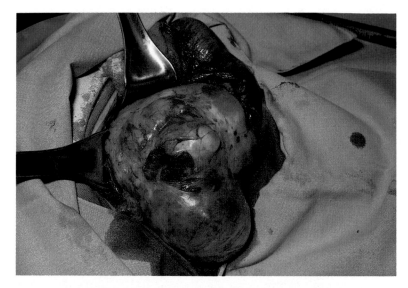

Figure 12.82 The tumor is dissected free and is about to be delivered from the abdomen.

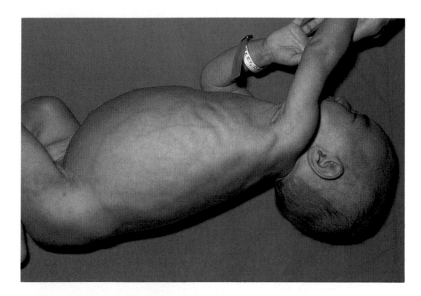

Figure 12.80 Retroperitoneal Abdominal Teratoma This 6-month-old presents with massive abdominal distention and obstructive jaundice.

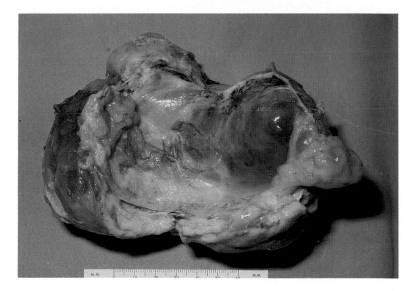

Figure 12.83 The cystic and solid elements of the teratoma are seen in the operative specimen. All three germ layers are demonstrated on microscopic evaluation of the tumor.

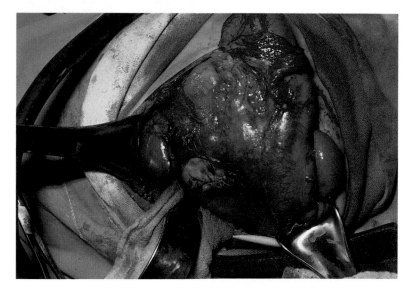

Figure 12.81 The huge right retroperitoneal mass compressing the extrahepatic bile ducts is a cystic and solid benign teratoma. It is being dissected from the adjacent liver, stomach, duodenum, and transverse colon.

Mediastinal teratomas may compress the trachea and lung, producing respiratory symptoms. Chest roentgenograms are usually sufficient to confirm the diagnosis. Surgical excision is performed through a lateral thoracotomy (see Figs 4.98–4.102).

Other thoracic teratomas include those of the pericardium and the myocardium. They require surgical excision, the latter by open cardiotomy.

Ovarian and testicular teratomas are discussed in Chapter 11.

Germ Cell Tumors

Malignant germ cell tumors usually arise from the gonads; rarely, they are found in the retroperitoneum, the mediastinum, or the sacrococcygeal area. They are composed of primitive cells, without differentiation into the three embryonic layers. Serum α-fetoprotein levels are often elevated in children with this tumor and may be used to monitor the patient for recurrence after resection. Chest radiographs or CT scans and radionuclide bone scans will help detect metastatic tumor.

Those that originate in the presacral area may grow rapidly and metastasize early (Figs 12.84–12.87). Complete excision, with removal of the coccyx, is the treatment for resectable tumors. Others may require chemotherapy to shrink the tumor before surgical resection. Chemotherapeutic agents that have been used to treat these tumors include actinomycin D, vincristine, cyclophosphamide, cisplatin, etoposide, and bleomycin.

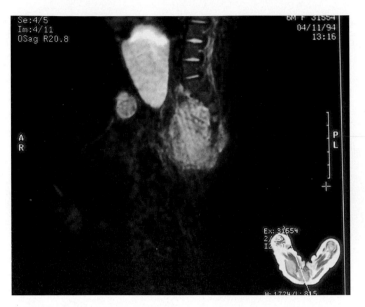

Figure 12.84 Germ Cell Tumor A mass in the right thigh was detected by the mother of this asymptomatic 6-month-old girl. A few days later, there is a swelling in the right groin. This magnetic resonance imaging study shows a large presacral tumor, with extension superiorly into the pelvis, and an anterior inguinal node metastasis.

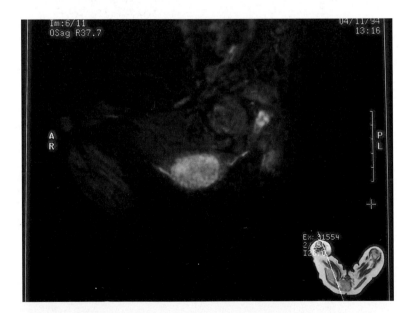

Figure 12.85 This lateral sagittal section of the magnetic resonance imaging study shows the extension of the presacral tumor into the right thigh.

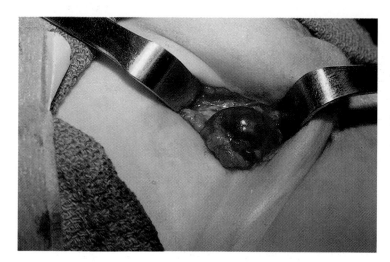

Figure 12.86 The inguinal node is found to be full of dark, friable tumor. It is excised for diagnosis. After 9 weeks of chemotherapy (four courses), the germ cell tumor is not detectable, grossly or on imaging studies. The coccyx is then excised and contains only a single microscopic focus of the tumor. She is tumor-free 3 years later.

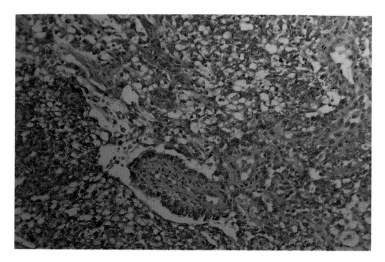

Figure 12.87 A microscopic section of the nodal metastasis shows the characteristic reticular pattern in the upper right and a Shiller-Duval body protruding into a vascular space in the lower part of the photomicrograph.

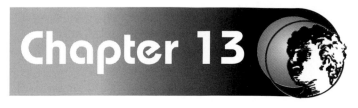

Chapter 13

Trauma and Child Abuse

Trauma is not only the primary cause of childhood deaths in the United States but also results in lifelong disability for approximately 100,000 young people each year. Safety and preventive measures, such as car seats and restraints, are reducing mortality and the incidence of some types of injuries. Immediate resuscitation and proper and prompt transportation are salvaging an increased number of trauma victims. The surgeon who is called on to treat trauma patients must be able to recognize and to deal effectively with injuries to children, both accidental and inflicted.

Characteristics of Pediatric Trauma

There are a number of characteristics that distinguish pediatric trauma, in general, from that suffered by adults. The etiology and nature of trauma to children is different. Blunt trauma is far more frequent than penetrating trauma, although there has been an unfortunate increase in weapon injuries among teenagers. Children are more often injured by being struck by vehicles as pedestrians and bicycle riders than as passengers. In the home, they suffer an inordinate number of falls, burns (both thermal and electrical), and ingestions of poisons, caustics, and foreign bodies. Sports injuries and drowning characteristically occur in the pediatric age group. Finally, children are the victims of a unique form of repeated physical and emotional trauma at the hands of their caretakers that is known as child abuse.

Physical and physiologic traits of children influence their response to trauma and must be considered in treating them. Young children have considerably narrower airways and less respiratory reserve than do adults. Their smaller blood volume makes fluid and blood losses more significant; a 10% loss of blood volume in a 10-kg child is only 75–80 mL. Hypothermia is a potential problem, as there is a high surface-to-volume ratio, leading to rapid heat loss. The child has a comparatively larger head and is subject to an increased number of head injuries. Infants and small children do not have the ability to communicate, making their evaluation more difficult.

Evaluation and Treatment of Trauma

Respiratory Trauma

Respiratory impairment can lead to the most serious consequences for the trauma patient; therefore, in major trauma, the respiratory status is evaluated first. Examination should include observation, palpation, and auscultation—front and back, unless there is a specific contraindication. Radiographs of the chest and neck are imperative for any suspected airway injury. The upper airway must be assessed for obstructing injuries and for bleeding that may flow into the tracheobronchial tree; nose, mouth, jaw (Fig 13.1), tongue, and larynx are visualized. The chest is especially flexible in children; compression may result in severe lung contusion (Fig 13.2) or mediastinal injury, even in the absence of rib or sternal fracture. When rib fractures are present in a traumatized child, injury to underlying organs must be suspected; the most common is pneumothorax (Fig 13.3). Bronchial disruption leads to massive pneumothorax and persistent air flow through the thoracostomy tube. Tracheal injury presents with subcutaneous and mediastinal emphysema (Fig 13.4). Multiple fractures of the same ribs, or of ribs on both sides of the sternum, produce a flail chest, recognized by the paradoxical motion of the chest wall with respirations. Penetrating wounds often result in an audible flow of air through the chest wall defect with each breath. Central nervous system (CNS) injuries may affect breathing by decreasing respiratory drive.

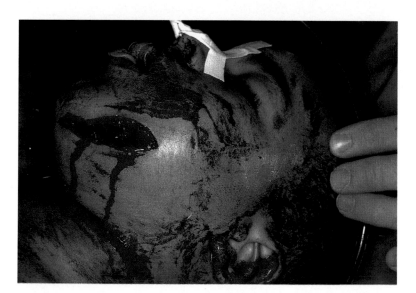

Figure 13.1 Respiratory System Trauma Hit by a car, this 4-year-old boy has an open fracture of the mandible, swelling of the neck, and swallowed blood—all interfering with respirations.

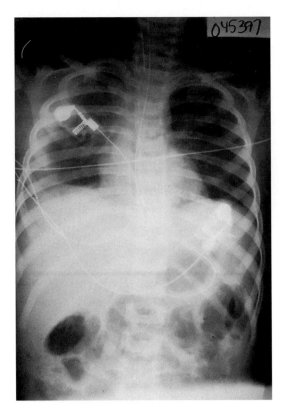

Figure 13.2 Bilateral lung contusions, greater on the child's right side, are the result of a crush injury.

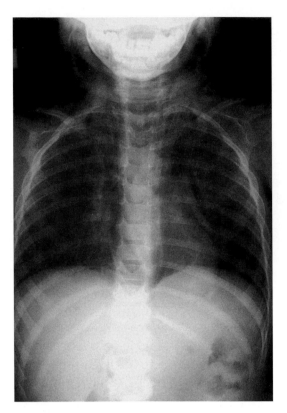

Figure 13.4 Mediastinal and subcutaneous emphysema in a 2-year-old results from his pulling a table over onto his chest. In this child, laryngeal trauma and a proximal esophageal laceration requires a tracheostomy, gastrostomy, and open drainage of a mediastinal abscess.

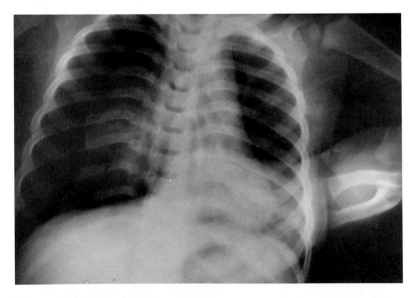

Figure 13.3 After suffering trauma as an unrestrained automobile passenger, this boy has many injuries; this radiograph shows a pneumothorax with multiple posterior rib fractures on the right.

If there is impingement on the airway, it must be cleared. The tongue should be displaced forward to keep it from blocking the oropharynx, especially in the supine patient. Secretions and blood are suctioned from the oropharynx and tracheobronchial tree. Airway maintenance and ventilatory support are given as indicated: a mask and oxygen for less severe problems; endotracheal intubation and positive-pressure ventilation for a flail chest or CNS trauma; and tracheostomy (see Chapter 1) for laryngeal fracture or tracheobronchial disruption.

Chest tubes are placed in the upper chest for pneumothorax and in the lower chest to drain a hemothorax; severely traumatized patients often need both. With proper tube placement, air will be evacuated through the water-seal chamber of a chest drainage set until a simple pneumothorax resolves; continuous and vigorous bubbling reflects a more severe lower airway injury. The rate of blood and fluid drainage from the chest determines volume replacement, as well as the need for surgical intervention. Monitoring of blood oxygen saturation by pulse oximetry is helpful. Serial determination of arterial blood gases is a better method of monitoring the adequacy of respiratory therapy in the patient with major injuries.

Cardiovascular Trauma

Hemorrhage, which may lead to hypoperfusion of organs and shock, is of major concern in the traumatized patient. It is especially important to be aware of occult blood losses into the pelvis, the retroperitoneum, and the thigh that may result from blunt trauma. Chest injury may lead to hemopericardium and tamponade, with rising venous pressure, falling arterial pressure, and narrowing pulse pressure.

In children, a change in pulse rate is a more sensitive index of cardiovascular status than is blood pressure. Determination of the rapidity of capillary filling following nail-bed compression provides a simple assessment of peripheral perfusion. Urine output is the gauge of renal perfusion; any child with severe injuries or in shock should have an indwelling bladder catheter. Serial determinations of hematocrit and monitoring of central venous pressure are additional clues to blood volume loss.

Initial resuscitation requires an adequate-sized intravenous cannula—two if the child is in shock or bleeding profusely. Blood is drawn and sent for type and crossmatch. Ringer's lactate in 5% dextrose is an excellent solution for immediate infusion. Whole blood or packed red cells may follow when available. In massive hemorrhage, O+ blood may be used if type-specific blood is not available. The object of therapy is restoration of normal tissue perfusion and control of the site of bleeding.

Abdominal Trauma

Blunt trauma to the abdomen may result in injury to one or more organs, with disruption of solid viscera and perforation of hollow ones. The nature of the injury and the necessity of surgical intervention are determined by careful clinical evaluation. Rupture of a hollow viscus, or persistent bleeding from a solid organ, is an indication for surgery. Penetrating injuries to the abdomen should lead, in general, to laparotomy, unless it can be determined by careful exploration of the wound that the peritoneum has not been entered.

Blood, bile, pancreatic juice, urine, and gastrointestinal contents all are irritating to the abdominal peritoneum. Abdominal distention, localized tenderness, and muscle guarding are important clues to acute peritonitis in the reactive patient. Peritoneal lavage, with insertion of the catheter through a tiny abdominal and peritoneal incision, is recommended when abdominal injury is suspected in the comatose or noncooperative patient. A peritoneal ef-

fluent containing gross blood, bile, or intestinal contents confirms significant visceral injury. Ultrasonography, computed tomography (CT), and nuclear scans all have their role in assessing abdominal trauma.

Spleen and Liver Trauma

A splenic disruption leads to bleeding, with tenderness and muscle spasm in the left upper abdomen. One third of patients have left diaphragmatic irritation and pleuritic pain, radiating to the shoulder, that increases with the patient in Trendelenburg position. Pallor and prostration out of proportion to the bleeding that has taken place are associated with splenic rupture. The white blood cell count tends to be elevated. Some patients have subcapsular bleeding that is contained for several days after the injury and then produces acute symptoms when the capsule ruptures, spontaneously or from minor trauma.

Liver lacerations are accompanied by right upper abdominal tenderness or tenderness over the lower rib cage. A fracture of a right lower rib raises the suspicion of liver damage (Fig 13.5). Like some splenic injuries, early subcapsular bleeding from the liver may spontaneously rupture into the abdominal cavity, producing sudden symptoms and peritoneal signs.

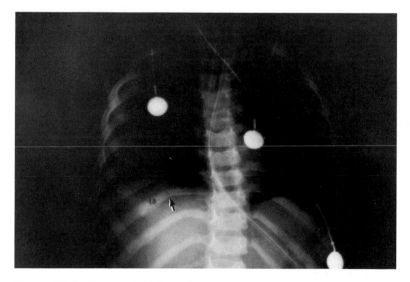

Figure 13.5 Liver and Spleen Trauma A fracture of the right 10th rib posteriorly is associated with a major liver laceration in this 2-year-old with lung contusions (see Fig 13.2).

Liver or spleen lacerations can often be localized by ultrasonography or CT (Fig 13.6). However, in the child younger than 2 years of age with low visceral fat stores, lack of differences in tissue density may make the CT unreliable. In that case, and when clinical suspicions are not adequately confirmed, nuclear liver–spleen scans are indicated (Fig 13.7).

Surgery for splenic injury in children (Fig 13.8) is always undertaken with the objective of possible repair, rather than removal, because the asplenic child is subject to the possibility of overwhelming and fatal sepsis. Splenic lacerations are sutured, and salvageable portions of a ruptured spleen are preserved. These maneuvers are possible because the spleen has a radial segmental blood supply. In suturing the spleen, large needles with a gentle curve are used, and ''bolsters'' of Dacron material or compressed hemostatic (gelatin [Gelfoam] or microfibrillar collagen [Avitene]) are placed between the suture and the splenic capsule to distribute the tension and avoid cutting into the splenic pulp.

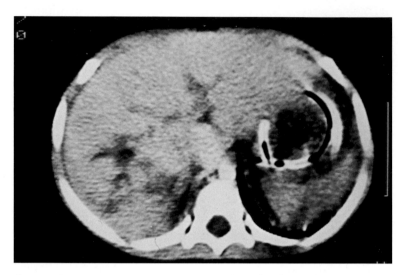

Figure 13.6 Computed tomography demonstrates multiple liver lacerations and a fractured spleen. This 4-year-old girl fell from a sixth story roof; she survived after surgery for repair of the lacerated liver and spleen.

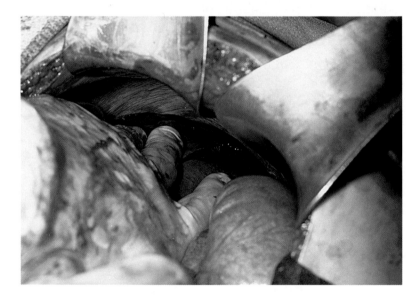

Figure 13.8 This deep splenic laceration is the result of a football injury in a 15-year-old boy. It is repaired with sutures.

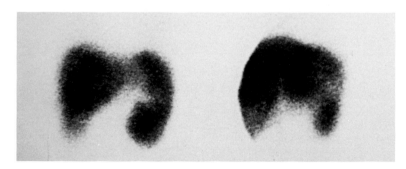

Figure 13.7 A liver–spleen radionuclide scan, with anteroposterior and lateral views, demonstrates a defect in the midspleen following abdominal trauma.

Liver lacerations with persistent hemorrhage (Fig 13.9) must be controlled by suture repair. Massive liver injuries require resection and debridement. Control of the hepatic systemic and portal blood supply and a knowledge of the segmental anatomy of the liver are essential for proper surgical management of these injuries.

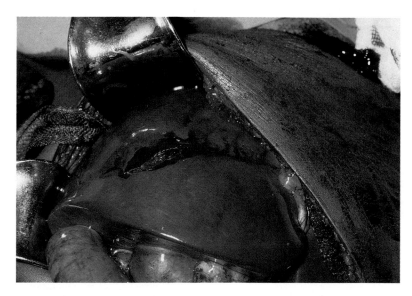

Figure 13.9 This extensive liver laceration is seen at surgical repair in the patient who is imaged by computed tomography in Figure 13.6.

In recent years, pediatric surgeons have recommended nonoperative treatment of spleen and liver injuries in the stable patient. Such treatment requires close observation and repeated frequent evaluation of the traumatized child, with immediate operative intervention for evidence of rapid or continuing bleeding; an estimated loss of 40% or more of the child's blood volume is an indication for operation. In most patients who have been treated nonoperatively, subsequent imaging studies have shown complete healing (Fig 13.10).

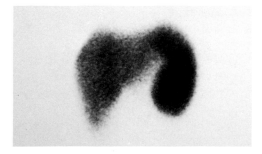

Figure 13.10 Six months after the radionuclide scan of Figure 13.7, this scan shows complete healing of the splenic laceration.

Intestinal Injury

Intestinal perforation is characterized by abdominal distention, tenderness, and evidence of pneumoperitoneum. The notable exceptions are perforation into the retroperitoneum (Figs 13.11, 13.12) and into the mesentery (Figs 13.13–13.15). Duodenal rupture into the retroperitoneum may present with lower abdominal pain, and early roentgenographic signs may be missed (Fig 13.16).

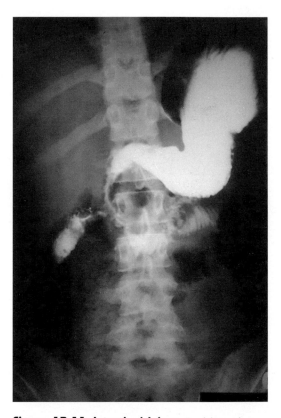

Figure 13.11 Intestinal Injury Sudden abdominal compression led to this 14-year-old girl's injury. Contrast material leaking from a perforation in the second portion of the duodenum is seen in the right retroperitoneum.

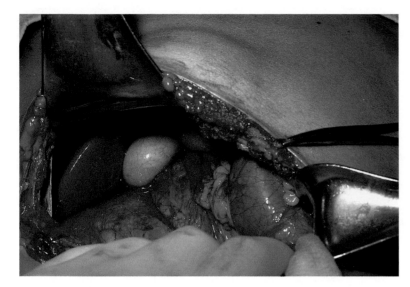

Figure 13.12 A "blowout" perforation of the duodenum, seen just below the pink gallbladder, is found at exploration.

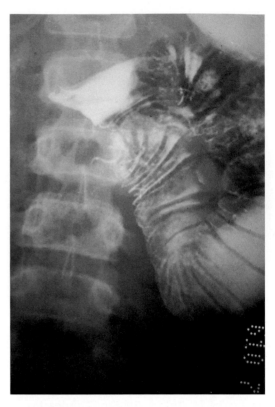

Figure 13.14 A close-up view shows a tiny thread of barium tracking caudad from the apparently obstructed jejunum.

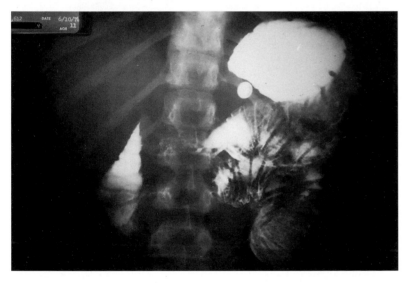

Figure 13.13 An upper gastrointestinal contrast study shows no passage of barium beyond the proximal jejunum. This 12-year-old boy presented with sudden, severe epigastric pain 5 days after jamming the handle of a hockey stick into his abdomen.

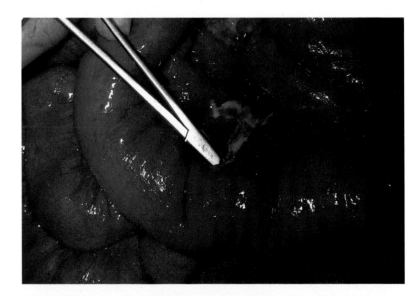

Figure 13.15 The tip of the hemostat shows a tiny jejunal perforation into the mesentery; it was contained for 5 days before eroding into the peritoneal cavity.

At surgery, the bile duct must be examined for injury. Repair of a duodenal tear can be difficult and may require unusual methods, such as serosal patch closure using adjacent jejunum (Fig 13.17). Duodenal hematoma commonly presents as a high obstruction 2–3 days after the abdominal injury (Fig 13.18); nasogastric decompression and observation have replaced operative intervention, with spontaneous resolution expected in 5–7 days.

Primary closure of a small perforation, or resection and anastomosis of an extensive laceration, is possible, especially in the small bowel. Multiple perforations, colonic perforations, and any with delayed diagnosis and subsequent widespread peritoneal contamination may require initial intestinal exteriorization and future closure.

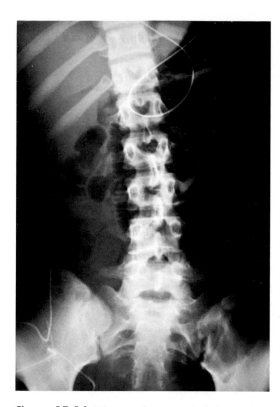

Figure 13.16 This is the initial abdominal radiograph of the patient represented in Figures 13.11 and 13.12. The flecks of air in the lower right side of the abdomen, which resulted from a duodenal perforation, were not originally appreciated to be in the retroperitoneum.

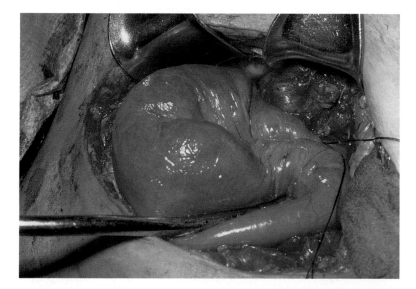

Figure 13.17 The jejunum is mobilized, and its antimesenteric serosa is used as a patch around the ragged duodenal perforation to effect closure. Duodenal mucosa will grow over the serosal patch.

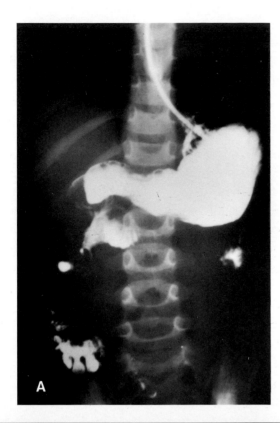

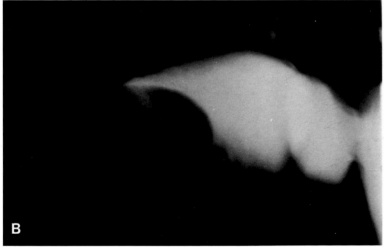

Pancreatic Injury

Pancreatic injuries occur when the organ is compressed against the vertebral column in the midline. The result may be contusion with traumatic pancreatitis, laceration, or complete transection. There is often an associated duodenal injury. Exquisite upper abdominal pain and tenderness are typical, with grunting respirations. An abdominal tap or peritoneal lavage yields a specimen high in amylase, and the serum and urinary amylase levels are elevated. Nasogastric decompression is begun—as is indicated in all severe abdominal injuries. Clinical or imaging evidence of pancreatic disruption must lead to exploration, pancreatic repair or partial resection, and drainage of the area of damaged pancreas. The resolution of traumatic pancreatitis is observed as diminished swelling on serial CT scans and a fall in amylase levels; in the clinically stable patient, the nasogastric tube is then removed, and the patient is fed. Pancreatic pseudocyst is a potential complication, discussed in Chapter 9.

Figure 13.18 Duodenal Hematoma A. A 2-year-old girl has persistent vomiting after a fall onto her abdomen. The barium study shows evidence of partial duodenal obstruction. **B.** A close-up view of the barium study demonstrates the negative shadow of a hematoma in the duodenal wall.

Urinary Tract Injury

Hematuria is the primary sign of trauma to the urinary tract. Kidney injury may lead to flank swelling, and bladder perforation produces suprapubic tenderness and possible urinary ascites. Urethral disruptions, often associated with pelvic fractures, are characterized by swelling, tenderness, and ecchymotic discoloration in the perineum, and gross blood at the urethral meatus.

Bladder catheterization is performed initially, unless a urethral tear is suspected. Ultrasonography may be helpful, especially in visualizing the kidneys; most often intravenous pyelography (IVP) or infusion pyelography, cystourethrography (Fig 13.19), or computed tomography (Fig 13.20) is needed to localize the injury. Complete nonvisualization of one kidney following administration of intravenous contrast material is indicative of renal vascular disruption; surgical exploration is indicated, unless congenital renal agenesis can be confirmed.

The majority of kidney injuries may be handled nonoperatively, because Gerota's fascia will contain and tamponade the bleeding. Disruptions of the urinary drainage system or bladder need to be repaired and drained.

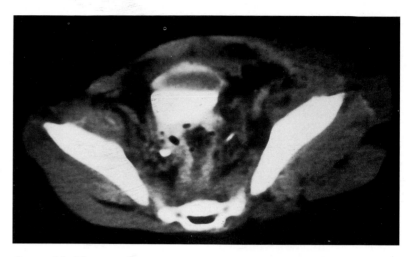

Figure 13.20 A computed tomogram of the pelvis shows the bladder injury and extravasated contrast material.

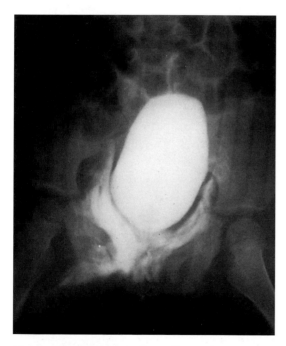

Figure 13.19 Urinary Tract Trauma A laceration of the bladder neck allows contrast to leak into the pelvis on cystourethrography in this child with a pelvic fracture.

Central Nervous System Trauma

The primary method of clinical evaluation of trauma to the brain and spinal cord is repeated observation and testing of the level of responsiveness. In relation to head trauma, it is the level of consciousness that is critical; for spinal injuries, peripheral sensation, motor function, and reflexes are most important. Table 13.1 is a modification of the Glasgow Coma Scale, which has been devised to standardize the assessment of CNS injury.

Imaging studies include neck films, skull films, and CT. Cervical vertebral fracture or subluxation, with potential cord damage, must be suspected in any major trauma to the head and face and in all rapid-deceleration injuries; traction and immobilization of the neck are indicated until such injuries can be ruled out. It is important to see all seven cervical vertebrae on the lateral neck film for complete assessment. If the neurologic examination shows a peripheral deficit, despite normal spine films, immobilization is maintained, and myelography or magnetic resonance imaging studies may be indicated.

In head trauma, it is increased intracranial pressure that is of concern. Epidural and acute subdural hematomas require neurosurgical decompression. Severe brain contusion leads to massive cerebral edema. Therapeutic measures to reduce brain swelling include administration of oxygen, controlled respirations and maintenance of a low PCO_2 (in the range of 20 torr), intravenous corticosteroid (dexamethasone, 1 mg/kg), and infusion of mannitol. Serial arterial blood gases are obtained, and intracranial pressure monitors are used by some to guide therapy.

Extremity Trauma

Survival of the limb and preservation of function are the major considerations in treating traumatic injuries to the extremities. Deformity indicates fracture or dislocation. Open wounds are noted, and distal circulation, sensation, and motion evaluated.

Hemorrhage is controlled first. Circulation must then be restored, by correcting a bony deformity—as in an anteriorly displaced supracondylar humeral fracture—or by direct anastomosis of severed vessels. Swelling of traumatized muscle within its fibrous sheath may impair its own circulation (compartment syndrome); fasciotomy may be needed to prevent muscle fibrosis or atrophy. When there is extensive traumatic tissue damage, the repair of nerves and tendons is best delayed. Fractures are reduced and immobilized. Tetanus prophylaxis must be considered for all open wounds if the immunization history is unknown or incomplete, or if it is more than 5 years since the last dose of toxoid. All these factors must be considered in the replantation of a severed, or almost-severed, extremity (Figs 13.21–13.24).

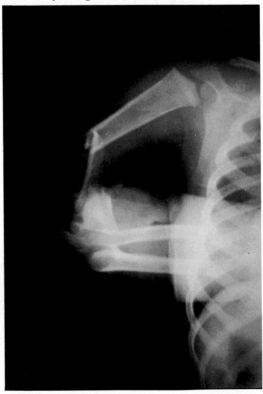

Figure 13.21 Extremity Trauma The left arm is almost amputated in this 18-month-old boy. The injury has divided the humerus, brachial artery, basilic and cephalic veins, and median and radial nerves.

Table 13.1

Eyes Open	
Spontaneously	4
To speech	3
To pain	2
None	1
Verbal Response	
Oriented	5
Confused	4
Inappropriate	3
Incomprehensible	2
None	1
Motor Response	
To commands	6
Localizes pain	5
Withdrawal	4
Flexion to pain	3
Extension to pain	2
None	1

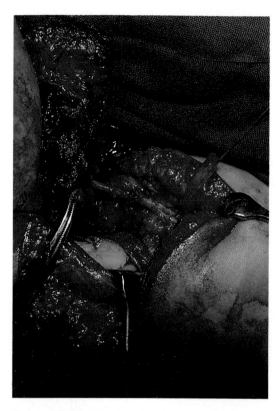

Figure 13.22 The brachial artery anastomosis is seen. The veins are approximated, and a rod secures the humeral ends. The nerves will be repaired at a future time.

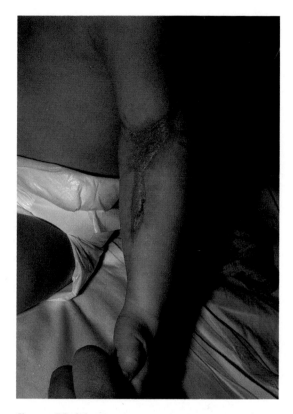

Figure 13.24 The healed repair is seen 6 weeks after injury.

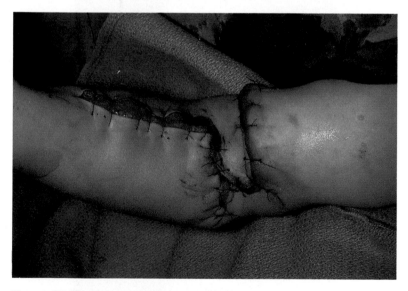

Figure 13.23 The operation is completed, using local skin flaps to cover the antecubital defect.

Burns and Scalds

In evaluating and treating burns and scalds in children, one must be aware of certain anatomic and physiologic differences, such as their high surface-to-volume ratio, large head size, and narrow airways. Children have relatively more skin surface and higher evaporative water loss than adults. The head constitutes 18% of the child's surface area, compared with 9% in adults. Respiratory burns in a child may have devastating effects, as mucosal edema narrows an airway of small diameter; early intubation and ventilation are indicated when there is evidence of such a burn.

The surface area involved and depth of burn determine therapy. Superficial burns (first degree), with mild cutaneous erythema, may be treated symptomatically. Partial-thickness burns (second degree) that involve less than 10% of body surface in infants and less than 15% in children older than 2 years of age may be treated on an outpatient basis; unruptured bullae are left intact, and antiseptic ointment (silver sulfadiazine) is applied regularly to prevent infection of the open areas. More extensive partial-thickness burns are better treated in the hospital (Figs 13.25–13.27) with intravenous fluid

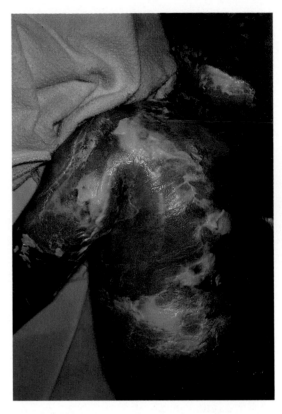

Figure 13.26 Silver sulfadiazine is applied to the burn surface to prevent infection.

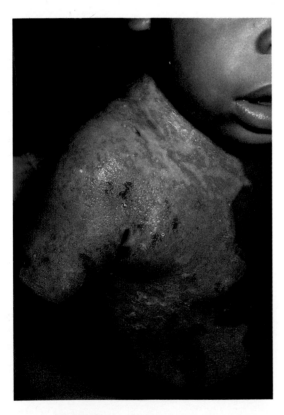

Figure 13.25 Burns There is an extensive second-degree burn of the shoulder, chest, and back of this 1-year-old.

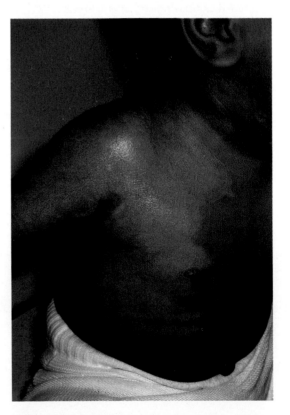

Figure 13.27 The burn heals spontaneously, without scarring.

resuscitation and support, as determined by the extent of the burn and the child's physiologic response. Infants and young children with perineal burns may be hospitalized because of the difficulty in keeping the area clean. Some children are admitted for "social" reasons: the inability of parents to give proper care, or the suspicion of child abuse.

Full-thickness involvement (third-degree burn) requires hospital care in almost every case, and children with involvement of more than 30% of the body surface are best treated in a burn center. Initial therapy requires ventilatory support when indicated, rapid intravenous fluid resuscitation, monitoring of urine output, and escharotomy for any restrictive circumferential burn. Most fluid resuscitation formulas are based on the early infusion of 5% dextrose in Ringer's lactate solution, 3–4 mL/kg multiplied by the percentage of body surface burned, in 24 hours; half of the volume is given in the first 8 hours, the remainder over the next 16 hours. Colloid, in the form of albumin or plasma, is given subsequently, as indicated. Changes are made on the basis of close monitoring of vital signs, urine output and specific gravity, hematocrit, peripheral perfusion, and central venous pressure. Adequate urine output is 0.7–1.0 mL/kg/h.

A topical antibacterial, such as silver sulfadiazine, is used to prevent burn wound sepsis. Systemic antibiotics are generally given for respiratory burns and as burn wound cultures dictate. Feeding, by mouth or nasogastric tube, is started early, because a major burn imposes markedly increased protein and calorie requirements. Hydrotherapy in a whirlpool bath, to loosen the eschar, and regular debridement are begun as soon as the patient's condition permits. Grafting of the burn area—with split-thickness autograft skin if possible, or allograft if the burn area is too large—is begun as soon as there is a satisfactory base of healthy granulating tissue. Recent ad-

vances in tissue engineering have resulted in the ability to grow sheets of skin cells that may be used for grafting and that will not be rejected by the recipient.

Deforming scars are major sequelae of deep burns. Sustained pressure with an elastic garment over the healing burn site has been shown to reduce scar thickness and to maintain greater skin pliability.

Electrical burns are sustained most often by infants and toddlers chewing on electrical wires or exploring electric outlets. The burn is commonly to the lips (Fig 13.28) and gums. Although some surgeons recommend early excision of the lip burn and primary repair, the extent of tissue damage is not always easy to determine, and some may heal satisfactorily without surgical intervention. Later reconstruction is occasionally necessary.

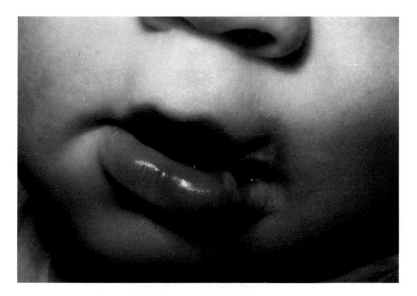

Figure 13.28 A full-thickness electrical burn of the lips is the result of this infant's chewing on a lamp cord. The necrotic tissue is allowed to slough before any surgical repair.

Child Abuse

The physician who deals with pediatric injuries, both minor and major, must be alert to the signs of child abuse. It has been estimated that 10% of the childhood injuries seen in hospital emergency departments are inflicted by a parent or other caretaker. Recognition of an abusive situation early in its course will allow intervention to prevent subsequent serious injury or even death.

Suspicion of abuse is raised by certain patterns of injury and by parental histories that are inconsistent with the physical findings. Multiple bruises of varying ages, or in an unusual location such as the perineum, are not consistent with a story that the child just fell down the stairs. Some objects leave irregular marks or characteristic bruises or abrasions, such as the loop of a folded electrical cord or a metallic belt buckle.

Burns

Burns associated with abuse may also have unusual characteristics. Round cigarette burns, especially on the hands, feet, and buttocks, are assumed to be inflicted. Immersion scalds of the hands and feet have a clearly demarcated "stocking" or "glove" distribution, frequently symmetrical, that is unlikely to be accidental (Fig 13.29). Symmetrical scalds of the buttocks and perineum or of both palms almost always represent abuse. Children do not voluntarily put both palms down simultaneously on a hot stove.

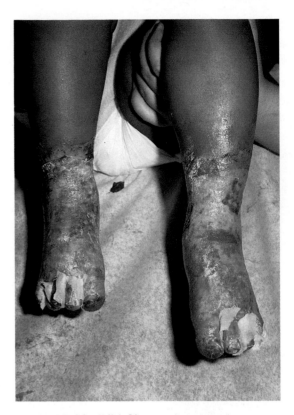

Figure 13.29 Child Abuse The "stocking" distribution of these symmetrical scalds of both feet and ankles belies the mother's description of the child accidentally stepping into a tub of hot water.

Fractures

The radiographic findings of multiple fractures in different stages of healing must raise the strong suspicion of abuse, unless the child is known to have a predisposing systemic illness, such as osteogenesis imperfecta. Spiral fractures of the long bones, especially in young children, are associated with twisting injuries, as are "bucket-handle" fractures of the epiphyses of long bones (Fig 13.30).

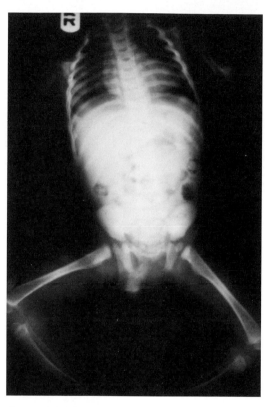

Figure 13.30 A left humeral fracture and bilateral "bucket-handle" fractures of the distal femurs are seen on the radiograph of this abused infant.

Abdominal Injuries

Abdominal injuries are similar to those suffered from any blunt trauma (Figs 13.31, 13.32). Occasionally a bruise of the abdominal wall indicates the site of trauma. It is usually the history, inconsistent with the nature or severity of the injury, that alerts the examiner to possible abuse.

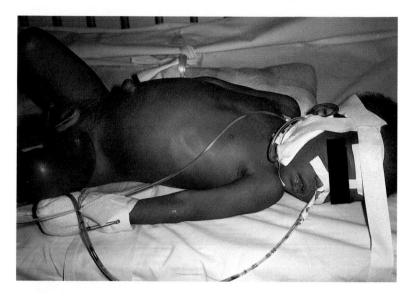

Figure 13.31 Abdominal distention and vomiting followed a kick to the lower abdomen of this abused 2-year-old girl.

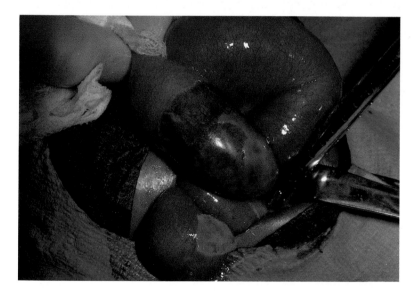

Figure 13.32 At exploration of the child in Figure 13.31, a gangrenous segment of the traumatized ileum is seen and resected.

Central Nervous System Trauma

Skull and central nervous system injuries may reflect either direct blows or the results of violent shaking. Subdural and subarachnoid hemorrhage may result, as well as "unexplained" skull fractures.

Malnutrition

Nutritional deprivation may result in generalized protein-calorie malnutrition (Fig 13.33) or specific deficiencies. In such children, there are often other signs of physical and emotional neglect.

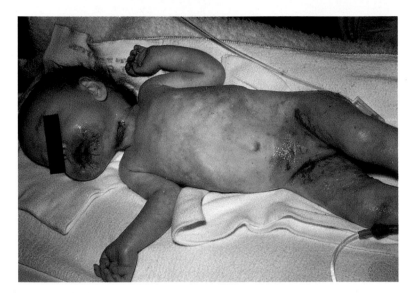

Figure 13.33 This emaciated infant with severe vitamin-deficiency dermatitis is a victim of severe nutritional neglect.

Sexual Abuse

Child sexual abuse is becoming widely recognized in our society, and help is available for the victim and the perpetrator. Subtle signs, such as perineal irritation or erythema, may go unnoticed initially. Vaginal discharge or recurrent urinary infections may have other causes. Bruises or lacerations of the perineum or vagina (Fig 13.34) are highly suspicious. However, the presence of syphilis, gonococcal infection, genital herpes, or condylomata (see Chapter 11) involving the vagina or rectum of a child is clear evidence of sexual abuse—as is sperm or acid phosphatase on the body or clothes of a child.

In all cases, there should be a thorough and gentle examination, swabs of the vagina and rectum for sperm and microorganisms, and consultation with the available professionals most experienced in dealing with child sexual abuse.

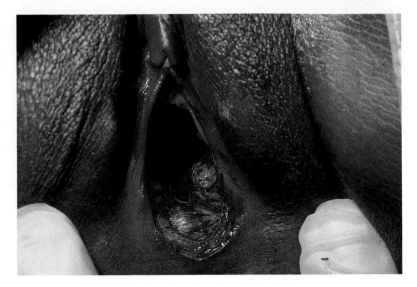

Figure 13.34 This 7-year-old allegedly fell onto a broom. The vaginal laceration is strongly suggestive of sexual abuse.

Care and Treatment of the Abused Child

Admission of abused children to the hospital is based not on their severity of injury but on the likelihood of abuse. In that setting, it is easiest to initiate both investigation and treatment of the family. The parent(s) must not be accused or threatened, or they and the child will disappear and be lost to further follow-up and help. All cases of suspected child abuse must—by law—be reported to the state or local child protection services. If the parental problems and stresses that lead to abuse can be ameliorated, the family unit can be preserved—a better solution for child, parent, and society than is a series of foster homes or an institution for the child.

Index

Note: Page numbers in *italics* indicate figures; those followed by t indicate tables.